Plagues and Politics

Global Issues Series

General Editor: **Jim Whitman**

This exciting new series encompasses three principal themes: the interaction of human and natural systems; cooperation and conflict; and the enactment of values. The series as a whole places an emphasis on the examination of complex systems and causal relations in political decision-making; problems of knowledge; authority, control and accountability in issues of scale; and the reconciliation of conflicting values and competing claims. Throughout the series the concentration is on an integration of existing disciplines towards the clarification of political possibility as well as impending crises.

Titles include:

Brendan Gleeson and Nicholas Low (*editors*)
GOVERNING FOR THE ENVIRONMENT
Global Problems, Ethics and Democracy

Roger Jeffery and Bhaskar Vira (*editors*)
CONFLICT AND COOPERATION IN PARTICIPATORY NATURAL RESOURCE MANAGEMENT

W. Andy Knight
A CHANGING UNITED NATIONS
Multilateral Evolution and the Quest for Global Governance

W. Andy Knight
ADAPTING THE UNITED NATIONS TO A POSTMODERN ERA
Lessons Learned

Graham S. Pearson
THE UNSCOM SAGA
Chemical and Biological Weapons Non-Proliferation

Andrew T. Price-Smith (*editor*)
PLAGUES AND POLITICS
Infectious Disease and International Policy

Michael Pugh (*editor*)
REGENERATION OF WAR-TORN SOCIETIES

Bhaskar Vira and Roger Jeffery (*editors*)
ANALYTICAL ISSUES IN PARTICIPATORY NATURAL RESOURCE MANAGEMENT

Global Issues Series
Series Standing Order ISBN 0–333–79483–4
(*outside North America only*)

You can receive future titles in this series as they are published by placing a standing order. Please contact your bookseller or, in case of difficulty, write to us at the address below with your name and address, the title of the series and the ISBN quoted above.

Customer Services Department, Macmillan Distribution Ltd, Houndmills, Basingstoke, Hampshire RG21 6XS, England

Plagues and Politics

Infectious Disease and International Policy

Edited by

Andrew T. Price-Smith

Assistant Professor
Department of Political Science and Public Administration
and
Director of the Program on
Environment, Health and Human Security
University of North Dakota

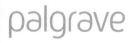

First published 2001 by
PALGRAVE
Houndmills, Basingstoke, Hampshire RG21 6XS and
175 Fifth Avenue, New York, N.Y. 10010
Companies and representatives throughout the world

PALGRAVE is the new global academic imprint of
St. Martin's Press LLC Scholarly and Reference Division and
Palgrave Publishers Ltd (formerly Macmillan Press Ltd).

ISBN 0–333–80066–4

This book is printed on paper suitable for recycling and
made from fully managed and sustained forest sources.

A catalogue record for this book is available
from the British Library.

Library of Congress Cataloging-in-Publication Data
Plagues and politics : infectious disease and international policy /
edited by Andrew T. Price-Smith.
        p. cm.
    Includes bibliographical references and index.
    ISBN 0–333–80066–4
    1. Communicable diseases—Political aspects. 2. World health.
    3. World politics—Health aspects. 4. Epidemics—Prevention.
    I. Price-Smith, Andrew T.
    RA643 .P675 2000
    614.4—dc21
                                                            00–066878

10   9   8   7   6   5   4   3   2   1
10   09 08 07 06 05 04 03 02 01

Printed and bound in Great Britain by
Antony Rowe Ltd, Chippenham, Wiltshire

I dedicate this book to my sister Adrienne Price Smith, my mother Cynthia Smith-McLeod, my step-father Jack T. McLeod and my father Richard Price-Smith, for all their support through the years.

Contents

List of Boxes, Figures, Tables and Maps

Acknowledgements

This book is the result of the nascent Program on Health and Global Affairs that was based at the Centre for International Studies (CIS) at the University of Toronto. I am particularly grateful to both Louis Pauly (Director) and David A. Welch (Assistant Director) of the CIS for their support of a research agenda that was regarded as being 'ahead of the curve' during the late 1990s. This book grew out of a CIS conference at the University of Toronto in the latter part of 1998. I am grateful to the Connaught Foundation of the University of Toronto for providing financial assistance for that initial assemblage of contributors to this volume. CIESIN at Columbia University provided me with generous financial assistance in the form of a post-doctoral fellowship for 1999–2000 that allowed me to put the finishing touches to this volume. I am grateful to both Marc Levy and Roberta Miller of CIESIN for their support of this initiative. Furthermore, I would also like to thank both Geoffrey Dabelko and P.J. Simmons of the Environment and Security project in the Woodrow Wilson Center of the Smithsonian for financial support of this initiative. My most sincere gratitude to Christina Greenough for her exceptional diligence in copy preparation and proofreading. I would also like to thank the entire team at Macmillan, particularly Alison Howson and Sally Crawford, for their continuing support of the project. Finally, I owe a debt of gratitude to my family who contributed both financial and moral support during those mad years of graduate school at the University of Toronto.

Permission to reprint the following material that has been published elsewhere has been kindly granted: Chapter 2 originally appeared in *Emerging Infectious Diseases*, vol. 1 (1), online journal; Chapter 3 is reprinted from *Consequences*, vol. 3, no. 2, 1997; Chapter 5 is reprinted with the permission of the Population Council, from *Population and Development Review*, vol. 23, no. 4 (December 1997), 693–728; Chapter 6 was originally published as a working paper by the Centre for International Studies of the University of Toronto, June 1998; Chapter 8 was originally published in the *International Journal*, vol. 54, no. 3, summer 1999; Chapter 9 is reprinted by permission of *Foreign Affairs*, vol. 75, no. 1, 1996. Copyright © 1996 by the Council on Foreign Relations, Inc; Chapter 13 of this book is informed by David P. Fidler's book *International Law and Infectious Diseases* (Oxford: Clarendon Press, 1999).

ANDREW PRICE-SMITH

Notes on the Contributors

Simon Carvalho, at the time of writing, is Associate Researcher in the Institute for International Relations at the University of British Columbia.

Robert Davis is lecturer in the Department of Economics at Seattle University.

Paul R. Epstein is Associate Director of the Center for Health and the Global Environment, and Instructor in Medicine, both at the Harvard Medical School.

David P. Fidler is Associate Professor of Law at the Indiana University School of Law – Bloomington.

Laurie Garrett is a medical and science reporter for *Newsday* magazine, and recipient of the Pulitzer, Polk and Peabody prizes in journalism.

Sara Glasgow is doctoral candidate in the Department of Government and Politics at the University of Maryland, College Park.

Loch K. Johnson is Professor in the Department of Political Science, University of Georgia.

Ann Marie Kimball is Associate Professor of Health Services and Epidemiology and Adjunct faculty to the Department of Medicine in the School of Medicine at the University of Washington.

Stephen S. Morse is Associate Professor of Epidemiology in the Mailman School of Public Health at Columbia University.

Dennis Pirages is Professor in the Department of Government and Politics, and Director of the Harrison Program on the Future Global Agenda, at the University of Maryland – College Park.

Andrew T. Price-Smith, at the time of writing, is Adjunct Assistant Professor in the School of International and Public Affairs, and

Post-Doctoral Research Scientist at CIESIN, also at Columbia University. He is currently Assistant Professor in the Department of Political Science and Public Administration at the University of North Dakota.

Diane C. Snyder, at the time of writing, is Adjunct Faculty in the Department of Government at Princeton University.

Simon Szreter is University Lecturer in the Faculty of History at Cambridge University.

Jim Whitman is Lecturer in the Department of Peace Studies, Bradford University, co-editor of the *Journal of Humanitarian Assistance*, and general editor of the Palgrave Global Issues series.

Mark Zacher is Professor in the Department of Political Science, and former Director of the Institute of International Relations at the University of British Columbia.

1
Introduction

Andrew T. Price-Smith

This volume sits at the cutting edge of interdisciplinary scholarly innovation. It reveals fresh approaches to problems that are just beginning to penetrate the public consciousness.

Of recent general developments in the social sciences, the newest and most striking is the recognition of the close relationship between health, prosperity and state stability. There is a growing awareness of the interconnections between epidemiology, political conflict, prosperity and the wellness/illness of populations. Around our troubled globe it is increasingly apparent that the wealth of nations depends on the health of nations.

In the post Cold-War era, the fast-changing pace of innovations in science and technology opens up vast new realms of opportunity. But humanity is also confronted by growing spectres derived from our continuing hubris and miscalculations, namely the long-term degradation of the Earth's biosphere and our continuing unwillingness to adequately address entrenched poverty throughout the developing world. It is precisely this combination of increasing environmental disruption and deep inequities in the global distribution of wealth that has generally contributed to the current resurgence of infectious disease on a global scale. As the articles collected for this volume attest, the return of infectious disease has enormous downstream implications for many aspects of human societies, including international development, international security and governance, and international law.

The global resurgence of disease is an intriguing story that illuminates the depth of our arrogance and ignorance when it comes to human interactions with the natural world. Early medical successes against infectious disease came in the form of Pasteur's heat-processing, Koch's identification of the cholera bacilli, Salk's development of the polio vaccine, and the early (and short-lived) victories over malaria through the use of vector-control agents such as DDT. Indeed, we have enjoyed some lasting victories over the microbes: polio has been generally eradicated from the Americas and Europe, and the once widespread killer, smallpox, is now confined to military research laboratories in the United States and Russia. Up until the mid-1970s, humanity had enjoyed triumph after triumph over the microbial world, to the extent that leading figures in the public health sciences began to comment that there was little, if any, need to continue to train physicians in the realm of infectious disease diagnosis and treatment.

Despite this premature celebration of victories over the microbial threat, there were early signs that pathogens would soon begin to reassert their normal ecological roles as the controlling agents of human populations. One early example of disease emergence came in the form of *Legionnella* (Legionnaire's disease), which gained notoriety for the mortality it generated. Meanwhile, immunity to vector-control agents (e.g. DDT) began to rise in arthropod populations,[1] just as the malaria parasites themselves began to develop increasing resistance to chemical prophylaxis such as quinine. Of course, the true wake-up call for humanity came in the form of the Human Immunodeficiency Virus (HIV) that causes AIDS, and which emerged in the early 1980s. At the start of a new century, the global HIV pandemic continues its relentless expansion across the globe, generating both record levels of new infections and HIV-induced deaths. HIV/AIDS is thoroughly entrenched in sub-Saharan Africa where upwards of 30 per cent of the adult populations of some states (for example, Zimbabwe, Botswana) are currently infected with the virus. The HIV pandemic is expanding rapidly throughout South Asia, particularly in India where an estimated 1 per cent of the aggregate population now tests positive for infection, and in the Indian province of Nagaland where over 7 per cent of the populace is now infected. HIV is also spreading rapidly throughout South-East Asia from its established foothold in Thailand, and Beijing has gone so far as to attempt to erect a disease wall in southern Yunnan province to keep the infection from spilling over into its population. While new HIV infection rates have recently begun to plateau in the developed world (Western Europe and North America), they are soaring in the former Soviet republics of Russia and Ukraine; there, in conjunction with the equally rapid proliferation of tuberculosis, we are likely to observe significant population morbidity and mortality in the near future.

After nearly 20 years of battling the HIV/AIDS pandemic there is still no vaccine for the virus and while drug cocktails (such as AZT, etc.)

have proven effective in prolonging the lives of patients, they cannot rid the patient of the virus completely. The greatest problem is that the provision of such anti-viral therapies and chronic care medical services are out of reach for the majority of the global population now infected with HIV. Peoples in the developing world have neither access to adequate health care infrastructures nor the fiscal resources required to purchase costly anti-viral medications.

Unfortunately, the one lesson that we can take away from the emergence of HIV and hepatitis, and the re-emergence of tuberculosis and cholera, is that the microbial world will continue to adapt to human-induced changes in the global ecology. Thus, the greater the degree of degradation that humanity visits upon fragile ecosystems, the more unpredictable the response from the microbial world as it is pushed to evolve faster to compensate for its changing environment. Indeed, the harder we attempt to push the microbes to the margin, the faster they will continue to evolve. Many prominent epidemiologists now warn that HIV/AIDS should be considered a shot across the bow, and that it is precisely because of the mechanics of biological evolution (and humanity's increasing ability to tamper with it) that we will continue to observe the emergence of new potentially virulent microorganisms. Given that microbial evolution is inevitable, it would be prudent to anticipate the emergence of lethal pathogens in the years ahead.

This book represents an attempt to bridge the disciplines, from the natural to the social sciences, and to generate a solid scientific foundation for future attempts to generate consilient knowledge.[2] Edward O. Wilson's eloquent plea for an increase in cross-disciplinary work recalls the endeavours of Sir Francis Bacon, who took all knowledge to be his province. Wilson argues for a new Renaissance in the pursuit of scientific knowledge, positing that many of the greatest scientific discoveries are in fact likely to be found at the interstices between disciplines. It is through the gradual aggregation of interdisciplinary knowledge that we will be able to emerge from the recesses of scientific compartmentalisation and the charade of inter-disciplinary rivalry. Recognising the fundamental value of interdisciplinary endeavour, this book represents an intellectual excursion into the realms of consilient knowledge.

As the following chapters document, the emergence of disease has conditioned the structure of international law over the centuries, has had negative effects on international trade and economic development, and is a growing threat to national security in both the developing and developed world. This volume brings together a number of writings concerning the impact of infectious disease on disparate facets of human society, ranging from the formation of international law, to international trade, national economic development and national security. It also includes contributions that place the phenomena of emerging and re-emerging disease within the context of human inter-actions with the biosphere. Thus, it is a preliminary step in the genera-tion of cross-disciplinary knowledge, and one that will help us to comprehend the socioeconomic and legal ramifications of emerging infections for the future of human societies. To that end, I have gath-ered together commissioned chapters as well as reprinting several seminal essays for inclusion in this volume, such that it may serve as a vehicle for the transmission of new consilient knowledge. It is my hope that the chapters herein will help to inform the reader of both the gravity of the biological issues that the human species will face as the century proceeds, and the complexity involved in dealing effect-ively with these new (and resurgent) threats to human security and prosperity.

The book is structured in such a way that the reader begins with a general overview of ecological and biological processes involved in the emergence and re-emergence of infectious disease. Following this, the reader is guided through the impacts of disease on international trade, and on the historical and current patterns of economic development in various societies. The latter section of the volume deals with the concept of biosecurity or health security, wherein the emergence and re-emergence of infectious disease constitutes a direct threat to the lives and welfare of populations, endangering national security. Finally, the role of infectious disease as a causal agent in the historical formation of international regimes is explored.

Chapter 1, the Introduction, presents the basic premises of the volume, expounds upon the current trends in the proliferation of disease agents, and details the sequence of chapters in the rest of the volume.

In Chapter 2, Stephen S. Morse describes the myriad complexities involved in the emergence and re-emergence of various infectious disease agents. Morse details factors such as ecological, environmental and demographic variables that increase the likelihood of colonization by pathogens or enable the distribution of such pathogens throughout the human ecology.

Chapter 3 continues this examination of the interplay between human-induced environmental change and the transmission of disease agents throughout the human ecology. Paul Epstein argues that phenomena such as climate change, changing land use, increasingly rapid international travel and the inequitable distribution of economic resources (among other things) are contributing to the emergence and re-emergence of disease agents.

Chapter 4 examines the emergence of disease pathogens within the Pacific Rim area, and notes the negative economic consequences that disease emergence is likely to have on international trade. Kimball and Davis note the direct and indirect costs of disease to economies in the region, and argue that there is a need for improved disease surveillance throughout the region in order to mitigate disease-induced economic loss in the future.

In Chapter 5, Simon Szreter critiques the commonly-held assumption that economic growth automatically results in improved human health, and that the basal health of a population is the product of its economic productivity. Szreter argues that economic growth can actually undermine the health of populations and thus impede the downstream development of nations.

Chapter 6 illuminates the role that infectious disease plays in limiting the consolidation of human capital, and impeding the economic development of societies over the long term. Price-Smith argues that infectious disease has a profound negative effect on the economic productivity of entire societies, ranging from the microeconomic to the sectoral and macroeconomic levels. He posits that, as the global burden of disease continues to increase, we shall observe declining productivity and economic development in those regions of the planet where the burden of disease is greatest, namely the tropics.

In Chapter 7, Jim Whitman provides a detailed and stimulating reconceptualization of the concept of security, away from historically dominant statist paradigms towards the more holistic and increasingly pragmatic paradigm of 'human security'. Whitman argues that widely held theories of International Relations (as a subset of the political science literature) are increasingly archaic and of marginal utility in a world where global phenomena, such as infectious diseases, threaten the security of the species. He concludes by calling for greater levels of interdisciplinary work, bridging the gap between the natural and social sciences, and between the particular disciplines within each camp.

Chapter 8 stands as a premier example of one of the earliest contributions to deal with the concept of health security. In this chapter, Laurie Garrett reveals the threat that emerging and re-emerging infectious disease poses to the national security and broader 'national interests' of the United States. She cites the growing loss of American lives to disease and the increasing toll of disease on trade and interstate relations as examples of how infectious disease may contribute to chaos in the post-Cold War era. Garrett also notes the increasing threat of biological warfare.

Chapter 9 takes the argument for the concept of health security a step further by demonstrating that infectious disease has historically had a far greater destructive effect on populations than warfare. Price-Smith also argues that the proliferation of infectious disease will likely have significant negative ramifications for the effective governance of both societies and states. Thus, states that are experiencing surges in disease rates within their respective populations will be prone to increasing levels of social instability and political destabilization. In this manner, the proliferation of disease may threaten the stability of nascent democracies and contribute to regional instability in areas such as sub-Saharan Africa and South Asia.

In Chapter 10, Pirages and Glasgow develop the concept of 'microinsecurity'. They identify both historical and contemporary discontinuities in biological and sociocultural evolution that are increasing the microbial threat to human societies. The article concludes by focusing on the biological and socioeconomic causes and consequences of the AIDS epidemic in southern Africa.

Chapter 11, by Loch K. Johnson and Diane C. Snyder, puts forth the argument that the growing saliency of health security as well as rising levels of infectious disease that undercut both security and national interests require the collection of public health data by intelligence officers in the field. The reluctance of many states to publicise their actual public health situations (in terms of disease prevalence) necessitates the collection of accurate public health information by intelligence professionals where it is not readily available.

In Chapter 12, Mark Zacher and Simon Carvalho examine the role of infectious disease as a principal agent in the evolution of international legal regimes from the 1880s to the early 1990s. The authors focus on the development of regulations requiring states to notify others during disease outbreak events and to employ specified control measures. The chapter next examines country submissions to the World Health Organization that evaluate the utility of current regulations and note difficulties with their implementation. Finally, Carvalho and Zacher assess recent revisions of the international regulations in response to the accelerating proliferation of infectious diseases.

In Chapter 13, Fidler examines the role of infectious disease as a parameter that, over the centuries, has forged the outlines of international law. Using the analytical lens of *microbialpolitik*, he also examines the manner in which pathogen emergence and proliferation has been dealt with in the arena of international politics. Most importantly, Fidler examines the dynamic wherein advances in international law (dealing with emerging public health threats) have influenced the dynamics of microbialpolitik.

Of course, any undertaking such as this involves a whole host of individuals who contributed to the development of this book over the years. First and foremost I would like to thank Christina Greenough for her invaluable assistance in the preparation and formatting of the manuscript. Considerable acclaim must also go to the Center for International Studies at the University of Toronto which hosted the conference on infectious disease and international policy that spawned this volume. In particular, I would like to thank Louis Pauly, David A. Welch, Janice Gross Stein, Mary-Lynn Bratti, Joan Golding and Tina Lagopoulos for all their support during my years at the Program on Health and Global Affairs in the CIS. Many thanks are due to my family for their support during my years in graduate school.

CIESIN, at Columbia University, provided both the physical and intellectual space and, most importantly, the funding, to complete the manuscript. I am indebted to Marc Levy, Roberta Miller, Deborah Balk and Meredith Golden for their comments and support during my tenure at Columbia. Finally, I would like to thank Mark Zacher for his continual challenging and for his solid advice, Steve Morse for his exceptional vision, and Dennis Pirages for sparking the health security debate in the first place.

Notes

1. Examples of such arthropod vectors are disease-transmitting insects such as mosquitoes and flies.
2. Edward O. Wilson employs William Whewel's definition of *consilience* as the jumping together of knowledge across disciplines. See Edward O. Wilson, *Consilience: the Unity of Knowledge.* New York: Knopf, 1998.

2
Factors in the Emergence of Infectious Diseases

Stephen S. Morse

Infectious diseases emerging throughout history have included some of the most feared plagues of the past. New infections continue to emerge today, while many of the old plagues are with us still. These are global problems (William Foege, former CDC director now at the Carter Center, terms them global infectious disease threats). As demonstrated by influenza epidemics, under suitable circumstances, a new infection first appearing anywhere in the world could traverse entire continents within days or weeks.

We can define as emerging, infections that have newly appeared in a population, or have existed but are rapidly increasing in incidence or geographic range (Morse and Schluederberg, 1990; Morse, 1993). Recent examples of emerging diseases in various parts of the world include HIV/AIDS; classic cholera in South America and Africa; cholera due to *Vibrio cholerae* O139; Rift Valley fever; hantavirus pulmonary syndrome; Lyme disease; and haemolytic uraemic syndrome, a food-borne infection caused by certain strains of *Escherichia coli* (in the United States, serotype O157:H7).

Although these occurrences may appear inexplicable, rarely if ever do emerging infections appear without reason. Specific factors responsible for disease emergence can be identified in virtually all cases studied (Morse, 1990, 1991, 1993). Table 2.1 summarizes the known causes for a number of infections that have emerged recently. I have suggested that infectious disease emergence can be viewed operationally as a two-step process: (1) Introduction of the agent into a new host population (whether the pathogen originated in the environment, possibly in another species, or as a variant of an existing human infec-

Table 2.1 Recent examples of emerging infections and probable factors in their emergence

Infection or agent	Factor(s) contributing to emergence
Viral	
Argentine, Bolivian haemorrhagic fever	Changes in agriculture favouring rodent host
Bovine spongiform encephalopathy (cattle)	Changes in rendering processes
Dengue, dengue haemorrhagic fever	Transportation, travel, and migration; urbanization
Ebola, Marburg	Unknown (in Europe and the United States, importation of monkeys)
Hantaviruses	Ecological or environmental changes increasing contact with rodent hosts
Hepatitis B, C	Transfusions, organ transplants, contaminated hypodermic apparatus, sexual transmission, vertical spread from infected mother to child
HIV	Migration to cities and travel; after introduction, sexual transmission, vertical spread from infected mother to child, contaminated hypodermic apparatus (including during intravenous drug use), transfusions, organ transplants
HTLV	Contaminated hypodermic apparatus, other
Influenza (pandemic)	Possibly pig-duck agriculture, facilitating reassortment of avian and mammalian influenza viruses*
Lassa fever	Urbanization favouring rodent host, increasing exposure (usually in homes)
Rift Valley fever	Dam building, agriculture, irrigation; possibly change in virulence or pathogenicity of virus
Yellow fever (in new areas)	Conditions favouring mosquito vector

Table 2.1   Recent examples of emerging infections and probable factors in their emergence *(continued)*

Infection or agent	Factor(s) contributing to emergence
Bacterial	
Brazilian purpuric fever (*Haemophilus influenzae,* biotype *aegyptius*)	Probably new strain
Cholera	In recent epidemic in South America, probably introduced from Asia by ship, with spread facilitated by reduced water chlorination; a new strain (type O139) from Asia recently disseminated by travel (similarly to past introductions of classic cholera)
Helicobacter pylori	Probably long widespread, now recognized (associated with gastric ulcers, possibly other gastrointestinal disease)
Haemolytic uraemic syndrome (*Escherichia coli* O157:H7)	Mass food processing technology allowing contamination of meat
Legionella (Legionnaire's disease)	Cooling and plumbing systems (organism grows in biofilms that form on water storage tanks and in stagnant plumbing)
Lyme borreliosis (*Borrelia burgdorferi*)	Reforestation around homes and other conditions favoring tick vector and deer (a secondary reservoir host)
Streptococcus, group A (invasive; necrotizing)	Uncertain
Toxic shock syndrome (*Staphylococcus aureus*)	Ultra-absorbency tampons
Parasitic	
Cryptosporidium, other waterborne pathogens	Contaminated surface water, faulty water purification
Malaria (in 'new' areas)	Travel or migration
Schistosomiasis	Dam building

* Reappearances of influenza are due to two distinct mechanisms: annual or biennial epidemics involving new variants due to antigenic drift (point mutations, primarily in the gene for the surface protein, hemagglutinin) and pandemic strains, arising from antigenic shift (genetic reassortment, generally between avian and mammalian influenza strains).

tion); followed by (2) establishment and further dissemination within the new host population (adoption) (Morse 1991). Whatever its origin, the infection emerges when it reaches a new population. Factors that promote one or both of these steps will, therefore, tend to precipitate disease emergence. Most emerging infections, and even antibiotic-resistant strains of common bacterial pathogens, usually originate in one geographic location and then disseminate to new places (Soares *et al.*, 1993).

Regarding the introduction step, the numerous examples of infections originating as zoonoses (McNeill, 1976; Fiennes, 1978) suggest that the zoonotic pool introduction of infections from other species is an important and potentially rich source of emerging diseases; periodic discoveries of new zoonoses suggest that the zoonotic pool appears by no means exhausted. Once introduced, an infection might then be disseminated through other factors, although rapid course and high mortality combined with low transmissibility are often limiting. However, even if a zoonotic agent is not able to spread readily from person to person and establish itself, other factors (for example, nosocomial infection) might transmit the infection. Additionally, if the reservoir host or vector becomes more widely disseminated, the microbe can appear in new places. Bubonic plague transmitted by rodent fleas and rat-borne hantavirus infections are examples.

Most emerging infections appear to be caused by pathogens already present in the environment, brought out of obscurity or given a selective advantage by changing conditions and afforded an opportunity to infect new host populations (on rare occasions, a new variant may also evolve and cause a new disease) (Morse, 1991, 1993). The process by which infectious agents may transfer from animals to humans or disseminate from isolated groups into new populations can be called microbial traffic (Morse, 1990, 1991). A number of activities increase microbial traffic and as a result promote emergence and epidemics. In some cases, including many of the most novel infections, the agents are zoonotic, crossing from their natural hosts into the human population; because of the many similarities, I include here vector-borne diseases. In other cases, pathogens already present in geographically isolated populations are given an opportunity to disseminate further. Surprisingly often, disease emergence is caused by human actions, however inadvertently; natural causes, such as changes in climate, can also at times be responsible (Rogers and Packer, 1993). Although this discussion is confined largely to human disease, similar considerations apply to emerging pathogens in other species.

Table 2.2 summarizes the underlying factors responsible for emergence. Any categorization of the factors is, of course, somewhat arbitrary but is intended to be representative of the underlying processes that cause emergence. I have essentially adopted the categories developed in the Institute of Medicine in Washington's report on emerging infections (Institute of Medicine, 1992), with additional definitions from the Centers for Disease Control and Prevention (CDC) emerging infections plan (Centers for Disease Control and Prevention, 1994). Responsible factors include ecological changes, such as those due to agricultural or economic development or to anomalies in climate; human demographic changes and behaviour; travel and commerce; technology and industry; microbial adaptation and change; and breakdown of public health measures. Each of these will be considered in turn.

Ecological interactions can be complex, with several factors often working together or in sequence. For example, population movement from rural areas to cities can spread a once-localized infection. The strain on infrastructure in overcrowded and rapidly growing cities may disrupt or slow public health measures, perhaps allowing establishment of the newly introduced infection. Finally, the city may also provide a gateway for further dissemination of the infection. Most successful emerging infections, including HIV, cholera, and dengue, have followed this route.

Consider HIV as an example. Although the precise ancestry of HIV-1 is still uncertain, it appears to have had a zoonotic origin (Allan *et al.*, 1991; Myers, MacInnes and Korber, 1992). Ecological factors that would have allowed human exposure to a natural host carrying the virus that was the precursor to HIV-1 were, therefore, instrumental in the introduction of the virus into humans. This probably occurred in a rural area. A plausible scenario is suggested by the identification of an HIV-2-infected man in a rural area of Liberia whose virus strain resembled viruses isolated from the sooty mangabey monkey (an animal widely hunted for food in rural areas and the putative source of HIV-2) more closely than it did strains circulating in the city (Gao *et al.*, 1992). Such findings suggest that zoonotic introductions of this sort may occur on occasion in isolated populations but may well go unnoticed so long as the recipients remain isolated. But with increasing movement from rural areas to cities, such isolation is increasingly rare. After its likely first move from a rural area into a city, HIV-1 spread regionally along highways, then by long distance routes, including air travel, to more distant places. This last step was critical for HIV and facilitated today's global pandemic. Social changes, which allowed the virus to

Table 2.2 Factors in infectious disease emergence*

Factor	Examples of specific factors	Examples of diseases
Ecological changes (including those due to economic development and land use)	Agriculture; dams, changes in water ecosystems; deforestation/reforestation; flood/drought; famine; climate changes	Schistosomiasis (dams); Rift Valley fever (dams, irrigation); Argentine haemorrhagic fever (agriculture); Hantaan (Korean haemorrhagic fever) (agriculture); hantavirus pulmonary syndrome, southwestern US, 1993 (weather anomalies)
Human demographics, behaviour	Societal events: population growth and migration (movement from rural areas to cities); war or civil conflict; urban decay; sexual behaviour; intravenous drug use; use of high-density facilities	Introduction of HIV; spread of dengue; spread of HIV and other sexually transmitted diseases
International travel commerce	Worldwide movement of goods and people; air travel	'Airport' malaria; dissemination of mosquito vectors; rat-borne hantaviruses; introduction of cholera into South America; dissemination of O139 *V. cholerae*

Table 2.2 Factors in infectious disease emergence* *(continued)*

Factor	Examples of specific factors	Examples of diseases
Technology and industry	Globalization of food supplies; changes in food processing and packaging; organ or tissue transplantation; drugs causing immunosuppression; widespread use of antibiotics	Haemolytic uraemic syndrome (*E. coli* contamination of hamburger meat), bovine spongiform encephalopathy; transfusion-associated hepatitis (hepatitis B, C), opportunistic infections in immunosuppressed patients, Creutzfeldt–Jakob disease from contaminated batches of human growth hormone (medical technology)
Microbial adaptation and change	Microbial evolution, response to selection in environment	Antibiotic-resistant bacteria, 'antigenic drift' in influenza virus
Breakdown in public health measures	Curtailment or reduction in prevention programmes; inadequate sanitation and vector control measures	Resurgence of tuberculosis in the United States; cholera in refugee camps in Africa; resurgence of diphtheria in the former Soviet Union

* Categories of factors (column 1) adapted from Institute of Medicine, 1992, examples of specific factors (column 2) adapted from Centers for Disease Control and Prevention, 1994. Categories are not mutually exclusive; several factors may contribute to emergence of a disease (see Table 2.1, above, for additional information).

reach a larger population and to be transmitted despite its relatively low natural transmissibility, were instrumental in the success of the virus in its new-found human host. For HIV, the long duration of infectivity allowed this normally poorly transmissible virus many opportunities to be transmitted and to take advantage of such factors as human behaviour (sexual transmission, intravenous drug use) and changing technology (early spread through blood transfusions and blood products) (see Table 2.1, above).

Ecological changes and agricultural development

Ecological changes, including those due to agricultural or economic development, are among the most frequently identified factors in emergence. They are especially frequent as factors in outbreaks of previously unrecognized diseases with high case-fatality rates, which often turn out to be zoonotic introductions. Ecological factors usually precipitate emergence by placing people in contact with a natural reservoir or host for an infection hitherto unfamiliar but usually already present (often a zoonotic or arthropod-borne infection), either by increasing proximity or, often, also by changing conditions so as to favour an increased population of the microbe or its natural host (Morse, 1991, 1993). The emergence of Lyme disease in the United States and Europe was probably due largely to reforestation (Barbour and Kish, 1993), which increased the population of deer and the deer tick, the vector of Lyme disease. The movement of people into these areas placed a larger population in close proximity to the vector.

Agricultural development, one of the most common ways in which people alter and interpose themselves into the environment, is often a factor (Table 2.2, above). Hantaan virus, the cause of Korean haemorrhagic fever, causes over 100 000 cases a year in China and has been known in Asia for centuries. The virus is a natural infection of the field mouse *Apodemus agrarius*. The rodent flourishes in rice fields; people usually contract the disease during the rice harvest from contact with infected rodents. Junin virus, the cause of Argentine haemorrhagic fever, is an unrelated virus with a history remarkably similar to that of Hantaan virus. Conversion of grassland to maize cultivation favoured a rodent that was the natural host for this virus, and human cases increased in proportion to the expansion of maize agriculture (Johnson, 1993). Other examples, in addition to those already known (Morse, 1990; Johnson, 1993), are likely to appear as new areas are placed under cultivation.

Perhaps most surprisingly, pandemic influenza appears to have an agricultural origin, integrated pig–duck farming in China. Strains that cause the frequent annual or biennial epidemics generally result from mutation (antigenic drift), but pandemic influenza viruses do not generally arise by this process. Instead, gene segments from two influenza strains reassort to produce a new virus that can infect humans (Webster *et al.*, 1992). Evidence amassed by Webster, Scholtissek and others, indicates that waterfowl, such as ducks, are major reservoirs of influenza and that pigs can serve as mixing vessels for new mammalian influenza strains (Webster *et al.*, 1992). Pandemic influenza viruses have generally come from China. Scholtissek and Naylor suggested that integrated pig–duck agriculture, an extremely efficient food production system traditionally practised in certain parts of China for several centuries, puts these two species in contact and provides a natural laboratory for making new influenza recombinants (Scholtissek and Naylor, 1988). Webster has suggested that, with high-intensity agriculture and movement of livestock across borders, suitable conditions may now also be found in Europe (Webster *et al.*, 1992).[16]

Water is also frequently associated with disease emergence. Infections transmitted by mosquitoes or other arthropods, which include some of the most serious and widespread diseases, are often stimulated by the expansion in the number of standing water bodies, simply because many of the mosquito vectors breed in water (World Health Organization, 1989; Monath, 1993). There are many cases of diseases transmitted by water-breeding vectors, most involving dams, water for irrigation, or stored drinking water in cities. (See the section below for a discussion of dengue.) The incidence of Japanese encephalitis, another mosquito-borne disease that accounts for almost 30 000 human cases and approximately 7000 deaths annually in Asia, is closely associated with flooding of fields for rice growing. Outbreaks of Rift Valley fever in some parts of Africa have been associated with dam building as well as with periods of heavy rainfall (Monath, 1993). In the outbreaks of Rift Valley fever in Mauritania in 1987, the human cases occurred in villages near dams on the Senegal River. The same effect has been documented with other infections that have aquatic hosts, such as schistosomiasis.

Because humans are important agents of ecological and environmental change, many of these factors are anthropogenic. Of course, this is not always the case, and natural environmental changes, such as climate or weather anomalies, can have the same effect. The outbreak of hantavirus pulmonary syndrome in the southwestern United States in 1993 is an example. It is likely that the virus has long been present in mouse populations but an unusually mild and wet winter and spring in that area led to an increased rodent population in the spring and summer and thus to greater opportunities for people to come in contact with infected rodents (and, hence, with the virus); it has been suggested that the weather anomaly was due to large-scale climatic effects (Levins *et al.*, 1993). The same causes may have been responsible for outbreaks of hantaviral disease in Europe at approximately the same time (Le Guenno *et al.*, 1994; Rollin, Coudrier and Sureau, 1994). With cholera, it has been suggested that certain organisms in marine environments are natural reservoirs for cholera vibrios, and that large-scale effects on ocean currents may cause local increases in the reservoir organism with consequent flare-ups of cholera (Epstein, Ford and Colwell, 1993).

Changes in human demographics and behaviour

Human population movements or upheavals, caused by migration or war, are often important factors in disease emergence. In many parts of the world, economic conditions are encouraging the mass movement of workers from rural areas to cities. The United Nations has estimated that, largely as a result of continuing migration, by the year 2025, 65 per cent of the world population (also expected to be larger in absolute numbers), including 61 per cent of the population in developing regions, will live in cities (United Nations, 1991). As discussed above for HIV, rural urbanization allows infections arising in isolated rural areas – which may once have remained obscure and localized – to reach larger populations. Once in a city, the newly introduced infection would have the opportunity to spread locally among the population and could also spread further along highways and inter-urban transport routes and by aircraft. HIV has been, and in Asia is becoming, the best known beneficiary of this dynamic, but many other diseases, such as dengue, stand to benefit. The frequency of the most severe form, dengue haemorrhagic fever, which is thought to occur when a person is sequentially infected by two types of dengue virus, is increasing as different dengue viruses have extended their range and now overlap (Gubler and Trent, 1993). Dengue hemorrhagic fever is now common in some cities in Asia, where the high prevalence of infection is attributed to the proliferation of open containers needed for water storage (which also provide breeding grounds for the mosquito vector) as the population size exceeds the infrastructure (Monath, 1993). In urban environments, rain-filled tyres or plastic bottles are often breeding grounds of choice for mosquito vectors. The resulting mosquito population boom is complemented by the high human population density in such situations, increasing the chances of stable transmission cycles between infected and susceptible persons. Even in industrialized countries, as, for example, in the United States, infections such as tuberculosis can spread through high-population density settings (for example, day care centres or prisons) (Allan *et al.*, 1991; Krause, 1992; Bloom and Murray, 1992; Hoge *et al.*, 1994).

Human behaviour can have important effects on disease dissemination. The best known examples are sexually transmitted diseases; the ways in which such human behaviours such as sex or intravenous drug use have contributed to the emergence of HIV are now well known. Other factors responsible for disease emergence are influenced by a variety of human actions, so human behaviour in the broader sense is also very important. Motivating appropriate individual behaviour and constructive action, both locally and on a larger scale, will be essential for controlling emerging infections. Ironically, as AIDS prevention efforts have demonstrated, human behaviour remains one of the weakest links in our scientific knowledge.

International travel and commerce

The dissemination of HIV through travel has already been mentioned. In the past, an infection introduced into people in a geographically isolated area might, on occasion, be brought to a new place through travel, commerce or war. Trade between Asia and Europe, perhaps beginning with the silk route and continuing with the Crusades, brought the rat and one of its infections, the bubonic plague, to Europe. Beginning in the sixteenth and seventeenth centuries, ships bringing slaves from West Africa to the New World also brought yellow fever and its mosquito vector, *Aedes aegypti*, to the new territories. Similarly, smallpox escaped its Old World origins to wreak new havoc in the New World. In the nineteenth century, cholera had similar opportunities to spread from its probable origin in the Ganges plain to the Middle East and, from there, to Europe and much of the remaining world. Each of these infections had once been localized and took advantage of opportunities that arose to be carried to previously unfamiliar parts of the world.

Similar histories are being repeated today, but opportunities in recent years have become far richer and more numerous, reflecting the increasing volume, scope and speed of traffic in an increasingly mobile world. Rats have carried hantaviruses virtually worldwide (LeDuc, Childs and Glass, 1992). *Aedes albopictus* (the Asian tiger mosquito) was introduced into the United States, Brazil and parts of Africa in shipments of used tyres from Asia (Centers for Disease Control and Prevention, 1991a). Since its introduction in 1982, this mosquito has established itself in at least 18 states of the United States and has acquired local viruses including Eastern equine encephalomyelitis (Centers for Disease Control and Prevention, 1991b), a cause of serious disease. Another mosquito-borne disease, malaria, is one of the most frequently imported diseases in non-endemic-disease areas, and cases of airport malaria are occasionally identified.

A classic bacterial disease, cholera, recently entered both South America (for the first time this century) and Africa. Molecular typing shows the South American isolates to be of the current pandemic strain (Wachsmuth *et al.*, 1993), supporting the suggestion that the organism was introduced in contaminated bilge water from an Asian freighter (Anderson, 1991). Other evidence indicates that cholera was only one of many organisms to travel in ballast water; dozens, perhaps hundreds, of species have been exchanged between distant places through this means of transport alone. Examples of microbial adaptation and change include antibiotic-resistant bacteria (Soares *et al.*, 1993; Davies, 1994) and new bacterial strains, such as the recently identified *Vibrio cholerae* O139, or an epidemic strain of *Neisseria meningitidis* (Moore, 1992; Moore and Broome, 1994); Examples of microbial adaptation and change) have disseminated rapidly along routes of trade and travel.

Technology and industry

High-volume rapid movement characterizes not only travel, but also other industries in modern society. In operations, including food production, that process or use products of biological origin, modern production methods yield increased efficiency and reduced costs but can increase the chances of accidental contamination and amplify the effects of such contamination. The problem is further compounded by globalization, allowing the opportunity to introduce agents from far afield. A pathogen present in some of the raw material may find its way into a large batch of final product, as happened with the contamination of hamburger meat by *E. coli* strains, causing hemolytic uremic syndrome (Centers for Disease Control and Prevention, 1993). In the

United States, the implicated *E. coli* strains are serotype O157:H7; additional serotypes have been identified in other countries. Bovine spongiform encephalopathy (BSE), which emerged in Britain in the last decades of the twentieth century was likely to be an interspecies transfer of scrapie from sheep to cattle (Morse, 1990) that occurred when changes in rendering processes led to incomplete inactivation of scrapie agent in sheep by-products fed to cattle (Wilesmith, Ryan and Atkinson, 1991).

The concentrating effects that occur with blood and tissue products have inadvertently disseminated infections unrecognized at the time, such as HIV and hepatitis B and C. Medical settings are also at the front-line of exposure to new diseases, and a number of infections, including many emerging infections, have spread nosocomially in health care settings (Table 2.2, above). Among the numerous examples, in the outbreaks of Ebola fever in Africa, many of the secondary cases were hospital acquired, most transmitted to other patients through contaminated hypodermic apparatus, and some to the health care staff by contact. Transmission of Lassa fever to health care workers has also been documented.

On the positive side, advances in diagnostic technology can also lead to new recognition of agents that are already widespread. When such agents are newly recognized, they may at first often be labelled, in some cases incorrectly, as emerging infections. Human herpesvirus 6 (HHV-6) was identified only a few years ago, but the virus appears to be extremely widespread (Inoue, Dambaugh and Pellett, 1993) and has recently been implicated as the cause of roseola (*exanthem subitum*), a very common childhood disease (Yamanishi *et al.*, 1988). Because roseola has been known since at least 1910, HHV-6 is likely to have been common for decades and probably much longer. Another recent example is the bacterium *Helicobacter pylori*, a probable cause of gastric ulcers (Peterson, 1991) and some cancers (Nomura *et al.*, 1991; Parsonnet *et al.*, 1991). We have lived with these diseases for a long time without knowing their cause. Recognition of the agent is often advantageous, offering new promise of controlling a previously intractable disease, for example, treating gastric ulcers with specific antimicrobial therapy.

Microbial adaptation and change

Microbes, like all other living things, are constantly evolving. The emergence of antibiotic-resistant bacteria as a result of the ubiquity of antimicrobials in the environment is an evolutionary lesson on microbial adaptation, as well as a demonstration of the power of natural selection. Selection for antibiotic-resistant bacteria (Soares *et al.*, 1993; Davies, 1994) and drug-resistant parasites has become frequent, driven by the wide and sometimes inappropriate use of antimicrobial drugs in a variety of applications (Bloom and Murray, 1992; Cohen, 1992; Neu, 1992). Pathogens can also acquire new antibiotic resistance genes from other, often nonpathogenic, species in the environment (Davies, 1994), selected or perhaps even driven by the selection pressure of antibiotics.

Many viruses show a high mutation rate and can evolve rapidly to yield new variant. (Domingo and Holland, 1994). A classic example is influenza (Kilbourne, 1978). Regular annual epidemics are caused by antigenic drift in a previously circulating influenza strain. A change in an antigenic site of a surface protein, usually the haemagglutinin (H) protein, allows the new variant to reinfect previously infected persons because the altered antigen is not immediately recognized by the immune system.

On rare occasions, perhaps more often with nonviral pathogens than with viruses (Morse, 1994), the evolution of a new variant may result in a new expression of disease. The epidemic of Brazilian purpuric fever in 1990, associated with a newly emerged clonal variant of *Hemophilus influenzae*, biogroup *aegyptius*, may fall into this category. It is possible, but not yet clear, that some recently described manifestations of disease by group *A. streptococcus*, such as rapidly invasive infection or necrotizing fasciitis, may also fall into this category.

Breakdown of public health measures and deficiencies in public health infrastructure

Classical public health and sanitation measures have long served to minimize dissemination and human exposure to many pathogens spread by traditional routes such as water or preventable by immunization or vector control. The pathogens themselves often still remain, albeit in reduced numbers, in reservoir hosts or in the environment, or in small pockets of infection and, therefore, are often able to take advantage of the opportunity to re-emerge if there are breakdowns in preventive measures.

Re-emerging diseases are those, like cholera, that were once decreasing but are now rapidly increasing again. These are often conventionally understood and well recognized public health threats for which (in most cases) previously active public health measures had been allowed to lapse, a situation that unfortunately now applies all too often in both developing countries and the inner cities of the industrialized world. The appearance of re-emerging diseases may, therefore, often be a sign of the breakdown of public health measures and should be a warning against complacency in the war against infectious diseases.

Cholera, for example, raged in South America at the end of the twentieth century for the first time in that century (Glass and Libel, 1992) and Africa. The rapid spread of cholera in South America may have been abetted by recent reductions in chlorine levels used to treat water supplies (Moore, 1992). The success of cholera and other enteric diseases is often due to the lack of a reliable water supply. These problems are more severe in developing countries, but are not confined to these areas. The US outbreak of waterborne Cryptosporidium infection in Milwaukee, Wisconsin, in the spring of 1993, with over 400 000 estimated cases, was in part due to a nonfunctioning water filtration plant (MacKenzie *et al.*, 1994); similar deficiencies in water purification have been found in other cities in the United States (Centers for Disease Control and Prevention, 1993).

For our future

David Satcher discusses the history of infectious diseases and the many infections that, from the dawn of history to the present, have travelled with caravans and followed invading armies (Satcher, 1995). The history of infectious diseases has been a history of microbes on the march, often in our wake, and of microbes that have taken advantage of the rich opportunities offered them to thrive, prosper and spread. And yet the historical processes that have given rise to the emergence of new infections throughout history continue today with unabated force; in fact, they are accelerating, because the conditions of modern life ensure that the factors responsible for disease emergence are more prevalent than ever before. Speed of travel and global reach are further borne out by studies modelling the spread of influenza epidemics (Longini, Fine and Thacker, 1986) and HIV (Flahault and Valleron, 1990, 1992).

Humans are not powerless, however, against this relentless march of microbes. Knowledge of the factors underlying disease emergence can help focus resources on the key situations and areas worldwide (Morse, 1990, 1992) and develop more effective prevention strategies.

If we are to protect ourselves against emerging diseases, the essential first step is effective global disease surveillance to give early warning of emerging infections (Morse, 1990; Institute of Medicine; Henderson, 1993; Centers for Disease Control and Prevention, 1994). This must be tied to incentives, such as national development, and eventually be backed by a system for an appropriate rapid response. World surveillance capabilities are critically deficient. (Institute of Medicine, 1993; Henderson, 1993; Berkelman *et al.*, 1994). Efforts, such as the CDC plan (Centers for Disease Control), now under way in the United States and internationally to remedy this situation, are the essential first steps and deserve strong support. Research, both basic and applied, will also be vital.

References

Allan, J.S., Short, M., Taylor, M.E. *et al.* Species-specific Diversity among Simian Immunodeficiency Viruses from African Green Monkeys. *J. Virol.*, 1991; 65:2816–28.

Anderson, C. Cholera Epidemic traced to Risk Miscalculation [News]. *Nature*, 1991; 354:255.

Barbour, A.G. and Fish, D. The Biological and Social Phenomenon of Lyme Disease. *Science*, 1993; 260:1610–16.

Berkelman, R.L., Bryan, R.T., Osterholm, M.T. *et al.* Infectious Disease Surveillance: a Crumbling Foundation. *Science*, 1994; 264:368–70.

Bloom, B.R. and Murray, C.J.L. Tuberculosis: Commentary on a Reemergent Killer. *Science*, 1992; 257:1055–64.

Centers for Disease Control and Prevention. *Aedes albopictus* Introduction into Continental Africa, 1991a. *MMWR*, 1991; 40:836–8.

Centers for Disease Control and Prevention. Eastern Equine Encephalitis Virus Associated with *Aedes albopictus* Florida, 1991b. *MMWR*, 1992; 41:115, 121.

Centers for Disease Control and Prevention. Update: Multistate Outbreak of *Escherichia coli* O157:H7 Infections from Hamburgers in Western United States, 1992–1993. *MMWR*, 1993; 42:258–63.

Centers for Disease Control and Prevention. Assessment of Inadequately Filtered Public Drinking Water. Washington, DC, December 1993. *MMWR*, 1994; 43:661–3.

Centers for Disease Control and Prevention. *Addressing Emerging Infectious Disease Threats: a Prevention Strategy for the United States*. Atlanta, Georgia: US Dept of Health and Human Services, Public Health Service, 1994.

Cohen, M.L. Epidemiology of Drug Resistance: Implications for a Post-antimicrobial Era. *Science*, 1992; 257:1050–5.

Davies, J. Inactivation of Antibiotics and the Dissemination of Resistance Genes. *Science*, 1994; 264:375–82.

Domingo, E. and Holland, J.J. Mutation Rates and Rapid Evolution of RNA Viruses. In: S.S. Morse, ed. *The Evolutionary Biology of viruses*. New York: Raven Press, 1994, pp. 161–84.

Epstein, P.R., Ford, T.E. and Colwell, R.R. Marine Ecosystems. *Lancet*, 1993; 342:1216–19.

Fiennes, R.W. *Zoonoses and the Origins and Ecology of Human Disease*. London: Academic Press, 1978.

Flahault, A. and Valleron, A.J. A Method for Assessing the Global Spread of HIV-1 Infection Based on Air Travel. *Mathematical Population Studies*, 1992; 3:161–71.

Flahault, A. and Valleron, A.J. HIV and Travel, no Rationale for Restrictions. *Lancet*, 1990; 336:1197–8.

Gao, F., Yue, L., White, A.T. *et al.* Human Infection by Genetically Diverse SIVSM-related HIV-2 in West Africa. *Nature*, 1992; 358:495–9.

Glass, R.I., Libel, M. and Brandling-Bennett, A.D. Epidemic Cholera in the Americas. *Science*, 1992; 265:1524–5.

Gubler, D.J. and Trent, D.W. Emergence of Epidemic Dengue/Dengue Hemorrhagic Fever as a Public Health Problem in the Americas. *Infectious Agents and Disease*, 1993; 26:383–93.

Henderson, D.A. Surveillance Systems and Intergovernmental Cooperation. In: S.S. Morse, ed. *Emerging Viruses*. New York: Oxford University Press, 1993; 283–9.

Hoge, C.W., Reichler, M.R., Dominguez, E.A. *et al.* An Epidemic of Pneumococcal Disease in an Overcrowded, Inadequately Ventilated Jail. *N. Engl. J. Med.*, 1994; 331:643–8.

Inoue, N., Dambaugh, T.R. and Pellett, P.E. Molecular Biology of Human Herpesviruses 6A and 6B. *Infectious Agents and Disease*, 1993; 26:343–60.

Institute of Medicine. *Emerging Infections: Microbial Threats to Health in the United States* (J. Lederberg, R.E. Shope and S.C. Oaks Jr, eds). Washington, DC: National Academy Press, 1992.

Johnson, K.M. Emerging Viruses in Context: an Overview of Viral Hemorrhagic Fevers. In: S.S. Morse, ed. *Emerging Viruses*. New York: Oxford University Press, 1993; 46–7.

Kilbourne, E.D. The Molecular Epidemiology of Influenza. *J. Infect. Dis.*, 1978; 127:478–87.

Krause, R.M. The Origin of Plagues: Old and New. *Science*, 1992; 257:1073–8.

Le Guenno, B., Camprasse, M.A., Guilbaut, J.C. *et al.* Hantavirus Epidemic in Europe, 1993. *Lancet*, 1994; 343:114–15.

LeDuc, J.W., Childs, J.E. and Glass, G.E. The Hantaviruses, Etiologic Agents of Hemorrhagic Fever with Renal Syndrome: a Possible Cause of Hypertension and Chronic Renal Disease in the United States. *Annu. Rev. Public Health*, 1992; 13:79–98.

Levins, R., Epstein, P.R., Wilson, M.E. *et al.* Hantavirus Disease Emerging. *Lancet*, 1993; 342:1292.

Longini, I.M. Jr, Fine, P.E.M. and Thacker, S.B. Predicting the Global Spread of New Infectious Agents. *Am. J. Epidemiol.*, 1986; 123:383–91.

MacKenzie, W.R., Hoxie, N.J., Proctor, M.E. *et al.* A Massive Outbreak in Milwaukee of Cryptosporidium Infection Transmitted Through the Water Supply. *N. Engl. J. Med.*, 1994; 331:161–7.

McNeill, W.H. *Plagues and Peoples*. New York: Anchor Press/Doubleday, 1976.

Monath, T.P. Arthropod-borne Viruses. In: S.S. Morse, ed. *Emerging Viruses*. New York: Oxford University Press, 1993.

Moore, P.S. Meningococcal Meningitis in sub-Saharan Africa: a Model for the Epidemic Process. *Clin. Infect. Dis.*, 1992; 14:515–25.

Moore, P.S. and Broome, C.V. Cerebrospinal Meningitis Epidemics. *Sci. Am.*, 1994; 271(5):38–45.

Morse, S.S. and Schluederberg, A. Emerging Viruses: the Evolution of Viruses and Viral Diseases. *J. Infect. Dis.*, 1990; 162:1–7.

Morse, S.S. Regulating Viral Traffic. *Issues Sci. Technol.*, 1990; 7:81–4.

Morse, S.S. Looking for a Link. *Nature*, 1990; 344:297.

Morse, S.S. Emerging Viruses: Defining the Rules for Viral Traffic. *Perspect. Biol. Med.*, 1991; 34:387–409.

Morse, S.S. Examining the Origins of Emerging Viruses. In: Morse S.S., ed. *Emerging Viruses*. New York: Oxford University Press, 1993, pp. 10–28.

Morse, S.S. Toward an Evolutionary Biology of Viruses. In: S.S. Morse, ed. *The Evolutionary Biology of Viruses*. New York: Raven Press, 1994, pp. 1–28.

Myers, G., MacInnes, K. and Korber, B. The Emergence of Simian/Human Immunodeficiency Viruses. *AIDS Res. Hum. Retroviruses*, 1992; 8:373–86.

Neu, H.C. The Crisis in Antibiotic Resistance. *Science*, 1992; 257:1064–72.

Nomura, A., Stemmermann, G.N., Chyou, P-H. *et al. Helicobacter pylori* Infection and Gastric Carcinoma among Japanese Americans in Hawaii. *N. Engl. J. Med.*, 1991; 325:1132–6.

Parsonnet, J., Friedman, G.D., Vandersteen, D.P. *et al. Helicobacter pylori* Infection and the Risk of Gastric Carcinoma. *N. Engl. J. Med.*, 1991; 325:1127–31.

Peterson, W.L. *Helicobacter pylori* and Peptic Ulcer Disease. *N. Engl. J. Med.*, 1991; 324:1043–8.

Rogers, D.J. and Packer, M.J. *Vector-borne Diseases, Models, and Global Change. Lancet*, 1993; 342:1282–4.

Rollin, P.E., Coudrier, D. and Sureau, P. Hantavirus Epidemic in Europe, 1993. *Lancet*, 1994; 343:115–16.

Satcher, D. Emerging Infections: Getting Ahead of the Curve. In: *Emerging Infections Disease*, Vol. 1, No. 1, January–March 1995, available at http://www.cdc.gov/ncidod/eid/vol1no1/satcher.htm.

Scholtissek, C. and Naylor, E. Fish Farming and Influenza Pandemics. *Nature*, 1988; 331:215.

Soares, S., Kristinsson, K.G., Musser, J.M. and Tomasz, A. Evidence for the Introduction of a Multiresistant Clone of Serotype 6B *Streptococcus pneumoniae* from Spain to Iceland in the late 1980s. *J. Infect. Dis.*, 1993; 168:158–63.

United Nations. World Urbanization Prospects, 1990. New York: United Nations, 1991.

Wachsmuth, I.K., Evins, G.M., Fields, P.I. *et al.* The Molecular Epidemiology of Cholera in Latin America. *J. Infect. Dis.*, 1993; 167:621–6.

Webster, R.G., Bean, W.J., Gorman, O.T. *et al.* Evolution and Ecology of Influenza A Viruses. *Microbiol. Rev.*, 1992; 56:152–79.

Wilesmith, J.W., Ryan, J.B.M. and Atkinson, M.J. Bovine Spongiform Encephalopathy: Epidemiological Studies on the Origin. *Vet. Rec.*, 1991; 128:199–203.

World Health Organization. Geographical Distribution of Arthropod-borne Diseases and their Principal Vectors. Geneva: World Health Organization (WHO/VBC/89.967), 1989:138–48.

Yamanishi, K., Okuno, T., Shiraki, K. *et al.* Identification of Human Herpesvirus-6 as a Causal Agent for Exanthem subitum. *Lancet*, 1988; i:1065–7.

3

Climate, Ecology and Human Health

Paul R. Epstein

> Epidemics are like sign-posts from which the statesman of
> stature can read that a disturbance has occurred in the devel-
> opment of his nation – that not even careless politics can
> overlook.
>
> Dr Rudolf Virchow, 1848

There are many determinants of health and well-being, and they can
all interact with one another. Human biological and psychological
factors come into play on a personal level, but ecological and global
systems are also involved, as are economics and access to health care,
which determine the social vulnerabilities to disease. Recently, our
chief means of controlling infections – antibiotics and insecticides –
have themselves become a source of new, resistant microbes and
disease carriers, and the growing number of people with malnutrition
or depressed immune systems have helped select and disseminate these
emerging organisms.

Environmental conditions, interacting with the biology of disease
agents, can exert profound effects. Changes in how land is used affect
the distribution of disease carriers, such as rodents or insects, while
climate influences their range and affects the timing and intensity of
outbreaks. This chapter examines how our health is influenced by the
interplay of social conditions, local environmental factors and global
changes. The discussion focuses primarily on the environment, for –
given its scale and pace of change – this sometimes forgotten determ-
inant seems destined to play an ever-increasing role in determining
disease patterns in the future.

At any time and in any age, human health tends to follow trends in
both social systems and the natural environment. In periods of relative

stability – measured in the number and distribution of people, their use of natural resources, and their generation of wastes – natural, biological controls over pests and disease organisms (or pathogens) can function efficiently. In times of accelerated change – often associated with economic or political instability, natural disasters, or war – infectious diseases can spread. Today, an increasingly unstable climate, the accelerating loss of species and growing economic inequities, challenge the resilience and resistance of natural systems. Acting together, these elements of change are contributing to the emergence, resurgence and redistribution of infectious disease on a global scale (Map 3.1).

An expected redistribution of infectious disease is but one of the biological consequences of global environmental change. In some regions of the globe, warming may at first appear beneficial. Plants may be fertilized by warmth and moisture, an earlier spring and more carbon dioxide (CO_2) and nitrogen. But warming and increased CO_2 can also stimulate microbes and their carriers, and added heat can destabilize weather patterns.

The consequences for agricultural pests and crop yields, for the health of livestock and fisheries and for human illness, may be significant; and the costs of epidemics can cascade through economies and ripple through societies. The resurgence of infectious diseases thus poses threats, both to food and biological security, and to economic development.

Water, food and health are among our most basic needs. These requirements are also interrelated, and environmental changes now underway threaten all three. Maintaining health demands clean water, safe food and unpolluted air, and in the modern world the latter depends upon clean energy. In the past, widespread diseases that affect multiple continents – pandemics – have often precipitated social disruption and major shifts in human settlements. In other, more productive instances, the resurgence of infectious disease has inspired social and environmental reforms that addressed the underlying causes. What will be our course this time?

Background

A recent report of the United Nations' World Health Organization records that, since 1976, 30 diseases have emerged that are new to medicine. The reappearance of old diseases – once thought under control – is of equal concern: Drug-resistant tuberculosis, exacerbated by HIV/AIDS, now causes three million deaths annually, while child-

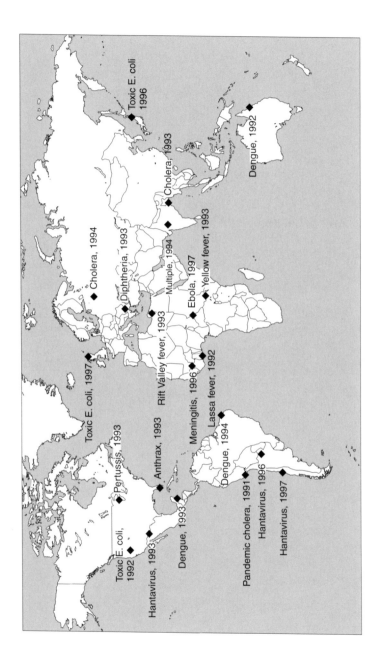

Map 3.1   Examples of emerging and resurgent infectious diseases in the 1990s.

hood diphtheria, whooping cough, and measles – which are also transmitted person-to-person – are also on the rise, particularly in those places where social systems have recently changed. Malaria, dengue (or 'breakbone fever', a severe, sometimes-deadly tropical disease transmitted by mosquitoes and accompanied by headache, rash and severe joint pain), yellow fever, cholera and a number of rodent-borne viruses, are also appearing with increased frequency. The distribution of the latter diseases, those that rely on animals or water as vehicles (or vectors) for transmission, reflect both environmental and social change. In 1995, US mortality from infectious disease attributed to causes other than HIV/AIDS rose 22 per cent above the levels of 15 years before, and 58 per cent in all.

The example of malaria

Malaria is an ancient, mosquito-borne disease that played a significant role in the history of Africa. For centuries, the presence of sickle cell and other types of red blood cell 'anomalies' limited the impact of malaria on native Africans. The disease also served to ward off foreign colonizers, who lacked these evolved defences, and helped deter deep penetration of the continent until the latter part of the nineteenth century. In the first phases of the scramble for African territory, Europeans selectively colonized highland regions to escape from swampy regions of malaria or 'bad air': a choice that also contributed to the separation of the races. For further protection, they drank water flavoured with quinine – a natural remedy, derived from the bark of the cinchona tree, discovered in Peru in the fifteenth century. To make the tonic more palatable, they added gin.

Eventually, control measures in Africa and the Americas, where malaria was also found, included environmental improvements and the application of insecticides, and by the 1950s there were dramatic drops in the incidence of the disease, worldwide. It was not conquered, however, but only held at bay. By the late 1970s, dwindling investments in public health programmes, growing insecticide-resistance, and prevalent environmental changes, such as forest clearing, contributed to a widespread resurgence. By the late 1980s large epidemics were once again the rule, often associated with the onset of warm, wet periods.

In the past five years, the worldwide incidence of malaria has quadrupled, influenced by changes in both land development and regional climate. In Brazil, satellite images depict a 'fish bone' pattern where roads have opened the tropical forest to localized development.

In these 'edge' areas, malaria has resurged. Temperature changes have also encouraged a redistribution of the disease: Malaria is now found in higher-elevations in central Africa and could threaten cities such as Nairobi, Kenya (at about 5000 ft, or the altitude of Denver, Colorado), as freezing levels have shifted higher in the mountains. In the summer of 1997, for example, malaria took the lives of hundreds of people in the Kenyan highlands, where populations had previously been unexposed.

The Anopheles mosquito that can carry malaria is present in the US, and, earlier this century, the disease was prevalent. After initially being brought under control, small outbreaks of locally-transmitted malaria have occurred in this decade in Texas, Georgia, Florida, Michigan, New Jersey and New York – and again, as in the 1980s, in California – primarily during hot, wet spells. A persistence of similar climatic conditions, combined with inadequate (or ineffective) control methods, could lead to further localized outbreaks.

Worldwide, up to 500 million people – roughly twice the present population of the US – contract malaria every year, and between 1.5 and 3 million, primarily children, die. Africa is most affected. Mosquito resistance to insecticides and parasite resistance to many drugs are widespread, and there are no operational vaccines, nor any foreseen in the near future. Ecological changes, along with increased weather variability and a warming trend, appear to be playing increasing roles in the spread of this disease.

Environmental change and opportunistic species

Regulatory mechanisms are a feature of all living systems. Some cells within the body stand guard to repel invading organisms or to reject cells that develop malignantly. In the environment, predators serve a similar role, keeping populations of pests under control.

Weeds, rodents, insects and microorganisms are opportunists that reproduce very rapidly. Rodents, for example, have huge broods, plus small body sizes, wide-ranging appetites, and well developed dispersal mechanisms.

In stable environments, large predators fare well and keep smaller, opportunistic species in check. But opportunists can readily colonize over-stressed environments, much as opportunistic infections take hold in patients with weakened immune systems.

Mosquito populations, for example, are naturally controlled by reptiles, birds, spiders, ladybirds and bats – as well as by pond fish that feed on mosquito larvae. Mosquitoes provide nourishment for these animals, but some carry malaria, yellow fever, dengue fever and several types of encephalitis. Similarly, owls, coyotes and snakes eat rodents; and rodents can devour grains and transport Lyme disease ticks, hantaviruses (a debilitating viral infection), arenaviruses (such as South American haemorrhagic fevers and Lassa fever), leptospirosis bacteria and human plague.

In the marine environment, fish, shellfish and sea mammals consume algae that form the base of the marine food web. A reduction in these plankton feeders as a result of overfishing or disease may thus contribute to blooms of harmful algae. Harmful algal blooms, or 'HABs', that despoil beaches and devastate shoreline birds and other animal life, can occur as oxygen-rich 'red tides', or as oxygen-poor or hypoxic 'brown tides'. Plankton blooms can also harbour cholera and other bacteria and threaten the health of swimmers, or those who consume affected fish and shellfish.

Environmental change and biological controls

Today, the activities of one species, humans, are reducing the diversity of all others and transforming the global environment. Ecosystems subjected to the stresses of 'global change' (including climate change and altered weather patterns, the depletion of stratospheric ozone, deforestation, coastal pollution and marked reductions of biological diversity), become more susceptible to the emergence, invasion and spread of opportunistic species. When subject to multiple stresses, natural environments can exhibit symptoms that indicate reductions in resilience, resistance and regenerative capabilities. Conversely, ecosystems have inherent flexibilities and survival strategies that can be strengthened by systematic stress, such as the seasonal battering they must endure in temperate latitudes. But their tolerance for abuse has its limits.

Several features of global change tend to reduce predators disproportionately, and in the process release prey from their biological controls. Among the most widespread are:

- fragmentation and loss of habitat
- dominance of monocultures in agriculture and aquaculture
- excessive use of toxic chemicals
- increased ultraviolet radiation, and
- climate change and weather instability

The breaking up of large tracts of forest or other natural wilderness into smaller and more diverse patches reduces the available habitat for large predators and favours many pests. Land and climate changes may act synergistically, as when constricted habitat frustrates a species' ability to migrate north or south to survive altered climatic conditions. Extensive deforestation and climate anomalies – such as the delayed monsoon rains that can result from El Niño – can also act synergistically, with costly results. A ready example is the massive haze from burning that covered much of South-East Asia in September and October 1998, causing acute and chronic respiratory damage as well as losses in trade, investment and tourism – the latter, a $26 billion a year industry.

The dedication of land to monoculture, that is, the cultivation of single crops with restricted genetic and species diversity, renders plants more vulnerable to disease. Simplified systems are also more suscept-ible to climatic extremes and to outbreaks of pests.

Over-use of pesticides kills birds and beneficial insects, as noted in 1962 by Rachel Carson. The title of her book, *Silent Spring*, made refer-ence to the absence of the chorus of birds in springtime, and the result-ing resurgence of plant-eating insects – that had also evolved a resistance to pesticides. The worldwide response to her message trans-formed agricultural policies and generated more enlightened pest man-agement. But today, the heavy application of pesticides still carries risks to both human health and natural systems. Over-use of pesticides in Texas and Alabama to control the boll weevil has alarmed farmers, for friendly insects such as spiders and ladybirds have died off and other plant pests have rebounded.

Ecosystem health

As noted earlier, one of 'nature's services' is to keep opportunistic species under control. Maintaining this service entails sustaining the health and integrity of ecosystems. One of the essentials is genetic and species biodiversity to provide alternative hosts for disease organisms. Another is sufficient stability among functional groups of species (such as recyclers, scavengers, predators, competitors and prey) to ensure the suppression of opportunists and preserve essential ecological functions. Habitat is crucial.

Stands of trees interspersed with agricultural fields, for instance, support birds that control insects; clean ponds with healthy popula-tions of fish serve to control mosquito larvae; and adequate wetlands filter excess nutrients, harmful chemicals and microorganisms.

As a case in point, in tidewater Maryland, buffer zones around farms and the restoration of wetlands and river-bed trees can absorb the flow of sediments, chemicals and harmful organisms into Chesapeake Bay, and thus reduce the emergence and spread of algae that are toxic to fish. Ecosystems are also interrelated: healthy forests and mangroves in Central America, for example, are crucial to coral reefs that spawn fish stocks, formed at the origin of the great Gulf Stream. Maintaining the integrity of natural environmental systems provides generalized defences against the proliferation of opportunistic pests and disease.

Population explosions of nuisance organisms, be they animals, plants or microbes, often reflect failing ecosystem health: a sign of systems out of equilibrium, in terms of the balance of organisms required to perform essential functions. The damage done, moreover, can be cumulative, for multiply-stressed systems are less able to resist and rebound when other stresses come along.

Rodents, insects and algae are thus key biological indicators of ecosystem health. Their populations and species compositions respond rapidly to environmental change – particularly to an increase in their food supply or a drop in the number of their natural predators. These indicator species are also linked to human health.

Impacts of a loss of biodiversity

The present rate of species extinctions around the world is a potential threat to human health when one considers the role that predators play in containing infectious disease. From the largest to the smallest scales, an essential element in natural systems for countering stress is a diversity of defences and responses. Thus, animals that seem redundant may serve as 'insurance' species in a natural ecosystem, providing a back-up layer of resilience and resistance when others are lost from disease, a changing environment or a shortage of food or water.

In 1996, the World Conservation Union reported that one-fourth of all species of mammals – and similar proportions of reptiles, amphibians and fish – are threatened. The current rate of extinctions (estimated at 100 to 1000 times the rate of loss in the pre-human era) falls heaviest on large predators and 'specialists', and thus may initially favour the spread of opportunistic species.

Environmental distress syndrome: monitoring global change

Some ecologists describe an evolving 'Environmental Distress Syndrome', with several recognizable symptoms that integrate local and global stresses. Such signals include the rapid decline (and wide-spread malformations) in frogs in 140 countries on six continents, which may be the result of habitat loss, toxic chemicals and increased ultraviolet-B radiation. Additional and more general symptoms of environmental distress are given in Box 3.1.

Monitoring these biological signs – as well as the populations of key biological indicator species such as rodents, insects and algae – can strengthen observing systems that currently track chiefly chemical and physical parameters, such as nitrogen flow into coastal waters and sea surface temperatures. Interactive geographical mapping that visually integrates the biological, chemical and physical measurements can help define and analyse the consequences, costs and the causes of global environmental change.

Climate and emerging diseases

Models of how the climate system will respond to enhanced green-house warming predict: (1) increased air temperatures at altitudes of two to four miles above the surface in the southern hemisphere; (2) a disproportionate rise in minimum temperatures (TMINs), in either daily or seasonally-averaged readings; and (3) an increase in extreme weather events, such as droughts and sudden heavy rains. There is growing evidence for all three of these tell-tale 'fingerprints' of enhanced greenhouse warming, and each of them is related to infectious diseases.

Persistent hot, humid weather spells can threaten the health of people who live in temperate latitudes. Farm animals are also adversely affected, especially when the air temperature remains uncommonly high throughout the night.

Box 3.1   An environmental distress syndrome

1. Emerging infectious diseases.
2. The loss of genetic and functional group species biodiversity.
3. Among animals, and birds, a growing dominance of 'generalists' that have wide-ranging diets (such as crows, Canada geese, and gulls) over 'specialists' (such as plovers) whose localized niches are disappearing.
4. A pronounced decline in one type of specialist – the pollinators (such as bees, birds, bats, butterflies and beetles) – whose activities are indispensable for the preservation of flowering plants, including crops.
5. Along coastlines, the proliferation of harmful algal blooms.

During the summer of 1995, excess deaths in Chicago and other large cities around the world were directly associated with heat waves, compounded by social isolation. In many instances, according to meteorologists, the key factor was the lack of relief at night. In the latter half of the twentieth century, TMINs over land areas have risen at a rate of 1.86° C per 100 years, while maximum temperatures have risen at 0.88° C per 100 years. Changed conditions in winter also bring problems: mild conditions and recurrent winter thawing can damage forests and can allow harmful insects (such as ticks) to survive.

Warmer temperatures and vector-borne disease

Changing social conditions, such as the growth of 'mega-cities', and widespread ecological change, are contributing to the spread of infectious diseases. But climate restricts the range in which vector-borne diseases (VBDs) can occur, and weather affects the timing and intensity of their outbreaks. Rates of insect biting and the maturation of microorganisms within them are temperature-dependent, and both rates increase when the air warms. Warming can also increase the number of insects, provided there is adequate moisture, although excessive heat can decrease survival of either microorganisms or their hosts. Between the limits of too hot and too cold is an optimum range of temperature in which warmer air enhances metabolism and the chances for disease transmission.

Most insects are highly sensitive to temperature change: ants even run faster in warmer weather. Findings from palaeoclimatic (fossil) studies demonstrate that changes in temperature (and especially in TMINs) were closely correlated with geographic shifts of beetles near the end of the last Ice Age, about 10 000 years ago. Indeed, fossil records indicate that when changes in climate occur, insects shift their range far more rapidly than do grasses, shrubs and forests, and move to more favourable latitudes and elevations hundreds of years before larger animals do. 'Beetles', concluded one climatologist, 'are better paleo-thermometers than bears'.

Computer models of global greenhouse warming project increased temperatures that will, in turn, favour the spread of VBDs to higher elevations and to more temperate latitudes. While 42 per cent of the globe presently offers conditions that can sustain the transmission of malaria, the fraction could rise to 60 per cent with a global increase of a few degrees centigrade.

Mosquitoes are hot weather insects that have fixed thresholds for survival. Anopheline mosquitoes and *Plasmodium falciparum* malaria transmission are sustained only where the winter temperature is kept above 16° C (61° F), while the variety of mosquito that transmits dengue fever, *Aedes aegypti*, is limited by the 10° C (50° F) winter isotherm. Shifts in the geographic limits of equal temperature (isotherms) that accompany global warming may extend the areas that are capable of sustaining the transmission of these and other diseases. The transmission season may also be extended in regions that now lie on the margins of the temperature and moisture conditions that allow disease carriers to reproduce. Similar considerations apply to cold-blooded agricultural pests, called stenotherms, that require specific temperatures for their survival.

Some of these projected changes, measured in montane regions, cool areas just below the tree line, may already be underway, for, as summarized in Box 3.2, there are now reports from several continents of new outbreaks of vector-borne diseases (VBDs) in mountainous regions – findings that are consistent with the recorded temperature increase, the general retreat of alpine glaciers and the reported upward displacement of temperature-sensitive plants.

The consistency among physical and biological indicators agrees with the 1996 consensus findings of the Intergovernmental Panel on Climate Change (IPCC) that climate appears to be changing, and that some of the anticipated impacts are now observable. The IPCC also concluded that human activities, including fossil fuel combustion and forest clearing and burning, are apparently contributing to these changes. There may be some positive impacts such as fewer winter deaths, or a drop in schistosomiasis in areas where excessive heat kills off the snails that can carry the parasite larvae. But overall, the current evaluation is that the impacts of an unstable and rapidly changing climate on human health are likely to be overwhelmingly negative.

The effects of climate variability on epidemics

Another significant climate trend that has been linked to systematic changes in temperature and precipitation is an increase in the variability, or extremes, of climate. This change in extremes can alter not only the intensity of individual events, such as storms and floods, but the

---

Box 3.2   Global change in montane regions

Both insects and insect-borne diseases (including malaria and dengue fever) are today being reported at higher elevations in Africa, Asia and Latin America. Highland malaria is becoming a problem for rural areas in Papua New Guinea and for the highlands of Central Africa. In 1995, dengue fever blanketed Latin America, and the disease or its mosquito vector, *Aedes aegypti*, are appearing at higher elevations. In addition, the displacement of plants to higher elevations has been documented on 30 peaks in the European Alps, and has also been observed in Alaska, the Sierra Nevada range in the US and in New Zealand. These botanical trends, indicative of gradual, systematic warming, accompany other widespread physical changes: Montane glaciers are in retreat in Argentina, Peru, Alaska, Iceland, Norway, the Swiss Alps, Kenya, the Himalayas, Indonesia and New Zealand. Some may soon disappear.

Since 1970, the lowest level at which freezing occurs has climbed about 160 metres higher in mountain ranges from 30°[#]N to 30°[#]S latitude, based on radiosonde data analysed at NOAA's Environmental Research Laboratory. The shift to higher levels on mountainsides corresponds to a warming at these elevations of about 1°C (almost 2°F), which is nearly twice the average warming that has been documented over the Earth as a whole. Notably, atmospheric models that incorporate observed trends in stratospheric ozone, sulfate aerosols and greenhouse gases, predict that, at least in the southern hemisphere, the warming trend at high mountain elevations should exceed that at the Earth's surface. Thus, mountain regions – where shifts in isotherms are especially apparent – can serve as sentinel areas for monitoring global climate change.

---

timing and spatial patterns of weather as well. Since the mid-1800s, the average surface temperature of the globe has risen about 0.4° C–0.6° C, and periods of persistent warming can, in general, be associated with increased variability. The IPCC projects that the warming trend may be accompanied by more intense heat waves and altered drought and rainfall patterns.

As reported in the first issue of the journal *Consequences* (Karl *et al.*, 1995), data from the National Climatic Data Center – the US's main repository for meteorological data – indicate that, since the 1970s, extreme weather events have indeed increased in the continental US. On average, periods of drought are systematically longer, and bursts of precipitation (greater than two inches of rain over 24 hours) are more frequent. A warmed atmosphere accelerates evaporation, and for every rise of 1° C, the air can hold 6 per cent more water. One consequence is that we are now receiving a greater percentage of precipitation in the form of sudden, intense bursts that are more typical, for example, in the tropics. Longer droughts and more heavy bursts of rain, accompanied by flash floods, were more common in the 1980s than in the 1970s, and more so in the 1990s than in the 1980s.

Extreme events – floods, storms, droughts and uncontained fires – can be devastating for agriculture, for human settlements and for health. An increase in brief cold snaps is also possible, and winter storms, like heat waves, bring an increase in cardiac deaths. Floods spread bacteria, viruses and chemical contaminants, foster the growth of fungi, and contribute to the breeding of insects. Prolonged droughts, interrupted by heavy rains, favour population explosions of both insects and rodents. Extreme weather events (often associated with the recurring climatic conditions that are initiated by large-scale changes in sea surface temperatures in the Pacific, known as El Niño/La Niña events) have been accompanied by new appearances of harmful algal blooms in Asia and North America, and – in Latin America and Asia – by outbreaks of malaria and various water-borne diseases, such as typhoid, hepatitis A, bacillary dysentery and cholera.

Disease clusters

In August 1995, the eastern, tropical region of the Pacific Ocean surface turned cold, initiating a La Niña event that would last until late 1996. Along the Caribbean coast of Colombia, a summer 1995 heat wave was followed by the heaviest August rainfall in 50 years, ending a long drought that accompanied the preceding, prolonged El Niño conditions of 1990–95. The heat and flooding precipitated a cluster of diseases involving mosquitoes (Venezuelan equine encephalitis and dengue fever), rodents (leptospirosis), and toxic algae (that killed 350 tons of fish in Colombia's largest coastal lagoon).

Prolonged anomalous conditions of the sort that applied in 1990–95, can also have cumulative biological consequences. In New Orleans, for example, five years without a killing frost was associated with an explosion of mosquitoes, termites and cockroaches. Termites persisted inside trees into the cold winter of 1995–96, and now threaten to destroy stands of New Orleans' fabled 'mighty oaks'. We may have only just begun to understand the true biological impacts of the persistent anomalous climate of the 1990s.

Rodents: synergies and surprises

Rodents are a growing problem in the US, Latin America, Africa, Europe, Asia and Australia. These pre-eminent opportunists are believed to be the fastest reproducing mammal and they eat everything humans do, thrive on contaminated water and food, and are extremely capable swimmers. Meadow voles, whose numbers are kept in check by predatory marsh hawks, can have up to 17 broods a year, for example, each of half a dozen offspring. Rodents consume 20 per cent of the world's grain, including almost a seventh in the US, and up to three quarters of what is grown and stored in some African nations. Rodents can also carry diseases.

A controlled experiment with Canadian snowshoe hares depicts how multiple factors can act synergistically to greatly increase the number of rodents. Excluding predators by confining the animals to cages led to a population doubling, compared to the fate of a number of similar animals in the wild. Augmenting food tripled hare density. Together, the interventions in the controlled experiment resulted in more than a ten-fold population explosion.

Rats, mice and the hantavirus

The story of the hantavirus illustrates a similar synergy in the case of microbial agents. A prolonged drought in the US southwest in the early 1990s reduced the populations of animals such as owls, coyotes and snakes that prey on rodents. When the drought yielded to intense rains in 1993, the grasshoppers and piñon nuts on which rodents feed became more abundant. The result, when combined with the drop in predators, was a ten-fold increase in rats and mice by June of that year. An outcome was the emergence of a 'new' condition called hantavirus pulmonary syndrome: from a virus – perhaps already present, but dormant – transmitted through rodent saliva, urine and droppings. Predators returned, however, and by summer's end the outbreak had abated.

Rodent-borne hantaviruses have resurged in several European nations, and most notably in the former Soviet Union and in Yugoslavia. In late 1996, hantavirus infection emerged in South America in western Argentina. Within the first few months, at least ten deaths resulted, frightening off tourists and threatening the economic livelihood of the region. Hantavirus Pulmonary Syndrome has now appeared in Bolivia, Brazil, Canada, Chile, Ecuador, Paraguay and Uruguay, with about 50 per cent mortality and several cases of person-to-person transmission.

Some other examples

Evidence of another rodent-borne disease – leptospirosis – is increasingly reported in US urban centres, in areas where the disposal of sewage and other measures to protect public health have declined. In 1995, there were substantial outbreaks of the disease in Central America and Colombia, as heavy La Niña rains, following the prolonged El Niño drought, drove rodents scurrying from their burrows. Although leptospirosis is treatable with antibiotics, in 1995, before the diagnosis was established, there were fatalities.

A combination of stresses has contributed to the sudden appearances of several rodent-borne viral haemorrhagic fevers in rural Latin America in the past several decades: junin in Argentina (1953), machupo in Bolivia (1962 and 1996), guaranito in Venezuela, and sabiá in Brazil. In Bolivia, systematic clearing of trees apparently shifted populations of a variety of disease-carrying mice, known as calomys, from forest to field settings where they became dominant. Heavy applications of DDT – meant to eradicate malaria – helped reduce their natural predators. When cats were reintroduced to the area in 1962, the epidemic of Bolivian hemorrhagic fever was abated, although not until it had killed 10 to 20 per cent of the inhabitants of the small villages in which the disease was present. Habitat loss and excessive use of toxic chemicals acted together in this case.

In southern Africa, rodent populations exploded as a consequence of climate variability, when heavy and then lighter rains came in 1993 and 1994, on the heels of six years of prolonged drought. When the rains came, rodents found themselves in a world where avian and land predators were virtually absent. Moreover, because so many drought animals had also succumbed, there was little tillage of the land and the underground burrows in which rodents live went largely undisturbed. After an initial successful harvest in 1993, the maize crop in Zimbabwe was decimated by rodents. Soon after, human plague broke out in Zimbabwe and on the borders of neighbouring Malawi and Mozambique, carried – as in the devastating plague of fourteenth-century Europe – by fleas on rats. Subsequently, a rodent-borne virus took the lives of 81 elephants in South Africa's Kruger Park, and plague returned in the summer of 1997.

Plague in India resurfaced in 1994, following a blistering summer when temperatures reached 124° F, leaving animals prostrate in the northern part of the country and fuelling the breeding of fleas in houses that held stored grain. The unusually heavy monsoons following the 1994 heat wave led to population crowding in Surat on the western coast, north of Bombay, and an apparent outbreak of pneumonic (person-to-person) plague. Cases of malaria and dengue fever also surged in the wake of flooding. Meanwhile, in Australia, rodents emerged as serious crop pests in 1995, accompanying the same prolonged El Niño of the early 1990s and the ensuing years of intense drought.

Current land-use practices and the overuse of chemicals to control pests may increase the chances for such 'nasty synergies'. Climate variability is also a key element in upsurges of pests – and were climate to become more unstable, it could exert an even greater influence on ecological dynamics and the patterns of infectious diseases in the future. A disturbance in one factor can be destabilizing; but multiple perturbations can reduce the resistance and the resilience of a entire system.

Marine coastal ecosystems

Seashores throughout the world are subject to increasing pressures from residential, recreational and commercial development. These stresses may become more severe, for human population in the vicinity of sea-coasts is growing at twice the inland rate. Some of the pressures that we exert on coastal ecosystems are summarized in Box 3.3. All can increase the growth of algae.

Among the possible consequences of disruption in almost any marine ecosystem is an increase in the opportunistic pathogens that can abet the spread of human disease, sometimes to widespread proportions. One example is cholera.

Cholera

We often think of our modern world as cleansed of the epidemic scourges of ages past. But cholera – an acute and sometimes fatal disease that is accompanied by severe diarrhoea – affects more nations today than ever before. The Seventh Pandemic began when the El Tor strain left its traditional home in the Bay of Bengal in the 1960s, travelled to the east and west across Asia, and in the 1970s penetrated the continent of Africa. In 1991, the cholera pandemic reached the Americas, and during the first 18 months more than half a million cases were reported in Latin America, with 5000 deaths. Rapid institution of oral rehydration treatment – with clean water, sugar and salts – limited fatalities in the Americas to about one in a hundred cases. The epidemics also had serious economic consequences. In 1991, Peru lost $770 million in seafood exports and another $250 million in lost tourist revenues because of the disease.

Box 3.3   Marine ecosystem stresses

1. An excess in coastal waters of dissolved mineral and organic nutrients, particularly from nitrogen overload – derived from sewage, agricultural fertilizers and acid precipitation – resulting in an environment that favours plant over animal life.
2. Reduced acreage of wetlands, that serve as 'nature's kidneys' to filter nitrogen and other wastes that flow from the coastal environment.
3. Overfishing, that can reduce the population of beneficial predators of algae and animal plankton (zooplankton).
4. Chemical pollution and increased penetration of UV-B radiation that may increase mutation levels in near-shore sea life of all kinds, and disproportionately harm zooplankton and fish larvae.
5. Warming of coastal waters – and the associated trend toward stable, thermal layers that inhibit vertical circulation – which increases the metabolism and growth of algae and favours more toxic algal species such as cyanobacteria and dinoflagellates. Warming may also reduce the immune systems of sea mammals and coral and encourage the growth of harmful bacteria and viruses in their tissues.

The microbe that transmits cholera, *Vibrio cholerae*, is found in a dormant or 'hibernating' state in algae and microscopic animal plankton, where it can be identified using modern microbiological techniques. But once introduced to people – by drinking contaminated water or by eating contaminated fish or shellfish – cholera can recycle through a population, when sewage is allowed to mix with the clean water supply.

Five years ago, in late 1992, a new strain of *Vibrio cholerae* – O139 Bengal – emerged in India along the coast of the Bay of Bengal. With populations unprotected by prior immunities, this hardy strain quickly spread through adjoining nations, threatening to become the agent of the world's Eighth Cholera Pandemic. For a time, in 1994, El Tor regained dominance. But by 1996, O139 Bengal had reasserted itself. The emergence of this new disease, like all others, involved the interplay of microbe, human host and environmental factors.

The largest and most intense outbreak of cholera ever recorded occurred in Rwanda in 1994, killing over 40 000 people in the space of weeks, in a nation already ravaged by civil war and ethnic strife. The tragedy of cholera in Rwanda is a reminder of the impacts of conflict and political instability on public health and biological security – just as epidemics may, in turn, contribute to political and economic instability.

Is the ocean warming?

Surface temperatures of the ocean have increased in the twentieth century and a gradual warming of the deep ocean has been found in recent years in oceanographic surveys carried out in the tropical Pacific, Atlantic and Indian Oceans, and at both the Earth's poles. These findings could be indicative of a long-term trend. Corresponding temperature measurements of the sub-surface earth, in cores drilled deep into the Arctic tundra, show a similar effect.

The water that evaporates from warmer seas, and from vegetation and soils of a warmer land surface, intensifies the rate at which water cycles from ocean to clouds and back again. In so doing, it increases humidity and reinforces the greenhouse effect. Warm seas are the engines that drive tropical storms and fuel the intensity of hurricanes. More high cloud can also contribute to warmer nights by trapping outgoing radiation.

Some biological impacts

A warmer ocean can also harm marine plankton, and thus affect more advanced forms of life in the sea. A northward shift in marine flora and fauna along the California coast that has been underway since the 1930s, has been associated with the long-term warming of the ocean over that span of time.

Warming – when sufficient nutrients are present – may also be contributing to the proliferation of coastal algal blooms. Harmful algal blooms of increasing extent, duration and intensity – and involving novel, toxic species – have been reported around the world since the 1970s. Indeed, some scientists feel that the worldwide increase in coastal algal blooms may be one of the first biological signs of global environmental change.

Warm years may result in a confluence of adverse events. The 1987 El Niño was associated with the spread and new growth of tropical and temperate species of algae in higher northern and southern latitudes. Many were toxic algal blooms. In 1987, following a shoreward intrusion of Gulf Stream eddies, the dinoflagellate *Gymnodimuim breve*, previously found only as far north as the Gulf of Mexico, bloomed about 700 miles north, off Cape Hatteras, North Carolina, where it has since persisted, albeit at low levels. Forty-eight cases of neurological shellfish poisoning occurred in 1987, resulting in an estimated $25 million loss to the seafood industry and the local community. In the same year, anomalous rain patterns and warm Gulf Stream eddies swept unusually close to Prince Edward Island in the Gulf of St Lawrence. The result, combined with the run-off of local pollutants after heavy rains, was a bloom of toxic diatoms. For the first time, domoic acid was produced from these algae, and then ingested by marine life. Consumption of contaminated mussels resulted in 107 instances of amnesic shellfish poisoning, from domoic acid, including three deaths and permanent, short-term memory loss in several victims.

Also in 1987, there were major losses of sea urchin and coral communities in the Caribbean, a massive sea grass die-off near the Florida Keys, and on the beaches of the North Atlantic coast, the death of numerous dolphins and other sea mammals. It has been proposed that the combination of algal toxins, chlorinated hydrocarbons like PCBs, and warming may have lowered the immunity of organisms and altered the food supply for various forms of sea life, allowing morbilliform (measles-like) viruses to take hold.

The 1990s

For five years and eight months, from 1990 to 1995, the Pacific Ocean persisted in the warm El Niño phase; this was most unusual, for since 1877 none of these distinctive warmings had lasted more than three years. Both anomalous phases – with either warmer (El Niño) or colder (La Niña) surface waters – bring climate extremes to many regions across the globe. With the ensuing cold (La Niña) phase of 1995–96, many regions of the world that had lived with drought during the El Niño years were now besieged with intense rains and flooding. Just as in Colombia, flooding in southern Africa was accompanied by an upsurge of vector-borne diseases, including malaria. Other areas experienced a climatic switch of the opposite kind, with drought and wildfires replacing floods. During 1996, world grain stores fell to their lowest level since the 1930s.

Weather always varies; but increased variability and rapid temperature fluctuations may be a chief characteristic of our changing climate system. And increased variability and weather volatility can have significant consequences for health and for society.

Decadal variability

The cumulative meteorological and ecological impacts of the prolonged El Niño of the early 1990s have yet to be fully evaluated.

In 1995, warming in the Caribbean produced coral bleaching for the first time in Belize, as sea surface temperatures surpassed the 29° C (84° F) threshold that may damage the animal and plant tissues that make up a coral reef. In 1997, Caribbean sea surface temperatures reached 34° C (93° F) off southern Belize, and coral bleaching was accompanied by large mortalities in starfish and other sea life. Coral diseases are now sweeping through the Caribbean, and diseases that perturb marine habitat, such as coral or sea grasses, can also affect the fish stocks for which these areas serve as nurseries.

A pattern of greater weather variability has begun and is expected to persist with the El Niño of 1997 and 1998. Since 1976, such anomalies in Pacific Ocean temperatures and in weather extreme events have become more frequent, more intense, and longer lasting than in the preceding 100 years, as indicated in records kept since 1877.

Discontinuities and instability

The common perception that the natural world changes only gradually can be misleading, for discontinuities abound. Animals switch abruptly between two states – awake and asleep – that are sharply divided and marked by qualitative differences in levels of activity in the central nervous system. Water can rapidly change from vapour to liquid to solid. Ecosystems have equilibrium states that are also at times abruptly interrupted. An extensive fire in an old growth forest, for example, can radically change the types of plants and animals within it.

Climate regimes can also change surprisingly fast. Recent analyses of Greenland ice cores indicate that significant shifts, called rapid climate change events (RCCEs), have taken place in the past in the span of as little as several years – not centuries, as was previously believed. While the oceans may serve as a buffer against sudden climate change, this mechanism may be limited, for some of the RCCEs seem to be associated with abrupt changes in ocean circulation.

The climate system exhibits equilibrium states as well, of which three may have been most common: when the poles of the Earth were covered with small, medium or large ice caps. The present, Holocene period of the last 10 000 years – with medium-size caps and an average global temperature of 15° C (about 60° F) – has been associated with the development of modern agriculture and advancing civilization. But our present climate regime may be becoming less stable. Increased variance – that is, more extreme swings – in natural systems is inversely related to how stable and balanced the systems are, and how sensitive they are to perturbations. Wider and wider variations can occur as a system moves away from its equilibrium state.

Trends in the twentieth century

The gradual warming that characterised the climate during the first four decades of the last century, for example, was accompanied by substantial temperature variability, as borne out in the record of degree-heating-days in the US grain belt. The ensuing cooling trend from 1940 to the mid 1970s showed less variability. From 1976 to the present day, the variability – apparent in hot and cold spells, drought and floods – has again increased. Greenland ice core records suggest that the last time the Earth warmed abruptly, ending the last Ice Age, there was also a pattern of increased variability.

The connection between human health and environmental stability increases our need for a better understanding of the present state of the global climate system. There are several unanswered questions regarding the system's stability. Was the drift toward earlier springtimes that began in this country in the 1940s indicative of the first minor readjustment in the climate regime? Are the more frequent and intense El Niño events since the mid 1970s another such indicator? Has the baseline of ocean temperatures shifted? Does the present climatic volatility – evident in altered weather and precipitation patterns – increase the potential for an abrupt 'jump' in the climate system? And might further stresses lead to abrupt discontinuities of the type found in the Greenland ice cores, when the last Ice Age rapidly came to an end?

The costs of climate variability and disease outbreaks

Regardless of what caused it, the recent rise in severe wind- and flood-related events worldwide has had extraordinary consequences for property insurers. In the US, for example, prior to 1989, no single-event insured loss had ever exceeded a billion dollars. Since then, annual insured losses have risen dramatically – from almost $1.6 billion annually in the 1980s to $10 billion in the 1990s: a jump that is only partially explained by more intensive exploitation of rivers and land and seashore property. Federal relief bills, chiefly from flooding, totalled $13 billion for the five years from 1994 to 1999, compared to $3.3 billion for the preceding five.

Because they combine exposure with weather-related events, the costs to the property insurance industry may be the most telling indicator of the non-sustainability of our interference with natural global systems. With continued extreme climate variability, health and environmental restoration costs may grow in a similar manner. It is significant that we are having difficulty insuring our future.

The economic impacts of disease in humans, livestock and food crops can also be severe and far-reaching. Today the white fly – whose numbers swell when there is drought – is injecting at least 18 types of geminiviruses into tomato, squash and bean plants throughout Latin America, depleting the primary source of protein for many who live there. Recently, a necrosis virus (vectored by soil-based fungi) that attacks rice has appeared in Colombia. Further spread of a disease of this staple food source could have enormous impacts on world food supplies.

While the 1991 cholera epidemic cost Peru over $1 billion in tourist income locally, international airline and hotel industries lost from $2 to $5 billion from the 1994 Indian plague. Cruise boats, quite understandably, have begun to avoid islands racked by dengue fever. In the Caribbean, this trend could threaten a $12 billion-a-year tourist industry that employs more than half a million people. The 1997, California floods left fungi and root rot that threatens that state's $22 billion citrus industry. Indeed, the global resurgence of malaria, dengue fever and cholera, and the emergence of relatively new diseases such as Ebola, toxic *Escherichia coli* and Mad Cow Disease – which are related to ecology and animal husbandry practices – affect not only the health of individuals but also of national economies.

An historical note on pandemics

Pandemics emerge out of social and environmental conditions and they can induce changes in both of them. At times, the resulting changes have been disruptive; in other instances they have stimulated significant social reform.

The rise and fall of infectious disease

From a long-term historical perspective, pandemics have often been associated with major social transitions and overtaxed infrastructure. Their impacts have been lasting and profound.

A pandemic, of debated cause but remembered as the Plague of Justinian, struck Europe in AD 541. It came as the Roman Empire was in decline, and it raged for two centuries, claiming over 40 million lives, in an era when the total population of the Earth was at most 300 million. Urban centres were abandoned and the plague helped drive population resettlement into rural, feudal communities before it disappeared.

After a 600-year hiatus, plague again appeared, in AD 1346 – at the depths of the Middle Ages – when growing urban populations had again outstripped the capabilities of cities to sustain sanitation and basic public health. Several other factors played compounding roles: human populations had migrated from East to West; the Medieval Warm Period of the twelfth and thirteenth centuries may have contributed to the proliferation of rats and fleas that carried bubonic plague; and cats had been killed in the belief that they were witches. In the ensuing five years of the so-called 'Black Death', about 25 million lives were taken – about one of every three persons who lived in Europe at the time. Throughout Europe, social relations and labour patterns were dramatically altered. A third outbreak of widespread epidemic disease, almost 300 years later, would seem to have had a more positive outcome.

In the course of the early Industrial Revolution, improvements that accompanied development led to a substantial decline in mortality from infectious disease. Then, in the 1830s, under the burgeoning weight of industrialization and the growth of population – seven-fold in London from 1790 to 1850 – the conditions in European cities described in the novels of Charles Dickens became breeding grounds for three major infectious diseases: cholera, smallpox and tuberculosis. Suddenly growth and development had outgrown infrastructure, and infectious diseases rebounded.

But the resurgence of infectious disease this time precipitated protests throughout the European continent, and ultimately led to constructive responses. In England, the Sanitary and Environmental Reform Movements were born; and the field of epidemiology ushered in modern public health principles and eventually, led to a national health programme. The epidemics abated in the course of several decades, three-quarters of a century before the advent of anti-microbials.

Recent history

By the 1960s, widespread improvements in hygiene, sanitation and mosquito control led most public health authorities to believe that we would soon conquer infectious diseases. In the 1970s, public health schools turned their attention instead to chronic ailments, such as heart disease, stroke, diabetes and cancer. But the so-called 'epidemiological transition' to diseases of modernity never materialized in many developing nations. And, in the 1980s, the global picture shifted dramatically.

According to the UN World Health Organization's 1996 report, drug-resistant strains of bacteria and other microbes are having a deadly impact on the fight against several diseases, including tuberculosis, malaria, cholera and pneumonia – which collectively killed more than 10 million people in 1995. Spread of resistant organisms resulted from antibiotic overuse, microbial mutations and the geographic movement of humans, insects, rodents and microbes. Ironically, our very means to control infectious disease – antibiotics and insecticides – are, themselves, rapidly driving the evolution of new and unaffected strains. Notably, two-thirds of antibiotic use is in animal husbandry, agriculture and aquaculture.

In the 1990s, diphtheria rose exponentially in the former USSR as the public health system deteriorated following political and economic changes. The incidence rose from 4000 cases in 1992, to 8000 in 1993, and 48 000 in 1994, claiming the lives of over 4000 residents since 1990. Incidence has risen in 15 nations of Eastern Europe, although recent immunization campaigns have begun to control this infection.

Dengue fever, for which no vaccine is yet available, had essentially disappeared from the Americas by the 1970s, but has resurged in South America, infecting over 300 000 people in 1995 – which was, notably, the warmest year of this century. '*Aedes aegypti* is now well established in all areas of the Americas except Canada and Chile', ran a recent editorial in the British medical journal *Lancet*.

Settlements that surround typical mega-cities, such as Mexico City or Bombay, where discarded non-biodegradable containers serve as ideal mosquito breeding sites, provide especially vulnerable settings; milder 'cold' seasons and weather extremes can both help precipitate large outbreaks. Additionally, previous exposure and a change in the type of viral dengue circulating may lead to dengue haemorrhagic fever, a fever that carries a 5 to 10 per cent mortality.

In 1995, the largest epidemic of yellow fever since 1950 – carried by the same mosquito that transmits dengue – hit the Americas. Peru and the Amazon basin were heavily impacted and there is a growing potential for urban yellow fever. While there is a yellow fever vaccine, the current supply may be inadequate for future needs.

In 1996, the largest epidemic ever recorded of meningitis struck West Africa, something that was associated with pervasive drought, since dry mucus membranes may aid the invasion of the colonizing organisms. Over 100 000 persons contracted the disease and more than 10 000 people died. A vaccine is available, but must be used early to stop an epidemic.

Who is at risk?

Conditions conducive to the spread of epidemic infectious diseases now exist worldwide, according to the WHO report; and domestic environmental and social conditions that favour the spread of these diseases are present in the US and elsewhere today. Infectious diseases that have emerged, such as hantavirus pulmonary syndrome, Lyme disease, and toxic *E. coli*, were not imported from other nations. *E. coli*, for example, spreads in cattle raised in close quarters.

The transmission of tuberculosis, another example, is facilitated in homeless shelters and in prisons. And while poorer populations are at greatest risk, outbreaks of infectious disease are not restricted to disadvantaged regions, for today's population movements facilitate 'microbial traffic' between nations and economic groups.

What can be done?

The concerns that have been elaborated here are not hopeless ones: there are solutions to all of them. The steps that are needed, moreover, would benefit our own and future generations regardless of the future course of climate or the inevitable environmental surprises that await us in years ahead. Solutions can be divided into three levels, ranging from tactical and immediate, to strategic and long-term, and all are within our present capabilities.

The first-level solution is improved surveillance and response capability for the public health sector; that includes the development of vaccines, better treatments and more widespread support, around the world, for public health measures.

The second is the integration of health surveillance as an element of environmental monitoring. We need to make greater use of remote sensing and climate forecasts – as for El Niño/La Niña occurrence – to develop health early warning systems to alert communities of conditions conducive to the outbreak of infectious diseases.

The third level is the evaluation of environmental and energy policies in the context of their impacts on human health and well-being. Maintaining the integrity of ecosystems, such as forest habitat and wetlands, can provide defence against outbreaks of the opportunists that carry disease and provide a buffer against climatic vagaries and extremes, whether or not there is any change in the overall climate regime. Early intervention can save money and lives.

A personal conclusion

There are more and more fingerprints of an impending change in the global climate, and ever more evidence of our own ecological footprint on natural systems. We are living in a period of accelerated social, ecological and climatic change. But will our global society react to the symptoms of environmental dysfunction in time to take corrective measures?

We are changing the chemistry of the air, and in the process altering the heat budget of the world. It is the multiple changes induced in the Earth's atmosphere – carbon buildup, sulfate accumulation and ozone depletion – that constitute a destabilizing array of forcing factors. Together they may already have begun to alter natural climatic modes, such as the frequency and strength of the El Niño-Southern Oscillation. These modifications – along with the changes in coastal ocean chemistry – have begun to affect biological systems and human health.

Behind these chemical, physical, and biological changes, is our ever-increasing use of the Earth's finite resources, and our generation of wastes at rates beyond which biogeochemical systems can adequately recycle them. These patterns of consumption are simply not sustainable and come at costs that are real, often very high, and not acknowledged by current systems of economic accounting. Practices affecting forestry, fisheries, petrochemicals and fossil fuels, need all to be examined in the light of their costs across the full range of their ultimate impacts, including their effects on biodiversity, climate and the global resurgence of infectious diseases. Some of these practices now facilitate the spread of diseases by altering the environment, and others by undermining social infrastructures. The global environment is most drastically at risk from changes in the climate that are almost certain to follow our escalating combustion of fossil fuels. Air pollution – by particles and smog from fossil fuel combustion – add to the health hazards of warming. Ultimately, according to the first IPCC report, the world must reduce present greenhouse gas emissions from 60 to 70 per cent to stabilize the concentrations in the atmosphere and, we can hope, allow natural systems to readjust. The UN-sponsored Framework Convention on Climate Change that addresses the burning of fossil fuels is an essential step, for the global carbon budget is key to all living systems.

The instability of many economies also jeopardizes public health. Population growth and the relocation of people, driven by economic, environmental and political factors, exert enormous pressures on the environment. Migration levels of the past two decades – within and between nations – surpass the great migrations of the 1800s. World

Bank figures, not surprisingly, confirm that the ability of a society to stabilize its population – and as a consequence, bring public health and environmental degradation under control – is directly related to the degree of equity of income within it.

Unfortunately, international burdens of debt, binding austerity programmes, unequal terms of trade and numerous subsidies, negate many of the policies, plans and projects designed to alleviate poverty, preserve the environment and stimulate economic growth and security. Short-term, microeconomic goals are hampered by stronger macroeconomic forces, creating social instability and ultimately retarding healthy development.

The global resurgence of infectious disease in the last quarter of the twentieth century – a backward step that few would have anticipated 20 years ago – is a clear consequence of combined and compounding changes in physical, chemical, biological and social systems. Greater disease surveillance and response capability are the first, essential, steps. But, viewed as a symptom, the resurgence of infectious disease across a wide taxonomic range may indicate that we may be vastly underestimating the true costs of 'business-as-usual'.

Fortunately, consciousness and values can change even more rapidly than do the natural systems we all depend upon. We face important decisions in the way we use and re-use the finite resources that are available to us. Perhaps we are also vastly underestimating the economic opportunities and employment benefits to society as a whole as we make the transition to use resources more efficiently, generate energy cleanly, and restore essential functions of the natural environment. Curbing our unhealthy addiction to fossil fuels may be the lever that opens the portal to a healthy and productive future.

Further reading

Buchmann, S.L. and Nabhan, G.P. *The Forgotten Pollinators*. Washington, DC: Island Press, 1996.

Garrett, L. *The Coming Plague: Newly Emerging Diseases in a World out of Balance*. New York: Farrar, Strauss and Giroux, 1994.

Grifo, F. and Rosenthal, J. *Biodiversity and Human Health*. Washington, DC: Island Press, 1997.

'Human Health and Climate Change'. Washington, DC: Conference report published by President's Office of Science and Technology Policy and IOM, 1996.

McMichael, A.J., Haines, A., Slooff, R. and Kovats, S. (eds). *Climate Change and Human Health*. Geneva, Switzerland: WHO/WMO/UNEP, 1996.

Peters, R.L. and Lovejoy, T. (eds) *Global Warming and Biological Diversity*. New Haven, MA: Yale University Press, 1992.

World Health Report 1996: Fighting Disease, Fostering Development. New York: World Health Organization, United Nations, 1997.

Wyman, R.L. (ed.) *Global Climate Change and Life on Earth*. New York: Routledge, Chapman and Hall, 1991.

Some technical references

Anderson, P. and Morales, F.J. The Emergence of New Plant diseases. In: M.E. Wilson, R. Levins and A. Spielman (eds). *Disease in Evolution*, New York: NY Academy of Sciences, 1993, pp. 181–94.

Barry, J.P., Baxter, C.H., Sagarin, R.D. and Gilman, S.E. Climate-related, Long-term Faunal Changes in a California Rocky Intertidal Community. *Science*, 1995; 267:672–5.

Billet, J.D. Direct and Indirect Influences of Temperature on the Transmission of Parasites from Insects to Man. In: A.E.R. Taylor and R. Muller (eds). *The Effects of Meteorological Factors Upon Parasites*. Oxford: Blackwell Scientific Publications, pp. 79–95.

Billings, D.W. What We Need to Know: Some Priorities for Research on Biotic Feedbacks in a Changing Biosphere. In: G. Woodwell and F.T. Mackenzie (eds). *Biotic Feedbacks in the Global Climate System*. New York: Oxford University Press, 1995, Ch. 22, pp. 377–92.

Bindoff, N.L. and Church, J.A. Warming of the Water Column in the Southwest Pacific. Nature, 1992; 357:59–62.

Bouma, M.J., Sondorp, H.E. and van der Kaay, J.H. Health and Climate Change. *Lancet*, 1994; 343:302.

Bouma, M.J., Sondorp, H.E. and van der Kaay, J.H. Climate Change and Periodic Epidemic Malaria. *Lancet*, 1994; 343:1440.

Burgos, J.J. Anologias agroclimatologicas utiles para la adaptacion al posible cambio climatico global de America del Sur. *Revista Geofisica*, 1990; 22:79–95.

Burgos, J.J., de Casas, S.I., Carcavallo, R.U. and Galindez, G.T. Global Climate Change in the Distribution of Some Pathogenic Complexes. *Entomologia y Vectores*, 1994; 1:69–82.

Centers for Disease Control and Prevention (CDC). Mosquito-Transmitted Malaria – Michigan, 1995. *Morbidity and Mortality Weekly Review*, 1996; 45:398–400.

CDC. Local Transmission of *Plasmodium vivax* Malaria – Houston, Texas, 1994. *Morbidity and Mortality Weekly Review*, 1995; 44:295–303.

CDC. Mosquito-Transmitted *Plasmodium vivax* Infection – Georgia, 1996. *Morbidity and Mortality Weekly Review*, 1997; 46:264–7.

Dahlstein, D.L. and Garcia, R. (eds). *Eradication of Exotic Pests: Analysis with Case Histories*. New Haven, CT: Yale University Press, 1989.

Davis, M.B. Lags in Vegetation Response to Greenhouse Warming. *Climatic Change*, 1989; 15:75–82.

DeMeillon, B. Observations on *Anopheles funestus* and *Anopheles gambiae* in the Transvaal. Publications of the South African Institute of Medical Research, 1934; 6:195–248.

Diaz, H.F. and Graham, N.E. Recent Changes in Tropical Freezing Heights and the Role of Sea Surface Temperature. *Nature*, 1996; 383:152–5.

Dobson, A. and Carper, R. Biodiversity. *Lancet*, 1993; 342:1096–9.

Easterling, D.R., Horton, B., Jones, P.D. *et al.* Maximum and Minimum Temperature Trends for the Globe. *Science*, 1997; 277:363–7.

Elias, J.A. *Quaternary Insects and Their Environments.* Washington, DC: Smithsonian Institution Press, 1994.

Epstein, P.R., Pena, O.C. and Racedo, J.B. Climate and Disease in Colombia. *Lancet*, 1995; 346:1243.

Epstein, P.R. and Chikwenhere, G.P. Biodiversity Questions (Ltr.). *Science*, 1994; 265:1510–11.

Focks, D.A., Daniels, E., Haile, D.G. and Keesling, L.E. A Simulation Model of the Epidemiology of Urban Dengue Fever: Literature Analysis, Model Development, Preliminary Validation, and Examples of Simulation Results. *American Journal of Tropical Medicine and Hygiene*, 1995; 53:489–506.

Gill, C.A. The Relationship between Malaria and Rainfall. *Indian Journal of Medical Research*, 1920; 8:618–32.

Gill, C.A. The Role of Meteorology and Malaria. *Indian Journal of Medical Research*, 1920; 8:633–93.

Grabherr, G., Gottfried, N. and Pauli, H. Climate Effects on Mountain Plants. *Nature*, 1994; 369:447.

Graham, N.E. Simulation of Recent Global Temperature Trends. *Science*, 1995; 267:666–71.

Haeberli, W. Climate Change Impacts on Glaciers and Permafrost. In: A. Guisan, J.I. Holton, R. Spichiger and L. Terrier (eds). *Potential Ecological Impacts of Climate Change in the Alps and Fennoscandanavian Mountains.* Geneva, Switzerland: Ed Conserv Bot Geneve, 1995, pp. 97–103.

Hales, S., Weinstein, P. and Woodward, A. Dengue Fever in the South Pacific: Driven by El Niño Southern Oscillation? *Lancet*, 1996; 348:1664–5.

Hastenrath, S. and Kruss, P.D. Greenhouse Indicators in Kenya. *Nature*, 1992; 355 (6360):503.

Intergovernmental Panel on Climate Change (IPCC), 1996: Climate Change '95: The Science of Climate Change. Contribution of Working Group I to the Second Assessment Report of the IPCC. Houghton, J.T., Meiro Filho, L.G., Callandar, B.A. *et al.* (eds). Chapter 3, p. 149 and Chapter 7, pp. 370–4. Cambridge: Cambridge University Press, 1992.

Jacobson, G.L., Jr., Webb, T., III and Grimm, E.C. Patterns and Rates of Vegetation Change during the Deglaciation of Eastern North America. In: W.F. Ruddiman and H.E. Jr. Wright (eds). *North America and Adjacent Oceans During the Last Glaciation. The Geology of North America.* Vol. K-3, 277–88. Boulder, CO: Geological Society of America, 1987.

Karl, T.R., Jones, P.D., Knight, R.W. *et al.* A New Perspective on Recent Global Warming: Asymmetric Trends of Daily Maximum and Minimum Temperature. *Bulletin of the American Meteorological Society*, 1993; 74:1007–23.

Karl, T.R., Knight, R.W., Easterling, D.R. and Quayle, R.G. Trends in US Climate During the Twentieth Century. *Consequences*, 1995; 1:3–12.

Karl, T.R., Knight, R.W. and Plummer, N. Trends in High-Frequency Climate Variability in the Twentieth Century. *Nature*, 1995; 377:217–20.

Karl, T.R., Nicholls, N. and Gregory, J. The Coming Climate. *Scientific American*, 1997; May, 78–83.

Kaser, G. and Noggler, B. Observations of Speke Glacier, Ruwenzori Range, Uganda. *Journal of Glaciology*, 1991; 37 (127), 313.

Lear, A. Potential Health Effects of Global Climate and Environmental Changes. *New England Journal of Medicine*, 1989; 321:1577–83.

Leeson, H.S. Longevity of *Anopheles maculipennis race atroparvus*, Van Theil, at Controlled Temperature and Humidity after One Blood Meal. *Bulletin of Entomological Research*, 1939; 30:103–301.

Lindsay, S. and Martens, P. Malaria in the African Highlands: Past, Present and Future. *Bulletin of the World Health Organization*, in press.

Loevinsohn, M. Climatic Warming and Increased Malaria Incidence in Rwanda. *Lancet*, 1994; 343:714–8.

Matola, Y.G., White, G.B. and Magayuka, S.A. The Changed Pattern of Malaria Endemicity and Transmission at Amani in the Eastern Usambara Mountains, North-Eastern Tanzania. *Journal of Tropical Medicine and Hygiene*, 1987; 90:127–34.

McArthur, R.H. *Geographical Ecology*, New York: Harper & Row, 1972.

Maldonado, Y.A., Nahlen, B.L., Roberto, R.R. *et al.* Transmission of *Plasmodium vivax* Malaria in San Diego County, CA, 1986. *American Journal of Tropical Medicine and Hygiene*, 1990; 42:127–34.

Martens, W.J.M., Jetten, T.H. and Focks, D. Sensitivity of Malaria, Schistosomiasis and Dengue to Global Warming. *Climatic Change*, 1997; 35:145–56.

Martin, D.H. and Lefebvre, M. Malaria and Climate: Sensitivity of Malaria Potential Transmission to Climate. *Ambio*, 1995; 24:200–9.

Mashell, R., Mintray, T.M. and Callandar, B.A. Basic Science of Climate Change. *Lancet*, 1993; 343:1027–31.

Matsuoka, Y. and Kai, K. An Estimation of Climatic Change Effects on Malaria. *Journal of Global Environment Engineering*, 1994; 1:1–15.

McMichael, A.J., Haines, A. and Slooff, R. (eds). *Climate Change and Human Health*. Geneva, Switzerland: World Health Organization, World Meteorological Organization, United Nations Environmental Program, 1996.

Molineaux, L. In: W.H. Wernsdorfer and I. McGregor (eds). *Malaria, Principles and Practice of Malariology* (volume 2). NY: Churchill Livingstone, 1998, pp. 913–98.

Overpeck, J.T., Bartlein, P.J. and Webb, T. III. Potential Magnitude of Future Vegetation Change in Eastern North America: Comparisons with the Past. *Science*, 1991; 254:692–5.

Parmesan, C. Climate and Species' Range. *Nature*, 1996; 302:765.

Patrilla, S., Lavin, A., Dryden, H. *et al.* Rising Temperatures in the Sub-Tropical North Atlantic Ocean over the Past 35 Years. *Nature*, 1994; 369:48–51.

Patz, J.A., Epstein, P.R., Burke, T.A. and Balbus, J.M. Global Climate Change and Emerging Infectious Diseases. *Journal of the American Medical Association*, 1996; 275:217–23.

Pauli, H., Gottfried, M. and Grabherr, G. Effects of Climate Change on Mountain Ecosystems – Upward Shifting of Alpine Plants. *World Resource Review*, 1996; 8:382–90.

Peters, R.L. Consequences of Global Warming for Biological Diversity. In: R.L. Wyman (ed.), *Global Climate Change and Life on Earth*. NY: Routledge, Chapman and Hall, 1996.

Reeves, W.C., Hardy, J.L., Boison, W.K. and Milby, M.M. Potential Effect of Global Warming on Mosquito-Borne Arboviruses. *Journal of Medical Entomology*, 1994; 31:323–32.

Reisen, W.K., Meyer, R.P., Preser, S.B. and Hardy, J.L. Effect of Temperature on the Transmission of Western Equine Encephalomyelitis and St. Louis Encephalitis Viruses by *Culex tarsalis* (*Diptera: Culicadae*). *Journal of Medical Entomology*, 1993; 30:51–160.

Regaldo, A. Listen up! The World's Oceans may be Starting to Warm. *Science*, 1995; 268:1436–7.

Retallack, G.J. Early Forest Soils and their Role in Devonian Global Change. *Science*, 1997; 276:583–5.

Roemmich, D. and McGowan, J. Climatic Warming and the Decline of Zooplankton in the California Current. *Science*, 1995; 267:1324–6.

Rozendaal, J. Assignment Report: Malaria. World Health Organization. Pt. Moresby. Papua New Guinea. Geneva: World Health Organization, 1996.

Santer, B.D., Taylor, K.E., Wigley, T.M.L. *et al.* A Search for Human Influences on the Thermal Structure of the Atmosphere. *Nature*, 1996; 382:39–46.

Shope, R. Global Climate Change and Infectious Disease. *Environmental Health Perspectives*, 1991; 96:171–4.

Some, E.S. Effects and Control of Highland Malaria Epidemic in Kenya. *East African Medical Journal*, 1994; 71(1):2–8.

Suarez, M.F. and Nelson, M.J. Registro de altitud del *Aedes aegypti* en Colombia. *Biomedica*, 1981; 1:225.

Susskind, J., Piraino, P., Rokke, L. *et al.* Characteristics of the TOVS Pathfinder Path A data set. *Bulletin of the American Meteorological Society*, in press.

Sacherst, R.J. Impact of Climate Change on Pests and Diseases in Australasia. *Search*, 1990; 21:230–2.

Thompson, L.G., Mosley-Thompson, E., Davis, M. *et al.* 'Recent warming': Ice Core Evidence from Tropical Ice Cores with Emphasis on Central Asia. *Global and Planetary Change*, 1993; 7:145.

Thwaites, T. Are the Antipodes in Hot Water? *New Scientist*, 1994; 12 November, 21.

Travis, J. Taking a Bottom-to-Sky 'Slice' of the Arctic Ocean. *Science*, 1994; 266:1947–8.

World Health Organization. The World Health Report 1996: Fighting Disease, Fostering Development. Geneva, Switzerland: WHO, 1996.

Yoon, C.K. Warming Moves Plants up Peaks, Threatening Extinction. *The New York Times*, 1994, 21 June, C4.

Zucker, J.R. Changing Patterns of Autochthonous Malaria Transmission in the United States: a Review of Recent Outbreaks. *Emerging Infectious Diseases*, 1996; 2:37.

4

The Economics of Emerging Infections in the Asia-Pacific Region: What Do We Know and What Do We Need to Know?

Robert Davis and Ann Marie Kimball

Recently, the Asia Pacific Economic Cooperation (APEC) joined a number of other trading cooperations and communities in making the issue of emerging infectious diseases a priority. Although there is a perception that epidemics are costly, description or quantification of these costs has not been systematic. We reviewed published and unpublished information about the costs of epidemic disease activity in the 19 Asia Pacific Economic Cooperation economies and other regional economies to establish the economic costs over the past ten years. Our own study did not include a number of direct or human costs related to the occurrence of major infectious diseases. These costs include treatment costs and lost income as well as other costs related to social changes brought about by the onset of an infectious disease. Rather, we focused on loss in revenues and costs of regulation and trade and travel dislocation to economies. Our findings are: (1) measurement of economic impact of infectious diseases has been haphazard, and information is therefore uneven; (2) due to the sparcity of information, it proved impossible to quantify a total cost figure for the APEC economies due to epidemic activity impact on trade and travel; (3) a case study approach allows the most useful consideration of such activity; (4) describing risk factors for economic loss may prove useful; (5) more systematic prospective monitoring would be useful to quantify the impact of epidemic activity.

Since World War II, the value of merchandise trade on a global basis has increased by over 1000 per cent (World Trade Organization, 1995). This trend has been especially important for the Asian economies where trade more than doubled just between the years of 1984 to 1994 (World Trade Organization, 1995). Many nations within APEC rely on trade to ensure growth in their economies. Most importantly for disease transmission, trade in agricultural products between 1961 and 1991 has been substantial (Figure 4.1). The growth rate of agriculture trade within Asia has been 7 per cent annually between 1990 and 1994, and by 1994, nearly 20 per cent of all agriculture exports came from Asia. In fact, the economic vitality of trade for these economies is evidenced by the creation of the Asia Pacific Economic Cooperation itself – as a vehicle to liberalize trade in the region.

Along with increased trade (and migration), the pace of emergence and transmission of infectious diseases has apparently increased, particularly within the developing nations of APEC (Map 4.1). The costs of these incidents are unclear, with press accounts relying largely on sources within trade ministries and industry representatives to measure the costs. The economic impact of most epidemic events in the region have not been studied. In reviewing the major epidemics reported for the region either through the PROMED alert system or through the World Health Organization's Weekly Epidemiological Record, we were unable to locate economic studies for the large majority of clusters or outbreaks.

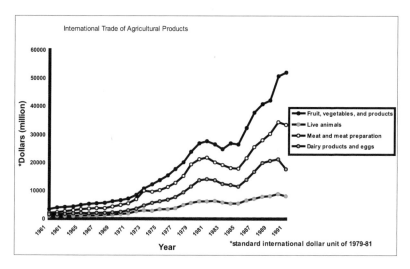

Figure 4.1 International trade of agricultural products.
Source: World Agriculture: Trends Indicators, 1961–91; Market Competition Branch, Agricultural Trade and Analysis Division and Economic Research Service.

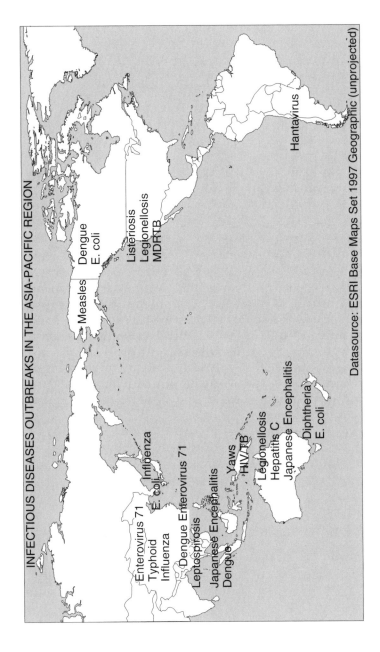

Map 4.1 Microbial threats in the Asia-Pacific region, 1998–99.
Source: Pro-Med

The economic literature is no more complete than the biomedical literature in this regard. Only one emergent infection – HIV/AIDS – has been studied to any extent. There have been a number of conflicting studies on the possible impact of the epidemic on economic growth rates of various nations, using two basic techniques. The first technique (Kambou, Devarajan and Over, 1992; Cuddington, 1993a, b; Cuddington and Hancock, 1994), involves modelling the economy of interest and simulating the effect of AIDS on, for example, growth in per capita gross domestic product. First applied to the economic effects of disease (Barlow 1967), it takes parameters from actual economies (for example, the percentage of cases that involves the skilled rather than the unskilled work-force), and uses those values in established economic models to project the effects of the epidemic. The effect of AIDS on growth in these models varies from a loss of 2 percentage points per year (Kambou, Devarajan and Over, 1992) to three-tenths of a percentage point per year (Cuddington and Hancock, 1994).

The second technique (Bloom and Mahal 1997) uses econometrics to measure the actual effects of the epidemic on economic growth. Bloom and colleagues applied this method in a large study of 51 countries during the period 1980 through 1992. A standard model of growth is used and includes a measure of AIDS prevalence for study countries over the period 1980 through 1992. AIDS prevalence is measured by the EPIMODEL, which is estimated along with the rest of the model. The findings are that although AIDS has a statistically significant effect on growth in the economies before any other determinants of growth are added, after these other determinants are added, the effect becomes statistically insignificant.

Why do the results from the two techniques differ so much? In part because the results using econometrics are statistical in nature and cannot really be compared to the results of simulations, which do not include standard errors. However, both techniques may prove useful in examining the costs of other epidemics reviewed in this paper. In particular, it may be useful to evaluate the economic impact of the 1991 cholera epidemic in Peru using either of these techniques in the future.

It is notable that despite the rapidly increasing incidence and prevalence of HIV/AIDS in the Asia Pacific region, few systematic studies have been carried out. UNDP sponsored a series of research papers early in the Asian epidemic that included a detailed study of the Thai economy, a sectoral study on the Thai transportation sector and a study of the impact on overseas contract workers from Philippines (Bloom and Lyons, 1993). Each of these areas is pertinent to the liberalization of trade and travel envisioned by APEC. Using the Interagency Working Group model to model the future epidemic, Michai Viravaidya and colleagues (1991); estimated Thailand's potential economic loss at US$ 7.3 billion by the year 2000, a figure which drew high level political attention to the crisis. In fact, in testimony during a 1992 US Congressional forum, this same group of researchers placed the potential loss as high as US$ 8.7 billion. This estimate was based on an estimated total of more than 3.4 million infections, 650 000 cases of AIDS and 500 000 deaths. However, due in part to the subsequent vigorous national prevention programme, as of 1997, WHO estimates that just 780 000 infections have occurred, with 260 000 clinical cases of AIDS and 230 000 deaths. This suggests that the actual experience in Thailand will demonstrate less economic impact, but follow-up studies have not been done.

The sectoral study suggested that the transportation sector of Thailand should be affected by the epidemic, given the behaviours and infection rate of truckers (Giraud, 1994). The study of overseas guest workers included very limited data on actual infection, but demonstrated that risks of wage earners abroad could profoundly affect the economy at home (Salon and Barrozo, 1995) – an example of cause and effect which we found was echoed in other economies and with other diseases.

In the United States and Canada, studies of economic impact have been carried out. In Canada, Hanveldt and colleagues documented a loss of wealth production due to HIV/AIDS deaths of $2.11 billion for the period 1987–91 (Hanveldt, Ruedy and Strathdee, 1994). Recent work in the United States has measured the loss of QALYs (quality adjusted life years) rather than lost wealth *per se*, and direct costs have increased with new therapies while QALY's have decreased due to increased years of healthy survival (Holtgrave and Pinkerton, 1997).

WHO estimated an annual infection rate in Asia of 1.7 million and a total of 6 million people infected with HIV (1997 figures) (UNAIDS, 1997), and yet few economies have attempted to quantify their losses in direct, indirect trade and travel-related costs as the epidemic has matured in the region. Thus, 'external' losses are unknown; domestic impacts only have been measured.

Methodology for this study

We found four epidemics that affected the economies of the region for which adequate information was available to begin to look at such losses: the 1991 Cholera epidemic in Peru, the 1993 pneumonic plague epidemic in India, the 1996 Japanese *E. coli* outbreak in Sakai, and the

1997 Avian flu epidemic in Hong Kong. We then evaluated the costs experienced by the economies in which these events occurred. Information has been compiled into summary case studies below. Based on the case studies, we have proposed an outline of potential economic risk factors, gleaned from the above events. Such a risk framework may prove useful to policy makers when deciding how to prioritize the expenditures necessary to prevent infectious diseases.

Case study descriptions of four epidemics

Cholera in Peru

In 1991, Peru experienced its first cholera epidemic that century (Emling, 1991; Gorman, 1991; Holman, 1991; Levinson, 1991; Lynn, 1991a, b; Cisternas, 1991; Associated Press, 1991). The epidemic began in Peru's northern ports in late January of that year and by the end of February had been blamed for more than a hundred deaths. By the end of 1991, there were over 300 000 cases of cholera in Peru and nearly 3000 deaths as a result (Pan American Health Organization, 1995). The epidemic continued through 1995 with another 300 000 cases and another 1500 deaths in Peru (Ibid.). Additionally, the disease spread throughout Latin America causing over 1 million cases and 10 400 deaths between 1991 and 1994.

As required by the International Health Regulations, Peru identified the epidemic and reported it to the World Health Organization in February of 1991. By the end of February, Peru's economy began to experience trade-related costs due to the epidemic. In particular, Peru experienced a drop in tourism as well as a loss in trade as a result of cancelled orders of fresh fruit and seafood (Lynn, 1991b). Tourism dropped between 60 and 70 per cent in the first quarter of 1991 from a year earlier (Holman, 1991). Export costs, including cancelled orders, delayed sales, deterioration in prices of exports and increased inspection costs were set at as high as $700 million dollars in 1991 (Associated Press, 1991).

The Peruvian cholera epidemic can be characterized as the emergence of a known pathogen in a previously unaffected geographic area. Its emergence in part is attributable to a decade of severe economic decline of Peru between 1981 and 1992. During this period, national production fell 23.5 per cent and per capita production dropped 28.9 per cent. Real per capita production in 1992 was no better than it had been in 1960. Inflation had reached a high of 7650 per cent in 1990 but had been reduced by economic measures at the time of the outbreak. As a result of this decline, real per capita social expenditure in

Peru fell from US$ 49.50 in 1980 to US$ 9.10 in 1991 (in 1985 dollars). In 1990, the Government's social expenditure for education, health and, housing and employment came to only 28 per cent of 1980 levels. This under-expenditure was reflected in a major shortfall in sanitary and water infrastructure for the population. The National Drinking Water and Sewerage Program reported that in 1992 only 76.5 per cent of the urban population was supplied with drinking water services and 60.5 per cent had sewerage services; in rural areas 23.7 per cent had access to drinking water services and 17.4 per cent to sewerage services (PAHO, 1992, 1994).

Pneumonic plague in India

In the middle of September 1994, an outbreak of pneumonic plague occurred in the western Indian city of Surat. By the middle of October, at least 50 deaths were blamed on the disease along with as many as 2500 other cases (Bureau of National Affairs, 1994; Dow Jones, 1994; Hattangadi and Dawley, 1994; McDonald, 1994; Sidhva, 1994; Wagstyl and Cookson, 1994; Wagstyl, 1994). By all accounts, this outbreak of a known and highly contagious and mortal pathogen was accompanied by general panic in the population (despite the fact that plague is endemic in much of the subcontinent). Poor diagnostic capacity of many laboratories compounded confusion about the extent of the infection (Fritz *et al.*, 1996). The occurrence of the disease led to a well-publicized exodus of workers out of Surat (Asian Wall Street Journal, 1994), a phenomenon not seen in the Peruvian scenario described above.

Subsequently, a number of trade and travel restrictions were placed on India, most of which were lifted by the end of October. The Indian government spent millions of dollars in a campaign to limit the losses due to the trade restrictions (Hattangadi and Dawley, 1994).

The cost of the plague epidemic in India has been put at over $1.3 billion (Bureau of National Affairs, 1994). These costs include lost trade revenue as well as lost tourism (Hattangadi and Dawley, 1994). Additional costs may have occurred because of lost revenues from the forced return of Indian migrant workers from the middle east, as well as some lost or delayed foreign direct investment. Finally, there was loss in diamond trade due to the massive migration of diamond workers out of Surat after the discovery of the disease (Ibid.).

E. coli O157:H7 in Japan

On July 13 1996, the Public Health Department of Sakai City received notification from Sakai City Hospital that 10 elementary school children had been admitted complaining of bloody diarrhoea and cramps. On July 14 *E. coli* O157:H7 was isolated from a further 20 cases. This agent proved to be the cause of the subsequent massive epidemic. Over the following weeks a total of 14 153 symptomatic cases were reported to the authorities with three fatalities (Task Force [Sakai City], 1997).

Sakai City is located in Osaka prefecture and is a densely populated (pop. 979 421/137 sq. km.), highly urbanized area. Through an extensive epidemiologic and microbiologic investigation, radish sprouts in school children's lunches were identified as the most likely vehicle of the infection. This conclusion was supported by three facts: (1) school children were disproportionately affected by the epidemic and radish sprouts were the only uncooked item served in the school lunches in affected districts; (2) school children absent on the day the radish sprouts were served were not infected; and (3) molecular studies suggested that the agent was the same in sprouts and in the cases. Despite very high hygiene levels within households, secondary cases did occur.

Costs from the outbreak included: (1) local costs in prevention, care, screening and outbreak investigation (although these costs have not been quantified, Table 4.1 gives an idea of the scale of activity which occurred during this outbreak); (2) 'cost shifting' in compensation to the victims of the epidemic:

> In view of the fact that this case of mass food poisoning was caused by school lunches and that the city accepted the fact that these supposedly safe lunches caused harm to many school children and even resulted in death, those who were directly victimized and those who were the victims of secondary infection were eligible for compensation. (Task Force [Sakai City], 1997)

To date, no quantification of these compensations has been carried out, nor has there been any estimates of indirect costs within Japenese society. Costs continue as: (3) decrease in imports of radish sprouts from the United States. This also represents a cost to the United States, and demonstrates the impact of epidemics on trading partners. As shown in Figure 4.2, the total value of radish seeds for sowing shipped to Japan from the United States fell from a high of $3 933 675 in 1995, to $2 225 619 in 1996, and to $1 393 643 in 1997. Thus there was a two-year decrease of $1 540 032 in the value of this trade. Costs finally include: (4) the radish manufacturer in Japan who imported the seeds from the United States and sprouted them in Japan reportedly sued the

Table 4.1 Summary of economic loss from epidemic disease

Date, epidemic event, country	Source of economic loss described	Dollar amount by source
1991 Cholera, Peru (extension of known pathogen into new area)	Trade restrictions Increased inspection costs (fishing and produce) Lost tourism	Between $ 700 million and $1.5 billion
1994 Pneumonic plague, Surat, India (occurrence of outbreak of known highly contagious and lethal pathogen in endemic area)	Trade restrictions Lost tourism Forced return of migrants to other economies Loss of diamond revenues	Approximately $1.3 billion
1996 E. Coli O157:H7 in Japan (extension of a known pathogen into a new area)	Local costs of screening, inspection Loss of import market Litigation and compensation	At least $1.5 million in lost import market. Other costs unknown.
1997 Avian Influenza with human transmission, Hong Kong (occurrence of human transmission of known avian pathogen in new area)	Trade restrictions (on imports), alternate purchasing of poultry Increased testing, regulation of poultry Loss of locally preferred breeds	Difficult to measure accurately but it includes at least $13 million in lost produce.

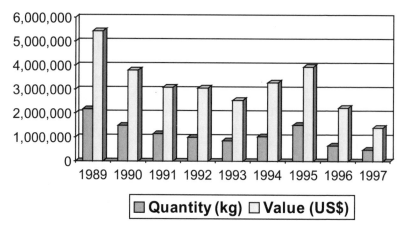

Figure 4.2   Impact of the Sakai epidemic on the radish seed trade with the US.

Japanese government for 50 000 000 yen (US$263 000) and the 19 manufacturers in the Japanese Radish Sprouts Association sued for 45 000 000 yen (US$200 000) for lost market. These suits have not been settled.

Japan is not the only economy in the region to suffer from *E. coli* O157:H7 epidemic disease. The United States has experienced outbreaks due to contaminated hamburgers served in fast food establishments (Bell *et al.*, 1994), and unpasteurized apple juice (Odwalla, 1996). In fact, the US experienced major beef recalls due to contamination with the agent that involved millions of pounds of product (USDA, 1997). However, we chose to study the Japanese outbreak because of its proximate relationship to trade; a linkage that was less apparent in the US experience.

Hong Kong avian flu

In May 1997, Hong Kong experienced its first human fatality from a flu that was believed to have been contracted from chickens (Milwaukee Journal Sentinel, 1998). Although this was a single case, it was unprecedented for an avian flu strain to directly infect a human, and this biological fact caused alarm worldwide. Normally, influenza viruses pass from fowl through pigs prior to circulating in humans. Concern that this agent (H5N1) represented a major shift in flu virulence, and a highly pathogenic one for humans was compounded by the subsequent occurrence of additional human cases. A total of 18 human cases and six fatalities were recorded in the outbreak (Hong Kong Health Department, 1997).

The government of Hong Kong halted imports of chickens from mainland China in late December 1997 and proceeded to slaughter the entire population of chickens on the island in early January of 1998. The total number of chickens lost was 1.3 million at an estimated cost of about $13 million. In addition, Hong Kong residents lost access to a particularly prized variety of chicken for up to two years. Another short-term cost to the residents of Hong Kong was the necessity of shifting consumption to expensive frozen chickens from Thailand for the months that fresh chicken was not available. Tourism was also affected by the epidemic (Dow Jones, 1998; *Chicago Tribune*, 1998; *New York Times*, 1998; *Dallas Morning News*, 1998; *Seattle Times*, 1998; Associated Press, 1998; *Financial Times*, 1998). The lost tourism reported as caused by the event was caused in part by travel warnings posted by Thailand and Taiwan. However, tourism to Hong Kong had already been reduced because of the economic situation in Asia as well as by the change in government in Hong Kong.

As with the trade in United States radish sprouts to Japan, chicken exports from the People's Republic of China to Hong Kong stopped during the outbreak. This cost to the PRC has not been quantified.

Framework for evaluating risk of economic impact

Economic loss from epidemic disease is summarized in Table 4.1. Such infectious disease events were made worse by failures of local sanitation, timely disease investigation, pest control or food inspection systems. To some extent, therefore, the trade and tourism losses can be attributed to inadequate investment in public health (Kimball *et al.*, 1998). It is of note that when we analysed the total health expenditure of selected APEC economies and compared the growth in this expenditure over time to the growth in trade volume, we found that health expenditure did not appear to keep pace (Figure 4.3, above). Previous studies of public health projects have proposed establishing the 'counterfactual' – that is, establishing the costs of not doing the project and comparing them to the costs of doing the project (Hammer, 1993, 1997). In addition to the costs discussed in this chapter regarding the demand for the services provided by the project, the following framework should help determine the possible trade- and tourism-based costs of failing to provide adequate public health facilities.

Trade and food-borne agents

Food-based infectious diseases (cholera, cyclospora, hepatitis A, *E. coli*) often lead to trade restrictions. Thus the dependency of a given economy on food or agricultural exports or imports will determine its risk of losses from foodborne infections.

Trade restriction, law and politics

What kind of restrictions on exports should the policy maker expect if an epidemic occurs? International health regulations require that the least invasive or disruptive measures to control three notifiable diseases (cholera, plague and yellow fever) are the maximum allowable. However, even for these diseases, experience reinforces the impression that import restrictions are not based on science but rather on the political economy of trade. These restrictions, although in violation of the international rules, often last a number of months before being lifted. An additional risk parameter is therefore the extent to which the agricultural export sector competes with powerful rivals in the countries to which it exports those products. If there are such rivals, they may use the epidemic as a pretext to lobby for additional protection for their products by restricting imports from the affected economy.

Trade safety and public health

The state of food and water safety 'at home' among trading economies affects the risk of epidemics in their own economies, and the risk of economic impact to their trading partners. As was seen in Peru, the deferral of investment in public health systems was costly to Peru in lost dollars but also costly to economies that imported affected products from Peru. Conversely, if public health infrastructure in a trading partner is perceived to be weak and vulnerable to transmission of imported disease, that economy may be more willing to place restrictions on imports until adequate inspection controls are in place in the economy of origin. Timeliness in notification and investigation and resolution of an epidemic threat is a capacity of public health, dependent, in part, on investment. In turn, duration of an epidemic is a key factor in costs. Increasing the efficiency and timeliness of investigation will decrease costs that are due to longer (and therefore broader) transmission within the population.

Fate of affected product

The costs to an economy in terms of trade restrictions depends on what happens to the product that is not exported as the result of the epidemic. Can the product be sold at home? If so, then the price of the goods will fall at home, thus increasing consumer welfare even as it lowers industry profits. Additionally, the exporters might be able to sell the product in a third country that does not impose trade restrictions. These sales will be at either a higher cost or a lower price, but the lost profits for the industry will be lower than the cancelled sales numbers often reported in the press.

Inspection costs

Costs of inspection are also likely to increase as a result of an epidemic. These costs will increase export costs over the long term but are likely to have some positive effects as well. Hong Kong reportedly spent $1.92 million annually in enhanced inspection and testing to reinstate its live chicken trade with the mainland (Chin, 1998). To some extent, domestic food safety programmes can act as a substitute for export inspection programmes and they carry the obvious domestic health benefit as well.

Reliance on migrant labour and/or travel and tourism

Two possible costs illustrated by the plague event in India are lost tourism and loss of benefits of migrant labour (either lost income from restrictions on the outflow of labour or increased wages as a result of a decrease in the inflow of labour). In Hong Kong, an 11-per-cent decline in tourist arrivals was noted following the avian flu outbreak. As described above, Peru also experienced lost tourism. Economies that rely on either tourism or migrant labour, therefore, should factor these possible losses into public health infrastructure spending decisions.

Lost foreign direct investment

Multinational corporations make investments in developing economies in the expectation of receiving a return. Anything that might disrupt that return imperils foreign direct investment (FDI). Risk of lost business due to epidemic activity theoretically serves as a deterrent to foreign direct investment and although this matter has not been studied to date, there are two main effects:

1. This might hinder technology transfer, particularly in the agricultural sectors.
2. Multinational corporations might have problems getting employees to travel to some spots if the disease is a particularly virulent one. This effect is hard to quantify but it may be important nonetheless.

Cost trade-offs

Clearly, the costs of emerging infections in APEC nations has been significant. However, the costs of preventing such infections is also significant. In particular, many infectious diseases are either transmitted because of poor water safety or because of poor food safety. The costs of adequate food and water safety systems can be high, both in terms of initial capital costs and in terms of annual maintenance costs. The Pan American Health Organization (1995) estimates that Peru had nearly a decade of deferred capital investment in its water and sanitation systems at the time of the 1991 cholera outbreak.

The benefits of such projects include all of the benefits of improved health of the local population. These benefits have been included in project analyses. However, it is not clear that the 'external' costs due to lost trade and lost tourism from emerging infections have been taken into account. As the interdependency of economics increases within trading communities, counting such costs will become more and more important.

Conclusion

The human costs of epidemics in suffering, illness and death are high. In addition, existing information suggests that epidemic costs are high in economic terms. Costs of recent outbreaks in the Asia Pacific region include direct and indirect costs to the affected economy, losses to trading partner economies and losses due to tourism and travel restrictions. Consideration of risk of loss includes evaluation of the public health infrastucture within economies and evaluation of their ability to stem the transmission of new infections as well as insight into the political economy of trade within the region. Improving the information base prospectively for the study of the economics of epidemics could be beneficial in guiding policy in epidemic control and for mitigating the economic impact of future epidemics. For instance, local costs can be limited when timely and accurate disease investigation allows the definition of source and prevention of massive infection. The capacity to carry out such epidemiologic work is an important technology that should be accessible to all economies. Understanding the interplay of markets and how epidemics affect them will allow the minimization of real losses. Within the framework of the new APEC Initiative on Emerging Infections, such prospective economic studies should become a priority.

The World Health Organization is the primary international agency involved in the health sector of economies around the world. APEC crosses three WHO regional offices: the Western Pacific, the South-East Asia, and the Americas (PAHO). However, APEC embraces the economies that are linked in trade and travel, and these activities may increasingly define the risk and economic impacts of epidemics. Thus, improving the information base about such impacts, and promoting synergies among agencies such as WHO, WTO and regional trading groups such as APEC in orchestrating regional response, appears to be an important strategy.

References

Asian Wall Street Journal Remember the plague (editorial). 1994, p. 8.

Associated Press Cisternas, C. Ecuador says Cholera Continues to Spread; Death Toll at 26. 1991; Quito.

Associated Press Emling, S. Cholera Sweeps into Latin America. 1991; Guatemala City.

Associated Press WHO chief says cholera epidemic may cost Peru $1 billion. 1991.

Associated Press Lynn, B. Spread of Cholera Threatens Millions in Latin America. 1991a; Lima.

Associated Press Lynn, B. Cholera Epidemic Hurting Peru's Economy. 1991b; Lima.

Barlow, R. The Economic Effects of Malaria Eradication. *The American Economic Review*, 1967; 128–30.

Bell, B.P., Goldoft, M., Griffin, P.M. *et al.* A multistate outbreak of *Escherichia coli* O157:H7 associated bloody diarrhea and hemolytic uremic syndrome from hamburgers, the Washington experience. *JAMA* 1994, Nov. 2 272(17):1349–53.

Bloom, Lyons (eds). The economic Impact of AIDS in Asia. UNDP Regional Programme Division, Regional Bureau for Asia and the Pacific 1993; Chapters 2, 5 and 7.

Bloom, D.E. and Mahal, A.S. Does the AIDS Epidemic Threaten Economic Growth? *Journal of Econometrics*, 1997; 77:105–24.

Cheung, P. Farmers in Hong Kong face lengthy recovery from chicken slaughter. *Orange County Register* (from Associated Press) 1998; a21.

Chickens back in Hong Kong after officials end six-week ban. *Milwaukee Journal Sentinel*, 1998; 3.

Chin, J. Nandonet as reported in ProMED mail February 8, 1998.

China – Hong Kong tries to deal with desertion by tourists. *The Seattle Times*, 1998; 10.

Compensation for poultry industry. *Chicago Tribune*, 1998; 7.

Cuddington, J.T. and Hancock, J.D. Assessing the Impact of AIDS on the Growth Path of the Malawian Economy. *Journal of Development Economics*, 1994; 43:363–8.

Cuddington, J.T. Further Results on the Macroeconomic Effects of AIDS: the Dualistic, Labour-Surplus Economy. *The World Bank Economic Review*, 1993a; 7(3):403–17.

Cuddington, J.T. Modeling the Macroeconomic Effects of AIDS, with an Application to Tanzania. *The World Bank Economic Review*, 1993b; 7(2):173–89.

Dow Jones India's trade deficit swells; plague hits exports. 1994; New Delhi.

Financial Times Sidhva, S. Airlines resume flights to India. London 1994; 4.

Financial Times Wagstyl, S. and Cookson, C. Indian trade hit by plague panic. London 1994; 2.

Financial Times Wagstyl, S. Indian food exports hit by plague panic. London 1994; 3.

Fritz, C.L., Dennis, D.T., Tipple, M.A. *et al.* Surveillance for Pneumonic Plague in the United States During an International Emergency: a Model for Control of Imported Emerging Diseases. *Emerging Infectious Diseases*, 1996; 2(1):30–6.

Giraud, P. The Economic Impact of AIDS at the Sectoral Level: Developing an Assessment Methodology and Applying it to Thailand's Transport Sector. 1994; p. 71.

Hammer, J.S. The economics of malaria control. *World Bank Research Observer*, 1993; 8(1):1–22.

Hammer, J.S. The economic analysis for health projects. *World Bank Research Observer*, 1997; 12(1):47–71.

Hanveldt, R., Ruedy, N. and Strathdee, S. Indirect Costs of HIV/AIDS Mortality in Canada. *AIDS* 1994, October 8(10):F7–11.

Hattangadi, S. and Dawley, H. India's Plague takes an Economic Toll, Too. *Business Week International Editions*, 1994; 24.

HK poultry industry presses government for more compensation. Dow Jones International News, Hong Kong 1998.

Holtgrave, D. and Pinkerton, S. Updates of Cost of Illness and Quality of Life Estimates for Use in Economic Evaluations of HIV Prevention Programs. *Journal of Acquired Immune Deficiency Syndrome and Human Retroviruses* 1997, September 1 16(1):54–62.

Hong Kong acts to placate chicken owners. *New York Times Abstracts*, 1998; 7.

Hong Kong Health Department, 1997, http://www.info.gov.hk/dh/

India's exports have been hurt badly. Bureau of National Affairs International Trade Reporter 1994; 11:1662.

Kambou, G., Devarajan, S. and Over, M. The Economic Impact of AIDS in an African Country: Simulations with a Computable General Equilibrium Model of Cameroon. *Journal of African Economics*, 1992; 1(1):109–30.

Kimball, A.M. *et al. The Asia Pacific Economic Cooperation Emerging Infections Network* 1998; University of Washington, Seattle.

Lucas, L. Hong Kong airline shares hit by bird flu. *Financial Times*, London edn, Hong Kong 1998; 29.

McDonald, H. Surat's revenge: India Counts the Mounting Costs of Poverty. *Far Eastern Economic Review*, 1994; 76.

ODWALLA. From the Centers for Disease Control and Prevention outbreak of *Escherichia coli* O157:H7 infections associated with drinking unpasteurized commercial apple juice – British Columbia, California, Colorado and Washington, October 1996. *JAMA* 1996, Dec 18; 276(23):1865.

PAHO at Work Today: the Case of Cholera. *Pan American Health Organization Bulletin*, 1992; 26(4):294.

PAHO. Peru. *Health Conditions in the Americas*, 1994; 11:349–60.

Pan American Health Organization, Cholera situation in the Americas: 1991–1995. *Epidemiological Bulletin*, 1995; 16(2):12.

Recovery for Hong Kong chicken farmers may take years. *Dallas Morning News*, Hong Kong 1998; 11A.

Salon, O. and Barrozo, A. Overseas Contract Workers and the Economic Consequences of the HIV and AIDS in the Philippines. 1995; p. 111.

Task Force [Sakai City] on the Mass Outbreak of Diarrhea in School Children of Sakai City, Takatorige, T. *et al.* (eds). Report on the outbreak of *E. coli* O157 infection in Sakai City. Sakai City, 1997.

Time Gorman, C. Death in the Time of cholera. 1991; 58.

UNAIDS, WHO HIV/AIDS Epidemic, estimates published June 1997.

USDA, media reports 'Agriculture Department to Investigate Beef Slaughter Process' September 12, 1997 as reported in ProMED mail, September 19, 1997.

Viravaidya, M., Obrembsky, S. and Myers, C. The Economic Impact of AIDS on Thailand. 1991; p. 7.

Wall Street Journal Holman, R.L. Postscripts. 1991; A14.

Washington Post Levinson, J.I. Cholera: Lesson for Latin America. 1991; A19.

World Trade Organization. Trends and Statistics in International Trade, World Trade Organization, 1995.

5

Economic Growth, Disruption, Deprivation, Disease, and Death: On the Importance of the Politics of Public Health for Development

Simon Szreter

Over the long term, the processes of rapid economic growth seem to be strongly correlated with improvements in the prosperity and health of a society. Hence derives the commonplace notion that economic growth results in development. This essay argues that, contrary to this widely held opinion, economic growth entails critical challenges and threats to the health and welfare of the populations involved and does not, therefore, necessarily produce development.

Since the 1940s, economic and demographic historians, social scientists and policymakers have broadly accepted that each national trajectory of sustained economic growth has always been attended by a 'demographic transition', a process in which a pronounced fall in national mortality levels (and also fertility levels) occurs as a result of the gains to national wealth. In fact the idea of a demographic transition, both as a theory and as a general historical model, has been subjected both to fundamental conceptual criticism and to empirical refutation. Important counter-examples have been uncovered, such as, historically, in France, where there was a decline in fertility before either rapid economic growth or mortality decline, and contemporary states such as Kerala, Costa Rica, Sri Lanka and China, where mortality has declined in advance rapid wealth creation.[1] Although there has been significant dissent, a glib post-World War II consensus has remained largely unperturbed: that economic growth causes mortality decline, principally through an epidemiological transition – a decline of infectious and communicable diseases.[2]

The example of Britain's well-documented economic and epidemiological history during and after the industrial revolution has been repeatedly used as the empirical centrepiece of the most influential postwar models, which have proclaimed that the promotion of rapid economic growth and industrialization is the principal means to enhance the health, welfare and development of a nation. But an entirely different analysis of the history of the relationship between economic growth and the health of the British population during the nineteenth century is presented here, emphasizing the disruptive consequences of industrialization and the crucial importance of the politics of public health.

The argument developed here is that economic growth should be understood as setting in train a socially and politically dangerous, destabilizing, and health-threatening set of forces. These negative consequences of rapid economic growth may be conceptualized as a sequential model: the 'four Ds' of disruption, deprivation, disease and death. The four Ds are always potential outcomes of rapid economic growth, but only the first 'D', disruption, is a universal accompaniment of the process. By disruption is meant, first, disturbance in the physical and biological environment – the ecological relationship between humans and the habitat. Second, is the ideological foment involving the cultural negotiation of new values and norms. Third, is institutional and administrative destruction and construction. Fourth, is political conflict among the competing social groups involved, some of them relatively new social formations thrown up as the agents of economic change.

It is, of course, possible to point to very many countries' histories in which substantial economic growth has been achieved over a long secular period without suffering the full rigours of the four Ds. What is less well known, however, is that many of these same successful developed and developing economies also suffered significant setbacks or stagnations in the health and welfare of their populations for substantial periods during their earlier histories of rising economic growth when their politics proved unable to restrain and master the four Ds. This is becoming increasingly clear from recent historical research on body height and mortality rates, not only for the British case, which is explored in some detail below, but also, for example, for nineteenth-century Holland, Germany, France, Australia, Canada, the United States, and early-twentieth-century Japan.[3] In the twentieth century there were the infamous 'growth sacrifices' of the peoples of the Soviet Union in the 1930s and of China in the Great Leap Forward, 1958–61.

Furthermore, many developing countries today have vast urban *favelas* where the full force of the first three Ds is very much in evidence but where, because of the life-maintaining capacities of relatively cheap and often foreign-aid-subsidized medical technology, the final outrage of the fourth D – death – can usually be successfully staved off. Thus, the extent to which the sequence of the four Ds unfolds to its final, lethal conclusion in any particular country experiencing economic growth, and which parts of the population suffer most, are contingent on the political, ideological, social and institutional history of that country.

The crucial point is that nothing inherent in the process of economic growth provides protection against its unwanted consequences – the four Ds. In those cases where such growth has proceeded without untoward health and mortality implications, the character of the politically negotiated social and institutional responses to the ever-present multi-dimensional challenges of disruption has enabled these countries to manage their economic growth in such a way as to evade deprivation, disease and death.

Much of the remainder of this chapter will describe the course of the relationship between economic growth, the politics of public health, and the state of the nation's health, in nineteenth-century Britain. This follows a long line of commentators, analysts and historians, since the British historical case has always occupied a central place in the literature on economic growth and development. Because Britain was the epicentre of the world's first industrial revolution, the most influential thinkers who originally addressed and debated the key issues focused their theories and prescriptions upon Britain's experience. Adam Smith, David Ricardo and Robert Malthus, Alexander Hamilton (architect of the American Republic's successful protectionism for its infant industry against British competition), John Stuart Mill, Friedrich Engels and Karl Marx premised their diverse ideas primarily upon their understanding of the British economy.

Moreover, the British state and its provincial upper and middle classes were assiduous students of their own fast-changing economy and society, generating a rich body of literature and comment, but also a mountain of relatively high-quality economic, demographic and social statistical evidence.[4] As a result, three of the most influential postwar empirical social science models of modern economic and social change have been primarily based upon the British nineteenth-century historical evidence: the idea of demographic transition; W.W. Rostow's theory of 'take-off'; and Thomas McKeown's thesis on the role of nutritional improvement.[5] Each of these three models deployed independent bodies of empirical evidence from the British historical case, drawn from the demographic, the economic and the epidemiological record, respectively. These are the principal historically based theories that have appeared to support so strongly the conventional notions that economic growth should be seen as a benevolent prime mover that causes improvements in the health of nations and that produces 'development'.

However, as the reference to Marx and Engels suggests, alternative interpretations have always been offered. Indeed, until the 1820s, leading Enlightenment medical opinion assumed that expansion of trade, increased riches and greater 'luxury' must also bring an increased harvest of death through the 'diseases of civilization' (for instance obesity, gout and venereal diseases); and it was observed that inequality and destitution were afflictions of wealthy, commercial societies, rather than of subsistence communities.[6] Malthus gave the latter viewpoint its most apocalyptic rendering in his series of essays, *On the Principle of Population*, from the 1790s. His views were translated into policy in Britain in the year of his death, 1834, with the enactment of the infamous New Poor Law to discourage the poor from reckless overbreeding. Marx and Engels, by contrast, famously pronounced the system of industrial capitalism itself to be dysfunctional beyond repair and viewed the increasing plight of the poor in Britain as the necessary condition for a revolutionary dénouement. But, in addition to the economic apologists for the interests of property and the critical sociological opponents of capital, there was a third, liberal and social reformist voice, that corresponded to the institutional and political position of the public health movement.

The public health perspective endorsed neither the proposition that we should place our faith in the invisible hand of economic growth nor the opposed position that economic growth could only lead to the immiseration of the masses and required political revolution as its antidote. Despite important differences in social and etiological theory, the leading practitioners of public health, in France, Germany and Britain (where there were further significant distinctions between the Scottish school and the English), broadly concurred on an essentially reformist strategy. The increased wealth generated by economic growth held out the possibility of healthy 'progress' for the majority in society. But this favourable outcome was in no way inevitable. It had to be devised with the aid of medical science and fought for politically. It could only be achieved if the serious health challenges brought on by economic change, industrial wage labour and urban living, were met with the appropriate political resolution to implement far-reaching preventive health measures, requiring the deployment of substantial social and economic resources to protect and enhance the health of the populace. This view characterized the outlook and efforts of Villermé and Bérard in France, Virchow in Germany, Alison in Scotland and Chadwick, Duncan, Farr and Simon in England.[7]

Within the terms of reference of this centuries-old debate, this essay concurs up to a point with Marx and Engels in arguing that there is indeed something intrinsically dangerous and socially destabilizing in the wake of economic growth. However, it does not view the relationship between capital and labour as being purely antagonistic nor as being of overwhelming significance in determining the historical outcomes that are possible (although the relationship of 'competitive interdependence' between capital and labour is certainly a condition of primary importance in market-oriented economic systems).[8] The chapter focuses instead on the importance of the politics of the public health movement in determining historical outcomes. It is argued that Britain's historical evidence indicates that rapid economic change necessarily brings widespread and pervasive disruption.

Of all the dimensions of disruption mentioned above, the most important in influencing possible health outcomes is the scale and nature of political disruption. For it is this that critically determines the capacity of the society, the state, its citizens and its various associations and administrative units to devise successful strategies to manage the disruptions of economic change without incurring the other three Ds. Hence, this points to the essential importance of the history of the politics of public health in explaining how mere economic growth and its attendant 'four Ds' can come to be harnessed into economic and social 'development'.

Economic growth and the health of the populace in Britain, circa 1750–1870

Our knowledge of the course of economic and demographic change across the entire period of industrialization in Britain is now considered to rest on a relatively firm empirical foundation. Economic growth was occurring throughout the eighteenth century at a steady, if gradual, rate of approximately 0.67 per cent per annum. In the last two decades of the century the rate of growth doubled to about 1.35 per cent and thereafter continued on its upward trend, reaching a plateau of an average of approximately 2.5 per cent per annum, more or less sustained across the three decades of the secular boom from 1843 to 1873, before falling back slightly to an average rate of just under 2 per cent per annum over the ensuing four decades, 1873–1913.[9] On the demographic side, after a period of population stasis and severe mortality during the last half of the seventeenth and first three decades of the eighteenth centuries, England's population began a sustained rise from 1731, when the total stood at 5.3 million, exactly doubling by 1815, at the end of the Napoleonic Wars; and then doubling again over the subsequent 55 years, to reach 21.5 million by 1871.[10] Thereafter the rate of growth slowed only slightly, so that England's population had reached 35.5 million by 1911.

The trend and patterns of urbanization are, of course, somewhat more complex. Until 1700, the process of urbanization was almost synonymous with the growth of London, which housed at that time 11 per cent of the national population and was already the largest city in Europe. A century later, although London had almost doubled in size to just under a million inhabitants, even more significant was the fact that rapid urbanization was now occurring in the provinces, too. Whereas in 1700 there had been only six other towns with over 10 000 inhabitants (in fact all of them under 33 000 in size and none of them expanding rapidly), by 1801, there were 48 such towns and many of these had been growing fast since the 1740s, so that more of the nation's population now lived in these 48 towns (12.7 per cent) than in London (10.7 per cent).[11] However, none of these provincial towns had reached as many as 100 000 inhabitants by 1801, just before the spread of the new mode of production involving the centralization and concentration of work processes made possible by the steam-powered mechanization of industry. Even in the leading sector of cotton manufacture, Boulton and Watt's rotary steam engine was not first successfully harnessed to a spinning mule until 1795 (by McConnel and Kennedy in Manchester).[12] But by 1841, six English provincial cities and one Scottish city (Glasgow) recorded populations over 100 000, with Liverpool, Manchester and Glasgow each well over 200 000 and Birmingham, Leeds, Bristol and Sheffield above 100 000). Urbanization continued at such a rate that this new phenomenon, the growth of large provincial cities above 100 000 inhabitants, accounted for 30 per cent of the national total by 1901, over twice as many as then lived in London, although the imperial metropolis was still easily the biggest city in the world at that time.[13] The nineteenth century was, therefore, the era of industrializing urbanization in Britain on an unprecedented scale, in a manner that is historically analagous to the economic and urban growth that has since been experienced in so many other countries outside Europe during the twentieth century.

What, then, was the relationship between these patterns of economic, demographic and urban growth and the health and welfare of the populace? On the one hand, the many real-wage series that have been constructed, though imperfect, probably offer the best measure of the trends in the economic prosperity (e.g. the disposable income) of the majority of workers and families during this period. On the other hand, in order to evaluate the health of the populace, measures derived from contemporary death records (parish registers before 1837 and the national civil registration system thereafter) are agreed to provide the most reliable indicators.

Insofar as the urban, industrial population was concerned, there seems little doubt among historians that, in general, the real wages received by those adult males born in or migrating to the centres of manufacturing in the eighteenth and nineteenth centuries were consistently higher than those paid to rural workers, and that for most workers, real wages were tending to rise, albeit spasmodically, throughout the period.[14] Undoubtedly there were large groups in the population whose real wages did not exhibit such a strong secular upward trend. These were principally agricultural labourers and their families from the south of England, a large minority of the labouring poor at the start of the period in 1750, but thereafter a steadily shrinking proportion of the national total as the manufacturing workforces of the northern and midland towns swelled in numbers.[15] It is also likely that real wages in the London economy, although high in comparison with all other regions, did not rise much across the eighteenth and early nineteenth centuries and so were, in effect, 'caught-up' by the urban workers of the north and midlands.[16]

On the other hand, this apparently favourable general pattern, which the adult male real-wage evidence indicates, regarding the relationship between economic growth and the prosperity and welfare of the industrial working populace is complicated, if not flatly contradicted, by our other principal category of evidence: mortality trends. Where the health of the nation as a whole is concerned, Wrigley and Schofield's reconstruction of trends in the national average expectation of life at birth (e_0) provides the best summary measure. This shows a sustained improvement across the initial period of gradual economic growth and urbanization: from the 1730s, when national e_0 stood in the low 30s, to a point almost a century later in the 1820s, when it had risen to around

40–41 years.[17] Although these gains were not subsequently lost, there was no further significant increase in the national average for life expectancy at birth until the 1870s. In other words, the period of most impressive, rising economic growth rates, c. 1800 to 1870, ushered in little if any health improvements for the nation as a whole.

This mid-nineteenth-century discontinuity in the upward trend in the national series for life expectancy at birth is all the more significant, from the point of view of the relationship between economic growth, living standards and welfare, when the differential experience of urbanizing and rural populations is examined. It is not possible to compare life expectancy at birth for these different environments until the second quarter of the nineteenth century, when a number of vital calculations were made by contemporaries, most importantly the first official life tables compiled by William Farr, based on the relatively solid foundation of the census and vital registration statistics collated by the new General Register Office (GRO), created in 1837.[18] In addition to compiling a national life table based on the census year of 1841 and the deaths registered during the years 1839–42, Farr also published several extremely helpful sectional life tables. These were produced for the cities of London, Liverpool and Manchester; for a collection of rural parishes in Surrey; and for a selected set of the most healthy districts found in the country, relating to approximately 5 per cent of the population in 1851.[19] As a result of these contemporary studies, it is possible to form a relatively clear picture of the relationship between industrialization and health during the second quarter of the nineteenth century in England, after approximately a century of economic and demographic growth, rising real wages for the urban workforce, and improving national average life expectancy.

This evidence shows that at a time when the national e_0 was about 40 years, the population of London, at 37 years' life expectancy, was very close to the national average. This was especially remarkable considering the appalling levels of mortality that have been documented for London a century earlier; its life expectancy at birth may well have been little above 20 years during the second quarter of the eighteenth century.[20] Although Schwarz's research has confirmed that there had been only modest improvement in the capital's real wages during the intervening period, the health of its populace had apparently improved beyond recognition, despite continued urban expansion. Second, in the Surrey countryside, Farr found e_0 at 45 years and therefore significantly above the national average. This was also notable, considering the difficulties experienced by agricultural labourers' families in the south throughout the previous century of Enclosures – a procession of unemployment, falling incomes and immiseration that culminated in the wave of 'Swing' riots in 1830.[21] Third, in the selected group of rural communities composing the nation's Healthy Districts, e_0 in 1851 was already as high as 49 years, a figure not reached by the national average until the next century.

The story was quite different in the two largest provincial cities, the centres of the nation's new prosperity and of workers who enjoyed the most consistently rising real wages. Here Farr found an appalling situation. Average life expectancy at birth for the inhabitants of Liverpool in 1841 was a mere 28 years and in Manchester it was 27 years.[22] As Table 5.1 shows, the largest and fastest-growing industrial cities (those above 100 000 inhabitants in each decade) still had life expectancies in the neighbourhood of 34 years during both the 1850s and the 1860s and showed no significant improvement until the 1870s and 1880s. We can add to this official data, one other vital piece of high-quality demographic evidence: that for the industrial city of Glasgow (along with Manchester and Liverpool, one of the three biggest industrial cities at that time). From this evidence, it seems certain, first, that the problem of life expectancy being substantially below the national average in these largest industrial cities was already evident in the 1820s (when the earliest Glasgow data are available, showing life expectancy at birth to be 35 years) and, second, that the problem became particularly marked during the 1830s and 1840s, as Table 5.1, above, shows. Additional evidence indicates that the many smaller, but also fast-growing, industrial towns of Britain at this time experienced the same pattern of sharply deteriorating mortality conditions across the second quarter of the nineteenth century.[23] Other demographic historians have identified a rise in mortality from infectious diseases and sanitation diseases, especially at ages 3–24 months, strongly implicated in this pattern of rising urban mortality in the second quarter of the nineteenth century.[24]

Table 5.1 Estimates of expectation of life at birth in provincial cities (not London) above 100 000 inhabitants in England and Wales, 1810s–1890s

	1810s	*1820s*	*1830s*	*1840s*	*1850s*	*1860s*	*1870s*	*1880s*	*1890s*
Cities > 100 000	–	35	29	30	34	34	38	40	42
England and Wales	41	41	41	41	41	41	43	45	46

Source: Szreter and Mooney, *Economic History Reviews* 51 (February 1998).

There is, therefore, no doubt as to the basic nature of the relationship between rapid economic growth and the health of the industrial working population in Britain during its classic period of industrialization. For that ever-increasing proportion of the population directly involved in urban and industrial expansion, despite gradually rising disposable income, there appears to have been a marked deterioration in average life expectancy during the second quarter of the nineteenth century and persisting into the third quarter. It is worth noting, incidentally, that this conclusion is supported where studies of trends in other indexes of health, social security and personal welfare have been constructed, relating to urban crime, illegitimacy, literacy and children's height attainments.[25]

But what caused these problems to manifest themselves so strongly at this point in time, when many of these towns had been growing rapidly and industrializing for three-quarters of a century or so? A number of important dimensions to the evidence rule out some of the more straightforward hypotheses. First, the fact that deterioration is documented during the same two to three decades in towns of widely varying size and growth trajectories, from a Glasgow or a Liverpool, to a Carlisle, Wigan or West Bromwich, militates against any simple notion that deterioration was occurring as a lagged result of earlier expansion or was precipitated by crossing a certain threshold of density, size or speed of growth. Second, the relative immunity to this deterioration of the colossus of London, and of many of the older and non-industrial market towns, makes it implausible to envisage some kind of epidemiological wave or general climatic factor accounting for the trends. However, there are two important positive clues in the epidemiological evidence. First, the generally increasing importance of sanitation and crowding (infectious) diseases, in particular infant diarrhea and digestive tract problems, along with typhus, typhoid and cholera; and second, the specific evidence from the city of Glasgow that smallpox mortality actually returned to plague that city in the 1830s and 1840s, after it had almost been eradicated in the 1800s and 1810s following the introduction of Jennerian vaccination.[26]

Both of these developments suggest the possibility of a political and administrative breakdown in the second quarter of the nineteenth century specific to the fast-growing industrial towns and cities, rather than to towns in general. It seems that urban local authorities in industrial centres were failing in the management of their crowded environments at this point. Apparently, such towns had been sufficiently well-organized to have delivered an effective preventive health programme against smallpox in a city like Glasgow during the first two decades of the nineteenth century, a period when Britain was engaged in a war with Napoleon's France. But thereafter things seem to have been allowed to slip in Glasgow. There is corroborative evidence for this view, both in terms of the level of effective voluntary action and in terms of 'state' provision. For instance, on the voluntary side, the second half of the eighteenth century had seen the build-up of sufficient momentum in civic activism so that a large number of voluntary hospitals had been constructed in Britain's towns. Yet the first half of the nineteenth century saw little further addition to these resources, with serious consequences for the provision of urban medical services.[27] Meanwhile, the principal state 'welfare' institution, the Poor Law, was dramatically reformed in the 1830s in a way that rendered it insensitive to the needs of the growing urban industrial proletariat, whose primary collective cause of insecurity was the trade cycle.

But why should there have been a failure of effective urban social and health administration in this particular period; and why was it specific to Britain's industrial towns and cities? Why were London and Bristol relatively unscathed? In seeking an answer to this problem, certain critical political, social and ideological developments will be examined. It will be argued that these developments provide the true reasons why there was a failure at this point in Britain's industrial cities to respond to the challenge of the four Ds posed by rapid economic growth, and also why these same cities were subsequently, in the last quarter of the nineteenth century, successfully made into healthier, safer places to live.

Economic growth and urban deterioration in early-nineteenth-century Britain

In the fast-growing, industrial towns of the first half of the nineteenth century, environmental deterioration occurred through a configuration of three socially divisive forces, which were themselves intimately related to, indeed entailed by, Britain's pattern of economic growth. First, inequality of incomes and wealth was growing apace, through capital accumulation, the seizing by a fortunate few of commercial opportunities, and the extraction of rents of various kinds.[28] Second, the industrial town was continually receiving rural inmigrants, often in great surges during times of depression; and these inmigrants tended to fill the least-secure and lowest-paid jobs.[29] This reinforced, with an economic basis, quasi-ethnic divisions in self-identity, aspirations and language between the urbanites and the rural immigrant families (the latter often including a significant proportion of Irish Catholics). Third, in the larger cities, there was the process of residential segregation or 'suburbanization', as it has been termed.[30] Due to the social and cultural aspirations of the commercial bourgeoisie, the wish to avoid the soot of the smoke-belching factory and the crowding of the city centres, along with the commercial logic of speculative land development, there was a powerful, centrifugal residential movement of the wealthy toward the city's perimeter, and usually in an upwind, westward direction. While low-cost land on the urban periphery was lavishly developed into fine villas in the new suburbs, to the mutual profit of landowners, builders, lawyers and surveyors, the older residential buildings in the centre were simply rack-rented, predominantly by the same class, to the maximum density for the maximum profit, in return for the minimum outlay on upkeep. There was no point in improving or replacing these buildings because tenants could not be found for higher rents. This, as Dyos and Reeder were careful to point out, was a logical and functional entailment of a profit-maximizing, capital-accumulating, wage-minimizing economy: the availability of low-rent housing in central locations for low-paid workers was an essential condition for the perpetuation of this form of economic growth.[31] These inner-city slums festered until they were demolished for a railway, a widened arterial roadway, more commercial premises, or, eventually in the last quarter of the century, for reasons of public health and municipal reconstruction.[32]

These, then, were the three principal forces of urban socioeconomic differentiation, accompanying industrializing economic growth and urbanization, as they occurred in nineteenth-century Britain. During this period of its genteel abandonment, from 1830 to 1860, the image of the industrial city centre increasingly assumes its dark, brutalizing, frightening and unknown aspect in the imagination of the propertied and educated class, as reflected in the novels of Charles Dickens from the late 1830s and Mary Gaskell from the 1840s. The educated, literate elite no longer dared or cared to know its own cities firsthand, by living in their centres and walking their streets. The urban police force was created at this time, deputed to maintain law and order in place of the community's absent social leaders.[33]

However, these dynamic forces of economic and cultural differentiation were not, alone, responsible for the deprivation, disease and death that occurred in Britain's industrializing cities. It is necessary to ask why there was no effective political and administrative response at the national or local government level to the environmental and welfare problems occurring at this time. The reason for this failure of political response leads us back to the first 'D', disruption. Rapid economic growth entails the disruption of established social relations, ideologies and structures of authority. It was this that created a political and administrative paralysis in British cities during most of the second and third quarters of the nineteenth century. Britain's urban political history during the first half of the nineteenth century shows how such paralysis occurred.

To appreciate fully the novelty of urban social and political disruption, particularly during the second quarter of the nineteenth century, one needs to understand that many industrial towns had grown just as fast, in proportional terms, during the second half of the eighteenth century as during the first half of the nineteenth, while nevertheless retaining considerable social integrity, political unity and, according to the only reliable evidence that is available (for the town of Carlisle), reasonable salubrity.[34] Indeed, in many of the prospering eighteenth-century and early-nineteenth century towns, there had gradually coalesced, across the property divide, an increasingly coherent and unifying anti-aristocratic, anti-rentier urban politics of reform. A plebeian radical tradition had joined hands with the bourgeois liberal cause of Nonconformist Dissent (i.e. from the established Anglican Church), uniting the ranks of the self-styled 'productive classes' (urban employers, small master artisans and their employees, the workers) against the rural, landed *ancien régime* of 'unproductive', idle, nepotistic aristocrats – 'Old Corruption', as it was called by the reforming radicals. Most manufacturing and commercial employers in the 1810s and 1820s were still relatively small-scale: working and living cheek by jowl with their workmen even in the largest towns; this was an era before the residential move to the suburbs and the rapid expansion of the factory. With burgeoning commercial and industrial wealth as well as increasing proletarian numbers on their side, such a cross-class reform movement was, by the 1820s, becoming far too powerful to be ignored or resisted by the ruling class, the landed gentry. Accordingly they now conceded various constitutional reforms: the Test and Corporation Acts, which had disabled religious dissenters from political service, were repealed in 1828; Catholics were emancipated in 1829; the commercial bourgeoisie was electorally enfranchised by the Great Reform Act of 1832; the 1834 New Poor Law overhauled the nation's social security system in the interests of 'economy' and against the practices of traditionalist paternalists; and the 1835 Municipal Reform Act created representative local government in the towns with an electorate of small-scale property-holders.

Nevertheless, these substantial successes for the reform movement resulted in the disintegration of the political alliance of urban employers and proletarian employees, especially as the incumbent, aristocratic, governing class had ensured that the reforms politically enfranchised only the employers and the propertied class while excluding the property-less proletarians, thereby successfully driving a wedge between the two. These new political divisions between urban employer and wage labourer had many popular manifestations: above all, the Chartist movement, which unsuccessfully campaigned for working-class suffrage, 1837–48; but also the Factory movement, the Ten Hours movement, the anti-Poor Law and antipolicing campaigns. Political alignments became so fragmented that in the last two of these campaigns the phenomenon of Tory Radicalism was seen in parts of the country, representing a political alliance of the still-influential, paternalist landed class with the manufacturing artisans and workers against their erstwhile allies, the local businessmen and industrialists. Yet at the same time, the Anti-Corn Law League was campaigning in full force, representing a continuation of the battle between urban food-consumer interests and the landed agricultural producers. Consequently, although the constitutional and electoral reforms granted by the landed class conceded significant powers to the urban, nonconformist, liberal and commercial interests, from the mid-1830s through the late 1860s, local politics in the provincial, industrial towns was in fact predominantly characterized by debilitating internal divisions, cross-cutting interests, shifting alliances and stymied initiatives. As a result, stalemate ensued, in terms of the capacities of cities and their governments to respond to the environmental and health problems that they faced as their populations grew rapidly.

Furthermore, with the mid-century consolidation in the industrial towns of newly reformed self-governing, usually Liberal, corporations, supported by a predominantly petty bourgeois electorate, a new political force emerged in most towns, which became the major source of obstruction to municipal improvements over the ensuing two mid-Victorian decades of relative prosperity: the petty capitalist class, with their ratepayers' associations and obsessive concerns for economy.[35] The petty bourgeois ratepayers, who had the majority of the votes in the reformed municipalities after 1835, predominantly represented those who lived among the crowded poor in the industrial and commercial districts of the town's centre. Though better-off than most of their neighbours, they were unable to afford the suburban villas that would have offered them and their families partial protection from high urban mortality. Nevertheless, they could not be induced to vote for, still less campaign for, the expensive municipal measures that might have saved their own lives. By the late 1840s, this was certainly not out of simple ignorance concerning the health threats they faced: the alarming death rates of different cities were well known and increasingly well publicized in the local press, with the annual and quarterly reports issuing from the GRO.[36] The notion of a strong connection between cleanliness, both of streets and of person, and freedom from disease was a commonplace of educated opinion by the beginning of the nineteenth century. The problem was that the benefits to be gained from extremely expensive urban improvements to clean up the environment were too abstract, remote and speculative to carry conviction for this class of practical men, whose principal attention was consumed with week-to-week survival in trade and the avoidance of bankruptcy. A dramatically increased demand for local rates out of their pockets, to pay for an improved local environment, was an all too tangible and painful call on their limited balances.

Whereas in the eighteenth century a patrician oligarchy of local gentry and urban merchants had been able to implement without great objection their class's preferences for collective spending on town improvements and services, such that some historians refer to this period as one of an 'urban renaissance', the disruptive forces of rapid economic growth had now thrown up new forms of wealth and property, challenging and, by the late 1830s, toppling the patrician ascendancy. The problem now was that the new men represented such a wide diversity of interest, in terms of wealth levels, income sources, religious creeds and social origins, that there was no obvious consensus among them regarding the town's priorities; and no one section could easily assert its authority over any of the others. This resulted in grave difficulties in mobilizing agreement on the thorny issue of self-taxation and on questions of how to proceed with the large collective enterprises required to maintain the hard-pressed urban environment. It was much easier to agree to disagree, and for each to get on with minding his own business, in accordance with the liberal and libertarian precepts of the age.

Ideological conflict and its historical momentum certainly played an important role in accounting for the prolonged period of municipal inactivism from the 1830s until the 1870s. In this heyday of mid-

Victorian prosperity and global trading expansion, the commercial classes were now ideologically confident and committed to their class's radical and liberal virtues: individualism, nonintervention in the workings of the urban and industrial economy, and low levels of taxation (including low municipal and low Poor Law rates). In 1834 the New Poor Law dramatically cut the nation's expenditure on 'welfare' payments to the sick, old and poor from 2 per cent of national product (probably the highest proportion in Europe at that time) to only 1 per cent.[37] The principal way in which this momentum of ideological and political commitment manifested itself across the three mid-century decades was in the vigour with which the 'retrenchment' and 'economy' campaigns of radicalism–liberalism were pursued, at both national and local government levels, respectively, by William Gladstone and by the ratepayers' associations.[38]

That it would have been administratively, financially, logistically and technically within the capabilities of mid-century municipalities to have engineered the kind of comprehensive sanitary facilities only subsequently provided during the last quarter of the century is demonstrated, first, by the fact that during the 1840s and 1850s town councils proved quite able to think big and act big where rail communications were concerned. City centres were refashioned on a grand scale as land-hungry rail lines, stations and marshalling yards were driven through the centres of all large towns.[39] Unlike a comprehensive water supply and sewerage, the commercial advantages of rail connection were unanimously held to be incontrovertible. The railway was considered to be an absolute imperative for a town's prosperity in a nation of shopkeepers that had, by now, so thoroughly embraced the ethos of trade. Individual town councillors and factions of local elites were eager to be seen as the ones responsible for bringing the railway to their town.

Second, as to this society's capacity for understanding the importance of observing rigorous standards of hygiene, diet and collective cleanliness, especially in crowded conditions, the research of Philip Curtin on European troop mortality, of Shlomowitz, Haines and Brennan on maritime sanitary practices during this period, and of S. Ryan Johansson on the medical advice taken by the unusually long-lived upper classes during the late eighteenth century, all show that there was no deficit of effective knowledge or practices at this time.[40] Although the germ theory of disease had not yet been developed, this society had adequate knowledge and practical capacity to protect itself against the worst hazards of dense and crowded urban living. Thus, the following brief examination of the relevant aspects of the history of water supply and sanitation in the growing industrial cities of nineteenth-century England shows that, while the appropriate technology for water provision and for arterial sewering was well understood by the 1840s at the latest, it was the debilitating socio-political divisions, and their eventual resolution from the 1870s onward, that critically influenced the course of provision in this vital health sphere.

Water, health and the politics and economics of public health in British cities

Comprehensive water supply and sanitation for the urban poor is a classic problem in the economics of the provision of public goods.[41] The scale and dispersed nature of demand for clean water created by rapid urbanization are so great that the investment costs involved are beyond the financial logic of any commercial operation, so long as the majority of customers remain too poor to pay more than a token amount for their water. It therefore requires political will and collective organization to cope with the challenge of supplying the less-wealthy majority to ensure the health of all. That cities such as Manchester and Birmingham could have grown in size to the hundreds of thousands of inhabitants by 1861 and still not have secured a comprehensive water supply, let alone an integrated mains sewering system, seems scarcely credible. But, of course, many *barriada* slum populations in the world's largest cities today face similar problems. The manner in which British cities initially did not, and then, in due course, did, successfully supply themselves with adequate water and comprehensive sewering provides an accurate mirror of the changing nature and the importance of the socio-political relationships that governed the way in which the forces of economic growth were, and eventually were not allowed to wreak the havoc of the 'four Ds' on the expanding British urban population.

The first half of the nineteenth century witnessed a rapid increase in the number of private companies supplying water to those who could pay in the fast-growing towns: businesses and wealthier homes.[42] However, during the 1840s, the alarming urban death rates publicized by the GRO, prompted official inquiries into the state of Britain's industrial towns, which resulted in passage of the nation's first general Public Health Act in 1848. This included provisions to enable local authorities to borrow sufficient funds (subsidized loans from the central government Exchequer, which still had to be paid back out of the town's rates) to provide their populations with adequate water and sewerage facilities. A pattern of subsequent municipalization of the urban water supply did indeed occur, including buyouts of private companies in many cases.

But this was not quite the sanitary revolution it might appear to have been. As noted above, the mid-Victorian towns were in thrall to the economizing interests of the 'shopocracy' – the petty bourgeoisie enfranchised by the 1835 Municipal Reform Act. In the name of local self-government, a virtual rebellion among this class of ratepayers took place against those clauses of the 1848 Public Health Act that threatened to force towns to spend on improving their water supply. As a result, these clauses were rarely invoked and were subsequently rescinded by an Act of 1858. The municipalization of water that occurred after 1848 was pursued primarily for other than health-promotion purposes. J.A. Hassan has emphasized that the significance of water as an industrial raw material was often the primary consideration, with commercial demand consuming in many cases half of the extra urban water supply capacity created after 1848.[43] In other words, because of the particular disposition of powerful local political interests, the state in Britain at this time was unable to enforce sanitary improvement on the principal voting constituency of reluctant urban citizens; often only when key local businessmen could see a commercial advantage was an initiative taken.

The telltale sign of the industrial and commercial, rather than health-promoting, motivational forces behind the municipal expansion of water supply from the late 1840s until the 1870s lies in the partial manner in which Edwin Chadwick's 'Sanitary Idea', the inspiration behind the 1848 Public Health Act, was being acted upon during that period. Chadwick had envisaged every urban house connected both to a clean water supply and to a water-borne mains sewerage system. Increased volume of water supply was forthcoming during these decades, but sewering was not. Hassan shows that the volume of constant-pressure water supplied rose substantially in most towns; but there was remarkably little effort or expenditure devoted to the other half of the engineering blueprint laid down by Chadwick as the means to attain healthy cities. Plenty of new mains water supply pipes were laid under dug-up streets from the 1840s onward, but the Royal Sanitary Commission found as late as 1871 that most provincial cities were only just then beginning to build the integrated sewerage systems necessary to avoid contamination from wastes. This was despite the fact that in the epidemic of 1854, E.C. Snow had conclusively demonstrated the role of waste-contaminated water supplies (the Broad

Street pump in London) in transmitting that most dreaded affliction of the Victorian age, cholera. Furthermore, except where the wealthier residents paid for it in their suburban villas, little effort before the last quarter of the nineteenth century was devoted to connecting-up, en masse, individual homes to the enhanced urban water supplies, a development that would inevitably have also led to the need to link such homes to an arterial sewerage system.

From the late 1860s onward, however, the dawn of a more genuinely effective public health movement began to stir in Britain's industrial cities, leading over the next four decades to an accumulating momentum of substantial investments in domestic water supply and in sewerage.[44] From the late 1860s, there was the beginning of a widening appreciation of public health aims as a high priority among the rising generation of politicians, town officials and the political, voting class of the largest industrial cities. This was part of a new, religiously inflected civic consciousness and pride, a social movement in the town halls of Britain's new industrial cities that has been appropriately termed 'the civic gospel', a call to undertake public good works first preached in Birmingham by a number of charismatic Nonconformist ministers.[45] As a sense of pride began to grip the imaginations of the wealthier inhabitants of these great cities, explicit parallels began to be drawn by the confident city fathers with the cultural achievements of the city-states of classical Greece and Renaissance Italy, as models for the corporate conversion of mere industrial prosperity into positive human progress, civilisation, art and learning.[46] From the 1870s, positions of public leadership in Britain's provincial cities were increasingly sought by practical men of substance and vision as valued positions of honour.[47] The status of the activities involved in municipal services and administration was commensurately enhanced during this period, with the proper self-organization and professionalization of many of this growing range of public service officials. For instance, the key post of Medical Officer of Health now became a salaried statutory office in every local authority; vocational training in specialist courses became mandatory (Dublin and Cambridge Universities being among the first to offer the new Diploma in Public Health), and a national professional journal for Medical Officers of Health, *Public Health*, was founded.[48]

The civic gospel was part of a wider 'optimistic' intellectual movement sweeping Britain's upper and middle classes in the 1860s and 1870s. This can, perhaps, best be summarized as the flowering of the mid-Victorian faith in the possibility of social progress and the relinquishing of the profound misgivings and fears that had accompanied the first three-quarters of a century of bewildering, rapid change.[49] A more optimistic assessment of the 'improvable' character of the labouring classes prevailed among an influential section of the elite, including Prime Ministers Disraeli and Gladstone.[50] Consequently, an electoral constituency potentially much more responsive to the ambitious patrician plans in Britain's industrial cities, was now created.

The hold of the ratepayer 'economy' over municipal politics was broken in the late 1860s and 1870s when the voting power of the petty bourgeoisie, in command since the 1830s, was submerged in the new, wider national and local franchises following the Second Reform Act of 1867 and the collateral Municipal Franchise Act and Assessed Rates Act, both passed in 1869.[51] In consequence, the electorate approximately quadrupled in size at urban local government elections, bringing an influx of working men, comprising about 60 per cent of all proletarian males, the class that had been left out in the cold in the 1830s.[52] Furthermore, many of these new voters, being wage-labourers and tenants rather than homeowners, did not pay local rates directly (they were termed 'compounders' as it was deemed that they paid local rates indirectly, compounded into the rents that they paid their landlords). The results of these electoral reforms increasingly brought into the calculations of urban politicians, both in local and national elections, questions of how best to cultivate the interests of these, the respectable and more prosperous, but non-ratepaying segments of the manual working classes.

Joseph Chamberlain, Mayor of Birmingham for three consecutive years, 1873–76, was the first major political figure to exploit this by constructing a coherent programme of practical policies to satisfy this working-class constituency with his 'gas and water' 'municipal socialism'.[53] His was a political programme whose democratic novelty lay in its appeal to the urban consumer, not the producer or retailer interests. Chamberlain rhetorically undercut the traditional cry for economy by arguing that failure to spend on the town's environment was *false* economy, causing untold costs to the health and working efficiency of the town's populace; *true* economy required municipal investments, whose value should be assessed over the longer term. Such views commanded respect when they came from one of the city's most successful businessmen. Their chances of political success were, of course, assisted by the fact that they were addressed to an electorate many of whom were not faced with direct bills for the increased rates required. Following Chamberlain's lead, sustained efforts to improve the living conditions and the amenities of the urban working class came to be seen as potentially paying high political dividends. In this era of the civic gospel, a rivalry developed between the town halls of many of Britain's great 'city states' during the last quarter of the century, as they competed with one another for salubrity, provision of public services, and the lowest death rates.

Once this cross-class alliance between the urban patriciate and the urban plebeians had again taken hold (having been in abeyance since the 1820s) the political will could be committed to investment in the urban environment. The nature of the transformation in the quality and scale of municipal activity from around 1870 onward can be grasped immediately, in summary form, by noting that the amount requested by local authorities in subsidized (low-interest) loans for sanitary activities from the central Exchequer increased eightfold, from £11 million during the period 1848–70 to £84 million during 1871–97.[54] But this massive increase in the use of such loans was only one of three principal methods that urban councils used to free their ambitious plans from exclusive and direct dependence on the local rates levy on fixed property. There was an active search during the 1870s and 1880s for new fiscal mechanisms to achieve the electoral promises of urban improvements for the minimum current costs in rates, so as to avoid unduly provoking the ratepayers' associations, the still-feared pressure groups of the petty bourgeoisie.

Apart from Exchequer loans, the two other techniques evolved were to take out large, long-term, low-interest loans on the commercial money markets of the City of London (thereby deferring costs for current improvement onto future generations and avoiding immediate, dramatic hikes in the rates) and indirect taxation on the urban populace through 'municipal trading' – running local monopoly services, such as gas, electricity and trams, at a profit in order to create revenue for the city to fund improvements.[55] Millward and his colleagues have shown that by 1913, £190 million in municipal loans had been raised in stock issues in this way, representing a quarter of all local authority debt at that time.[56] They also found that by the opening years of the twentieth century, a sample of 25 borough towns were showing, between them, net profits on their municipal trading activities equal to their entire annual labour, maintenance and capital costs for all public health and police activities.[57]

Following the earlier and mid-nineteenth-century trend of deterioration and uncertain recovery in the mortality experience of Britain's largest cities, Table 5.1, above, indicates the positive impact that these new political developments and associated investments in facilities and services were having on urban health and welfare during the last three decades of the Victorian era. The historical epidemiological evidence for England and Wales has been the empirical centrepiece of the highly influential McKeown thesis, which argued that municipal improvements could be assigned only a minor role in accounting for mortality decline in nineteenth-century Britain and that nutritional improvements delivered by rising real wages should be seen as performing the principal role.[58] However, McKeown's thesis was always under challenge when comparative evidence from other countries was considered.[59] It has also now been shown that McKeown seriously misconstrued his own analysis of this valuable body of evidence and that in fact the research results he published support the opposite conclusions to those he himself drew. While improvements in quality and quantity of urban food supply and rising average real wages were no doubt important contributors, detailed reinterpretation of McKeown's analysis of the historical British epidemiological evidence shows that in fact it was primarily improvement in mortality caused by diseases affected by sanitation and by specific public health measures (typhus, typhoid, cholera and infant diarrhea, in the former category; smallpox in the latter category) that most unequivocally made the primary contribution during the period before the Great War. As with the timing of urban health trends, therefore, this strongly implicates the importance of the politics of public health and of municipal preventive health measures as having played the most significant role in reversing the health fortunes of the British population from the 1870s.[60]

In a recent contribution to this debate, Constance Nathanson compared the histories of public health measures related to maternal and infant care and to tobacco control in the United States and France to develop a framework for conceptualizing the principal factors involved in the politics of public health.[61] From this comparison of one country with a strong political culture of the unitary central state (France) and one with a particularly strong culture of individual liberty *from* the central state (the United States), Nathanson showed that in each case the rhetorical and social construction of a significant public health risk, and the nature of the response to it, were consonant with these pronounced national differences in political system and ideology. For instance, in France the perception by central state officials and the national political leadership of a military threat to the nation's survival resulted in the creation of a national set of maternal and infant care measures following France's defeat in the Franco-Prussian war of 1870–71. Whereas in the United States, under the nation's fragmented state system, the initiative for such services instead had to come from a protracted grassroots movement of women reformers and married women themselves, concerned about their own health prospects. Furthermore, their legislative successes were far from total because their schemes were opposed by another association of interested citizens, the mainly male members of the American Medical Association.

Nathanson's analysis demonstrated that the highly variable character of the history of public and preventive health measures is intimately related to the varying powers and character of the state, lodged in its distinctive political culture. Both in France and in the United States, it was this which constrained, first, the manner in which perception of a significant health risk could be institutionally constructed as being of sufficient importance to require action; and, second, how it could then be acted upon with effective organizational resources. Christopher Hamlin has documented this in the British case with respect to the science of water purity during the second half of the nineteenth century.[62] Hamlin shows that with the British central state declining to take an authoritative position, there was enormous cultural, institutional and legal space for decades of debate both in official and professional journals and in the courts of law between different water analysts and engineering specialists to dispute questions of water purity and the implications for the relative merits and costs of alternative sanitary engineering proposals advanced by their competing clients – the private water companies and the municipal authorities. Hamlin's research details the protracted, highly negotiated nature of the scientific debate over defining and measuring acceptable standards of water purity and the complex implications this could have for investment in the appropriate 'lumpy' and expensive technology.

Hamlin demonstrates the impossibility of holding to any straightforward scientific or technological determinist viewpoint that would attribute the dramatic increase in water and sanitary investment to a particular scientific breakthrough (the most obvious candidate being the germ theory of disease, although William Bynum long ago showed the dilatory nature of the acceptance of even this theory by the medical profession itself).[63] The wrangling over the science of water technology went on into the 1880s and 1890s. The conclusions to be drawn from Hamlin's account emphasize the highly political, ideological and commercially involved nature of the public health policy debate. While it is always a powerful rhetorical move to claim scientific authority for the implementation of any public health measure, those in opposition can prove themselves equally adept at creating scientific uncertainty over the precise practical implications, as Nathanson's account also shows. Thus, while strong scientific evidence and arguments are in no sense unimportant in the history of the politics of public health, they are more realistically viewed as the necessary, rather than the sufficient, sources of public health activism on any issue. Science and technology are only parts of the complex political alliance of social and ideological elements that is necessary to drive such a large-scale phenomenon as the public health movement.

In terms of this chapter's focus, therefore, Nathanson provides us with a framework for understanding the politically contingent range of factors involved in determining the capacities of different societies to respond to the health challenges, generated by economic growth, of the four Ds. The case study of Britain presented here emphasizes the likely salience and significance of one or two additional considerations that can be incorporated into the framework that Nathanson proposes. It suggests that in countries which are not so extreme as either France or the United States in their respective veneration of or aversion to the central state, a range of intermediary civil institutions and socio-political forces, which fall somewhere between the central state and the social movement, may also be important determinants of the politics and practice of public health. Nathanson clearly recognized that in some circumstances the politics of local government might be a critical factor in public health, and this seems to have been the case in Britain.[64]

Indeed, a nuanced, variable and perhaps even decentralized conception of the state may be required. Michael Mann's conception of the intrinsically variable 'polymorphous' state may be helpfully developed in this connection.[65] This formulation recognizes that the 'presence' of agencies of the central state in the provinces, and the state's capacity to enlist the services of genuine brokers to be its eyes and ears as well as its arms and legs, crucially affect the strength of the state in terms of its reach into society and its capacity to transmit the drive of its engine.[66] Mann's notion of the state can embrace much of what is more often termed 'civil society' and, perhaps misleadingly, thought of as separate from the state: something that is especially true of local government agencies, the voluntary sector and the public service professions. The professions, like local government structures, can be of particular significance because of their relative permanence and capacity for institutionalizing specific aims and interests, which may or may not correspond with those of the central state. (This can also, of course, be true of certain long-lived voluntary or philanthropic associations, as well as commercial corporations, as Nathanson's tobacco example and Britain's nineteenth-century private water companies illustrate.)

In the British case, the Victorian and Edwardian public health movement would certainly count as a social movement in Nathanson's terms, but it was an unusually long-lived one, and one that had, from early on, colonized certain important institutional resources *within* the structures of the polymorphous state. This was principally by virtue of its early 'capture' (1837–41) of the nation's primary social and economic intelligence system (the General Register Office, the office of state responsible for taking the decennial census), which it promptly used to launch a continuous flow of influential propagandist public health publications.[67] Also important was the creation (from 1848), of a public health medical department within central government, and the statutory establishment (from 1875), of a trained cadre of Medical Officers of Health in every local authority around the country. In developing countries today, the role of the World Bank and the World Health Organization, international aid agencies, and nongovernmental organizations would evidently all need to be acknowledged as additional institutional and political forces influencing the relationship between state and society. Indeed, it may well be that the political and institutional presence of these nonindigenous agencies, rather than their technical or financial inputs and advice, have sometimes had the greatest impact on the development of public and preventive health measures in such countries.

Conclusions: the importance of politics, the state and social capital

The British historical evidence indicates that rapid economic growth can directly cause critical social insecurities and health problems. It necessarily brings, as its immediate corollaries, not security and prosperity but disruption and deprivation – unless mediated by effective social and political responses – in terms of both disease and death.

This chapter has examined a well-documented, long-term historical example of rapid economic growth pursued according to the principles of economic liberalism, with minimal intervention from the central state: the case of nineteenth-century Britain, the first industrial nation. Even in a society that was well endowed with voluntary institutions (friendly and other self-help provident societies as well as philanthropic and medical charities) and a relatively effective welfare net (the Poor Law), which had functioned throughout the early modern era to protect the poor from the worst rigours of indigence and misfortune, serious and alarming health problems rapidly ensued within a single generation. The processes of economic growth and the blind laws of profit-taking that were unleashed in Britain's industrial towns and cities generated the problems of disruption and deprivation. The evidence presented in this essay shows that economic growth, in and of itself, in no way guarantees a nation's health and welfare, but, if given free rein, may lead directly to and cause the four Ds.

The clear perception of the disruptive entailments of rapid economic growth ought to prompt a thoroughgoing reappraisal among social scientists and policymakers of the value of such growth. It is not an unalloyed good. It is highly questionable whether it is wise for a government's policies to be aimed simply at the promotion of rapid growth as its top priority. Policies favouring more modest and well-diffused increases in prosperity, as a goal both for the nation and for individuals therein, may well provide a healthier and more viable, deliverable and stable agenda than the rhetoric of maximizing growth. Of course, the 'sustainable growth' school of thought also advocates the approach recommended here on the separate, but no less important, grounds that it is necessary for long-term environmental viability. Governments would be well advised to pay as much attention and concern to monitoring trends in their nations' income distribution and in the health of vulnerable sections of the population (backward regions, migrant workers and women, for instance) as to their GNP figures. The governments of vast developing societies, such as those of China and other South and East Asian countries, are responsible for the future wellbeing of colossal numbers of individuals. They are nations currently experiencing rapid economic growth and seeking to transform that growth into genuine development throughout this century. It is imperative that these governments realize that the lessons of history, from nineteenth-century Britain through to Eastern Europe in the 1990s, are that nothing needs such careful planning and continual management as a 'free market' economy, if the four Ds are to be avoided.[68]

There is, however, a chronic problem in the way of establishing this as a permanent priority in the public mind, a problem that seems to result from an iron law of public health history, such that each generation has to relearn this lesson. This problem lies in the unintended consequences of the public and preventive health movement's own historic successes, whereby populations habituate to successful and effective preventive health measures, many of which have become so normal and routinized in advanced societies that they have become politically invisible. Who, for instance, would now consider that the historical origins of hard-surface urban streets of a certain minimum width lay principally in public health, rather than efficient transit considerations? Another salient example has been the recent fate of the welfare states in some Western liberal democracies. These were the proud creation of a previous generation (some of whom are still alive thanks to its provisions!), valued for its unifying social security and health provisions open to all citizens, regardless of wealth. By the late 1970s, however, all this had come to be so taken for granted by a sufficient proportion of the electorate in both the United States and Great Britain that their citizens voted throughout the 1980s for governments promising the Fools' Gold of lower personal taxes in return for dramatic reductions in the provision of such public services. The ensuing retrenchments were premised on the stigmatizing argument that such public services were wasteful and parasitic (on the 'productive' economy) and on the further presumption that no important negative consequences would flow from the contraction of these services and their selective targeting.[69] Both electorates eventually voted out these governments, finding that the incipient dismantling of the social security and preventive health systems has in fact resulted in unpalatable social and health problems, such as homeless teenagers on the streets, rising proportions of children living below the official poverty line, rising class sizes in state schools, and the BSE and other food scares in Great Britain.

Of course, it cannot be expected that the four Ds will manifest themselves in exactly the same manner in the contemporary developing countries as in historical Britain. In particular, the sections of the population bearing the highest health costs in the developing economies of the early twenty-first century may well be found in the countryside and in remote regions rather than in the cities, or among prime working-age males rather than among women and children – both of these situations which appear to be the case in China, for instance.[70] It may be that it is often deprivation, rather than disease or death, that is now the principal price such populations pay. Even so, this does not negate the validity of the four Ds approach: it does not predict that the negative consequences must be experienced in the cities or among any particular section of the population or that the full sequence of all four Ds is inevitable.

In this conclusion, therefore, I suggest that Britain's nineteenth-century history of the relationship between economic growth, the politics of public health and 'development' exhibits at least four specific aspects that may have more general relevance and that may apply to the late twentieth century.

First, given that rapid economic growth necessarily involves disruption of extant sources of authority as new forms of wealth and sources of power emerge, it seems likely that the intra-elite conflicts and cross-cutting clashes of interests among holders of different grades and types of property, along with ethnic or denominational rivalries of the sort found in the British historical case, will typically characterize such rapid economic growth in most societies. This competitive socio-political situation can cause serious and prolonged health problems for deprived sections of the population (whether urban or rural) if, as occurred in Britain, political and administrative paralysis ensues. The necessarily politically negotiated bargaining to promote expensive environmental and social improvements can all too easily become bogged down for decades by sectional conflicts and defensive political standoffs. This point can be related to the perspective developed by Drèze and Sen.[71] They invoke the concept of 'cooperative conflicts' to characterize the social relations of communities under pressure, where negotiation is required to finesse the Prisoner's Dilemma predicament they face: that all could benefit from mutual cooperation but this will not arise from pursuit of sectional self-interests. British political and urban history in the second quarter of the nineteenth century shows that the severe disruption entailed by rapid economic growth was reducing the capacity of this society to resolve its many cooperative conflicts. Mutual suspicions and misunderstandings were instead too much the rule, as the different sections of the community pursued their diverse economic interests and separate denominational codes of loyalty and association.

Second, the British case indicates the great importance of constitutional arrangements and of political organization, particularly the extent to which the poorer sections of the community have an effective political voice. This is not, however, simply a matter of working-class votes, though they can be critically important in the right circumstances, as the period from the 1870s onward shows in Britain. Equally important at that point was an imaginative, neo-patrician political leadership provided by a section of the urban propertied elite among the business class, effectively focusing the energies of the working-class voters on backing a practical programme for alleviating their health and environmental problems. In Marxian or Weberian terms this was a cross-class political alliance. This shows that there is no simple relationship between the acquisition of voting power by the poor and their effective political representation, because this class is, almost by definition, deficient in autonomous political resources. It is therefore their relationship with elements of other, more privileged, social groups and the latter's ideologies that may be more critical in determining the consequences of their voting power.

Third, there is the complex issue of popular ideas and conceptions of property rights, property interests and legitimate forms of local and central state taxation and appropriation.[72] This is intimately connected to the issues that Amartya Sen has emphasized with his concepts of entitlements and capabilities, in that these popular perceptions, and the ideologies behind them, govern the legitimacy in different societies of varying balances between the acceptability of private appropriations and the public redistribution of the wealth that is generated by economic growth.[73] As the political history of late-twentieth-century Britain showed, as clearly as that of the mid-nineteenth century, the libertarian British, like Americans, can be peculiarly sensitive to central and local governments' direct appropriations in taxes and rates from their current income, which they resent as a compulsory forfeit of what they believe they have personally earned. Yet they can remain supine in the face of even quite sharp rises in indirect taxation (value-added taxes) on their consumption activities, because they view the latter as essentially voluntary and elective. Although different cultures vary in their attitudes in this respect, the generalizable implication is that, given the enormous costs of maintaining the health and environment of the populace during rapid economic growth, politically successful solutions will probably depend on treating property rights and associated fiscal sensitivities with great respect. Furthermore, the particular types and forms of taxes adopted can themselves have a range of positive or negative redistributional implications, not always immediately apparent to the electorate or even to the specialists devising them (if, for instance, too narrow or undiscriminating a framework for analysing their impacts on different kinds of family or household is adopted).

Fourth, the British historical case indicates the importance of the state and politics in determining the character of the response to the four Ds and, therefore, in determining the changing relationship between economic growth and the health of the population. Once it is accepted that political choices and social and cultural institutions are critical in determining this relationship, it becomes incumbent on demographic and epidemiological social scientists to turn their attentions to the politics of public health, as has been recently advocated by Constance Nathanson. It is also necessary to adopt a much wider and more flexible understanding of the 'state' as embracing a range of devolved agencies, mediating institutions and ideological influences. For instance, in the British historical case, local government, the public service professions and a section of the urban big business class each played crucial roles.

To conclude, the argument here is not a Luddite one, of simply being against economic growth. Rather, the thesis is that the causal relationship between economic growth, enhanced human welfare and development, is a dialectical one and therefore can appear to be para-doxical. Rapid economic growth must be viewed, in the long run, as a necessary condition for improvements in human health and welfare, through its provision of the material resources for this possible outcome. But in the shorter run, the direct consequences of the more unrestrained forms of economic growth have often been inimical to the health and welfare of the individuals living in a society subjected to these processes. As noted above, recent research is uncovering a number of examples in the European, North American and Japanese historical record that bear the same demographic footprint of the four Ds as in the British case: where the initial phase of rapid economic growth was accompanied by an interruption in a longer-term trend of improving conditions of health.[74] The crucial further point is that the punitive short term does not automatically turn into the more beneficial longer term simply through the passing of time: such is the pernicious myth of the invisible hand or trickle down metaphors that enable growth apologists to ignore, or treat as trivial, the key political and institutional questions involved in development. Robert Dorfman recently noted that 'both Rostow and I use the terms economic growth and economic development interchangeably', asserting that 'economic growth and development are so closely linked ... [that] ... distinguish-ing between the two concepts does not seem worthwhile'.[75] The thrust of the present essay is to argue, on the contrary, that this semantic conflation is profoundly misleading. Economic growth only becomes sustained economic development through the mediation of the social and institutional forces promoted by the politics of public health.

Development is really a much broader concept than economic growth. While it may be true that development cannot occur without growth, it is equally true that economic growth cannot persist without development. The problem perhaps lies partly in language. The biolog-ical metaphors used here invite us to think of development as the product of growth, insidiously implanting the idea that growth is the prior, causal force, and development is its consequential outcome. But this is highly misleading. For instance, the social development of an expanding and diversifying education system producing a more literate and numerate population is both a product of the fruits of increasing national wealth (though high levels of education can also be delivered in nonindustrialized countries) and simultaneously a vital condition for that society's achievement of continuing economic growth. This is equally true of the relationship between economic growth and the health and welfare of the population. Given that it is the quality of the human working parts and their institutional relationships which determine the productivity of any economy, it is an unhelpful fiction to view growth of the economy as being prior to or independent of the accompanying changes in social institutions. Like the two strands of DNA's double helix twisting around each other, they are mutually dependent for their perpetuation.

Development therefore comprises a range of institutional changes that vary considerably in their manifestation in different countries, depending on each society's political and ideological inheritance and its familial and social structures. The importance of this fact is increasingly being recognized by growth and development economists and sociologists, among whom Cold-War notions of economic and social convergence toward a single kind of modern political economy have fallen out of favour. Instead, they have begun to envisage the salience of distinct models of market-oriented societies, such as 'American', 'European Social Market', 'British' and 'Japanese'.[76] At the same time, the 1990s have seen a growing acceptance of 'new growth theory' among economists, who recognize that there are serious limitations in the dominant, neoclassical 'growth accounting' model of economic growth, dating from the 1950s, and that the very different performances even of advanced economies since World War II indicate that social and cultural institutions play a much more formative role in economic affairs than has previously been acknowledged.[77]

The recent conceptual elaboration and empirical critique and application of the concept of social capital (as distinct from both financial capital and human capital) appear to offer a highly promising way forward for those exploring the relationship between economic change, social institutions, the state, the politics of public health and health outcomes.[78] The set of concepts related to social capital provides a methodology for specifying and studying the changing economic and political implications of social and cultural institutions influencing relationships of trust, honour, friendship, social equality and civic participation. Empirical research is beginning to explore the way in which social capital is vital both for good communications and the efficient functioning of economic organizations and for the promotion of positive health across societies.[79] The idea of social capital, along with other, related conceptual work on the embeddedness (in society and polity) of economic exchange relations, radically undermines the distinction, sacrosanct in the approach of neoclassical economics, between the state and the market (or, even more misleadingly, between the state and civil society).[80] Hence recent, comparative empirical work, critically developing the idea of social capital, has produced evidence of the importance of 'co-production' across the 'public–private divide', involving detailed negotiation and cooperation between state, voluntary and market agencies in bringing about positive economic developments in Taiwan, Kerala, Brazil and China, while also explaining the difficulties encountered in Nigeria, Mexico and Russia.[81] This looks rather similar to the account offered here. In Britain's nineteenth-century industrial cities, an initial period of disruption and breakdown was followed by the rebuilding of social capital and of mechanisms for 'co-production'. The sequence of the four Ds was only redressed and economic growth translated into positive economic and social development when the relations of social capital in Britain's industrial communities were sufficiently strong that the politics of public health could direct collective resources toward the good of the community as a whole.

Notes

NB: An earlier version of this essay appeared as a Working Paper of the King's College, Cambridge Centre for History and Economics, entitled 'Rapid Population Growth and Security: Urbanisation and Economic Growth in Britain in the Nineteenth Century' (July 1995). It was originally presented to a conference in Cambridge on 17–19 February 1995 on Population and Security, supported by the Pew Global Stewardship Initiative. The author is grateful to participants at the conference and at numerous seminars during 1996 and 1997 in San Francisco and at various locations in Australia, London, Cambridge, Munich and Liverpool, who have commented on presentations of this and related material. He also thanks Hilary Cooper, John Powles, Paul Seabright, Barry Smith and Gianni Vaggi for their critical readings.

1. The theory's most influential progenitor, Frank Notestein, was aware of its empirical limitations by the early 1950s: D. Hodgson, 'Demography as social science and policy science', *Population and Development Review* 9 (1983): 1–34, p. 12, citing F.W. Notestein, 'Economic problems of population change', *Proceedings of the Eighth International Conference of Agricultural Economists* (New York: Oxford University Press, 1953). For a conceptual critique, see S. Szreter, 'The idea of demographic transition and the study of fertility change: a critical intellectual history', *Population and Development Review* 19 (1993): 659–701; and S. Szreter, *Fertility, Class and Gender in Britain, 1860–1940* (Cambridge: Cambridge University Press, 1996), Ch. 1 and Ch. 10. On contemporary mortality declines in poor countries, see S.B. Halstead, J.A. Walsh, and K.S. Warren (eds), *Good Health at Low Cost* (New York: Rockefeller Foundation, 1985).

2. A.R. Omran, 'The epidemiological transition: a theory of the epidemiology of population change', *Milbank Memorial Fund Quarterly* 49 (1971): 509–38.

3. On Japan, see S.R. Johansson and C. Mosk, 'Exposure, resistance and life expectancy: disease and death during the economic development of Japan, 1900–60', *Population Studies* 41 (1987): 207–35. On the United States, see R.H. Steckel, 'Stature and the standard of living', *Journal of Economic Literature* 33 (1995): 1903–1940, p. 1920; and M.R. Haines, 'Health, height, nutrition and mortality: evidence on the Antebellum puzzle from Union Army recruits for New York State and the United States', in J. Komlos and J. Baten (eds), *The Biological Standard of Living in Comparative Perspective*, Vol. 1: *The Americas, Asia and Australia* (Stuttgart: Steiner Verlag, 1998). On the Netherlands, see E. Horlings and J.-P. Smit, 'The quality of life in the Netherlands 1800–1913: experiments in measurement and aggregation', in J. Komlos and J. Baten (eds), *The Biological Standard of Living in Comparative Perspective*, Vol. 2: *Europe* (Stuttgart: Steiner Verlag, 1998). On Germany, see S. Twarog, 'Heights and living standards in Germany, 1850–1939: the case of Württemberg', in R.H. Steckel and R. Floud, (eds), *Health and Welfare During Industrialisation* (Chicago: NBER, University of Chicago Press, 1997), pp. 285–330, esp. pp. 297–9 and 306–7. On France, see D.R. Weir, 'Economic welfare and physical well-being in France 1750–1990', in R.H. Steckel and R. Floud (eds), *Health and Welfare During Industrialisation* (Chicago: NBER, University of Chicago Press, 1997), pp. 161–200, esp. Figs. 5.8 and 5.10. On Australia, see G. Whitwell, C. de Souza, and S. Nicholas, 'Height, health and economic growth in Australia 1860–1940', in R.H. Steckel and R. Floud (eds), *Health and Welfare During Industrialisation* (Chicago: NBER, University of Chicago Press, 1997), pp. 379–422. On Canada, see F. Pelletier, J. Légaré, and R. Bourbeau, 'Mortality in Quebec during the nineteenth century: from the state to the cities', *Population Studies* 51 (1997): 93–103, esp. Table 2 and pp. 99–100.

4. M.J. Cullen, *The Statistical Movement in Early Victorian Britain: the Foundation of Empirical Social Research* (New York: Barnes and Noble, 1975).

5. W.W. Rostow, *The Stages of Economic Growth: a Non-Communist Manifesto* (Cambridge: Cambridge University Press, 1960); T. McKeown, *The Modern Rise of Population* (New York: Academic Press, 1976); on the dependence of the original formulation of demographic transition theory on the British

historical evidence, see S. Szreter, *Fertility, Class and Gender,* cited in note 1, pp. 9–21.

6. E.H. Ackerknecht, 'Hygiene in France, 1815–48', *Bulletin of the History of Medicine* 22 (1948): 117–55, p. 140; E.H. Ackerknecht, *Medicine at the Paris Hospital, 1794–1848* (Baltimore: Johns Hopkins Press, 1967), p. 156; W. Coleman, 'Health and hygiene in the *Encyclopédie*: a medical doctrine for the bourgeoisie', *Journal of the History of Medicine* 29 (1974): 399–421; K. Polanyi, *The Great Transformation* (New York: Rinehart, 1957; 1st edn 1944), p. 103.

7. On France, see W. Coleman, *Death Is a Social Disease: Public Health and Political Economy in Early Industrial France* (Madison: Wisconsin Publications in the History of Science and Medicine, 1982) and A.F. La Berge, *Mission and Method: the Early Nineteenth-Century French Public Health Movement* (Cambridge: Cambridge University Press, 1992). On Germany, see E.H. Ackerknecht, *Rudolf Virchow: Doctor, Statesman, Anthropologist* (Madison: University of Wisconsin Press, 1953) and S. Tesh, *Hidden Arguments: Political Ideology and Disease Prevention Policy* (New Brunswick, NJ: Rutgers University Press, 1988). On Britain, see M.W. Flinn, 'Introduction' to E. Chadwick, *Report on the Sanitary Condition of the Labouring Population of Great Britain* (Edinburgh: Edinburgh University Press, reprint, 1965); R. Lambert, *Sir John Simon 1816–1904 and English Social Administration* (London: MacGibbon and Kee, 1963); J. Eyler, *Victorian Social Medicine: the Ideas and Methods of William Farr* (Baltimore: Johns Hopkins Press, 1979); and C. Hamlin, *Public Health and Social Justice in the Age of Chadwick: Britain 1800–1854* (Cambridge: Cambridge University Press, 1997).

8. For the concept of the competitive interdependence of labour and capital, see M. Burawoy, *Manufacturing Consent* (Chicago: University of Chicago Press. 1979) and M. Burawoy, *The Politics of Production* (Verso UK, 1985).

9. Figures (rounded) from N. Crafts and C.K. Harley, 'Output growth and the British industrial revolution: a restatement of the Crafts–Harley view', *Economic History Review* 45 (1992): 703–30, p. 715; and C.H. Feinstein, *National Income, Expenditure and Output of the United Kingdom, 1855–1965* (London: Cambridge University Press, 1972). Of course, these average annual rates of growth are toward the lower end of what economists would categorise as rapid economic growth in the late twentieth century. Indeed, this modern perspective partly lies behind the currency of the historiographical notion of slow growth as characterising Britain's early, eighteenth-century stages of industrialisation, following Harley's celebrated revisionist article: C.K. Harley, 'British industrialisation before 1841: evidence of slower growth during the industrial revolution', *Journal of Economic History* 42 (1982): 267–89. The key historical point, of course, is that sustained economic growth at rates substantially above 1 per cent per annum for any length of time, let alone a period running into decades on end, was unprecedented in world history. If an economy today began to experience growth rates of about 15–20 per cent per annum, decade after decade, this would be a reasonable historical analogy to the revolutionary speed of sustained growth achieved by the British economy from c. 1800 onward.

10. E.A. Wrigley and R.S. Schofield, *The Population History of England, 1541–1871* (London: Edward Arnold, 1981), Table A3.1. These figures more or less represent England and Wales: in 1871 the population of Wales was about 1.3 million and in 1911 it was about 2 million.
11. P.J. Corfield, *The Impact of English Towns, 1700–1800* (Oxford: Oxford University Press, 1982), Tables I and II. In 1801, 70 per cent of the population still lived in an essentially rural environment (defined as a settlement of fewer than 2500 persons).
12. S.D. Chapman, *The Cotton Industry in the Industrial Revolution* (2nd edn, Houndmills, Basingstoke, Hampshire: Macmillan Education, 1987), p. 21. Of course, the factory method of workforce organization had already been pioneered before the application of the rotary steam engine, particularly from 1771 by Richard Arkwright at his water-powered cotton mills at Cromford, Derbyshire.
13. S. Szreter and G. Mooney, 'Urbanisation, mortality and the standard of living debate: new estimates of the expectation of life at birth in nineteenth-century British cities', *Economic History Review* 51 (February 1998): 84–112, Table 7. Outside England and Wales, the other major cities in Great Britain with over 100 000 inhabitants in 1871 were Edinburgh, Glasgow, Dundee, Dublin and Belfast.
14. M.W. Flinn, 'Trends in real wages 1750–1850', *Economic History Review* 27 (1974): 395–413; E.H. Hunt, *British Labour History 1815–1914* (London: Weidenfeld and Nicolson, 1981), Ch. 3; P. Lindert, 'Unequal living standards', in R. Floud and D. McCloskey (eds), *The Economic History of Britain Since 1700*, vol. 1: *1700–1860* (2nd edn, Cambridge: Cambridge University Press, 1994), pp. 368–72. The most recent research has revised downward to extremely modest rates the scale of likely real wage and real household income rises experienced before the 1840s by the population in general: C.H. Feinstein, 'Changes in nominal wages, the cost of living and real wages in the United Kingdom over two centuries, 1780–1990', in P. Scholliers and V. Zamagni (eds), *Labour's Reward: Real Wages and Economic Change in 19th- and 20th-Century Europe* (Aldershot, England: E. Elgar, 1995), pp. 3–36; S. Horrell and J. Humphries, 'Women's labour force participation and the transition to the male-breadwinner family, 1790–1865', *Economic History Review* 48 (1995): 89–117. However, it remains the case that urban, industrial workers and their families are believed to have been the main beneficiaries of the real wage and income rises that occurred throughout the period (see following note).
15. K.D.M. Snell, *Annals of the Labouring Poor* (Cambridge: Cambridge University Press, 1987), esp. Ch. 1.
16. L.D. Schwarz, 'The standard of living in the long run: London 1700–1860', *Economic History Review* 38 (1985): 26–41; E.H. Hunt, 'Industrialisation and regional inequality: wages in Britain, 1760–1914', *Journal of Economic History* 44 (1986): 935–66; E.H. Hunt and F.W. Botham, 'Wages in Britain during the industrial revolution', *Economic History Review* 40 (1987): 380–99; L.D. Schwarz, 'Trends in real wages, 1750–1790: a reply to Botham and Hunt', *Economic History Review* 43 (1990): 90–8.
17. Wrigley and Schofield, cited in note 10, Table A3.l; E.A. Wrigley, R.S. Davies, J.E. Oeppen, and R.S. Schofield, *English Population History*

from Family Reconstitution (Cambridge: Cambridge University Press, 1997), Table A9.1.

18. D.V. Glass carefully examined the technical reliability of Farr's early life tables, taking into account weaknesses of under-registration, especially of deaths, by the early vital registration system. He was nevertheless satisfied that there were no major problems with Farr's estimates and was prepared to cite them himself. Subsequently, Lee and Lam have noted minor technical problems with some of the early censuses but, again, their research would not indicate a need for any significant change in the figures calculated by Farr. D.V. Glass, 'Some indicators of differences between urban and rural mortality in England and Wales and Scotland', *Population Studies* 17 (1964): 263–7; R. Lee and D. Lam, 'Age distribution adjustments for English censuses 1821–1931', *Population Studies* 37 (1983): 445–64.

19. The national and sectional life tables based on the 1841 census were published in 1843 and 1845 in the 5th and 7th Annual Reports of the Registrar-General, while the Healthy Districts table, based on the 1851 census, was published in W. Farr, 'On the construction of life-tables, illustrated by a new life-table of the healthy districts of England', *Philosophical Transactions* 149 (1859): 837–78.

20. P. Laxton and N. Williams, 'Urbanisation and infant mortality in England: a long-term perspective and review', in M.C. Nelson and J. Rogers (eds), *Urbanisation and Epidemiologic Transition* (Uppsala: Uppsala University, Department of History, Family History Group, 1989), pp. 109–35; J. Landers, 'Age patterns of mortality in London during the "long 18th century"', *Social History of Medicine* 3 (1990): 27–60.

21. Snell, cited in note 15, Ch. 1 and Appendix, on southern agricultural incomes; E. Hobsbawm and G.F.E. Rudé, *Captain Swing* (London: Lawrence and Wishart, 1969).

22. Farr in fact produced figures that indicated values of 25.7 years for Liverpool and 25.3 years for Manchester. The slightly higher values cited in the text were calculated by Szreter and Mooney in order to reflect the full population of each city in 1841, including the 20–30 per cent of inhabitants resident in the somewhat healthier outer suburbs, a section excluded from Farr's original calculations: Szreter and Mooney, cited in note 13, Table 3 and footnote 25.

23. W.A. Armstrong, 'The trend of mortality in Carlisle between the 1780s and the 1840s: a demographic contribution to the standard of living debate', *Economic History Review* 34 (1981): 94–114; Szreter and Mooney, cited in note 13; P. Huck, 'Infant mortality and living standards of English workers during the industrial revolution', *Journal of Economic History* 55 (1995): 528–50, Table 1, examining infant mortality trends in West Bromwich, Sedgely and Walsall in the South Staffordshire Black Country and in Wigan and Ashton-under-Lyne in Lancashire.

24. R. Woods, 'On the historical relationship between infant and adult mortality', *Population Studies* 47 (1993): 195–219; Wrigley *et al.*, *English Population History*, cited in note 17. p. 260 and Figure 6.8.

25. On crime, see V.A.C. Gatrell, 'The decline of theft and violence in Victorian and Edwardian England and Wales', in V.A.C. Gatrell, *et al.* (eds), *Crime and the Law: the Social History of Crime in Western Europe since 1500*

(London: Europa Publications, 1980), pp. 238–370. On illegitimacy, see P. Laslett and K. Oostereven, 'Long-term trends in bastardy in England', *Population Studies* 27 (1973): 255–86. On industrial urban literacy, see R. Schofield, 'Dimensions of illiteracy, 1750–1850', *Explorations in Economic History* 10 (1973): 437–54. And on heights, see R. Floud, K. Wachter and A. Gregory, *Height, Health and History: Nutritional Status in the United Kingdom, 1750–1980* (Cambridge: Cambridge University Press, 1990); and P. Johnson and S. Nicholas, 'Health and welfare of women in the United Kingdom, 1785–1920', in Steckel and Floud, *Health and Welfare*, cited in note 3, pp. 201–50.

26. M.W. Flinn, *Scottish Population History from the 17th Century to the 1930s* (Cambridge: Cambridge University Press, 1977), pp. 388–95.

27. S. Cherry, 'The hospitals and population growth: the voluntary general hospitals, mortality and local populations in the English provinces in the eighteenth and nineteenth centuries', *Population Studies* 34 (1980): 59–75 (part 1), 251–66 (part 2).

28. H.J. Perkin, *Origins of Modern English Society* (London: Routledge, 1969), pp. 135–6, 419; H. Phelps Brown, *Egalitarianism and the Generation of Inequality* (Oxford: Oxford University Press, 1988), Chs 11.1, 14.3–14.4.

29. M.A. Anderson, *Family Structure in Nineteenth-Century Lancashire* (Cambridge: Cambridge University Press, 1971), esp. p. 157 and Table 43; C. Pooley and S. D'Cruze, 'Migration and urbanisation in north-west England circa 1760–1830', *Social History* 19 (1994): 339–58; see also S. King, 'Dying with style: infant death and its context in a rural industrial township 1650–1830', *Social History of Medicine* 10 (1997): 3–24.

30. H.J. Dyos and D.A. Reeder, 'Slums and suburbs', in H.J. Dyos and M. Wolff (eds), *The Victorian City: Images and Realities* (Boston: Routledge & Kegan Paul, 1978), Vol. 1, pp. 359–86, p. 369.

31. Ibid., p. 361.

32. J.R. Kellett, 'The railway as an agent of internal change in Victorian cities', in R.J. Morris and R. Rodger (eds), *The Victorian City: a Reader in British Urban History, 1820–1914* (London: Longman, 1993), pp. 181–208.

33. R.D. Storch, 'The policeman as domestic missionary: urban discipline and popular culture in northern England, 1850–80', in Morris and Rodger, cited in note 32, pp. 281–306.

34. Szreter and Mooney, cited in note 13: expectation of life at birth in Carlisle in the 1780s can be estimated at 38.7 years, which was actually above the national average of 36–37 years at that time.

35. E.P. Hennock, 'Finance and politics in urban local government in England, 1835–1900', *Historical Journal* 6 (1963): 212–25; D. Fraser, *Urban Politics in Victorian England: the Structure of Politics in Victorian Cities* (Leicester: Leicester University Press, 1976).

36. S. Szreter, 'The GRO and the public health movement 1837–1914', *Social History of Medicine* 4 (1991): 435–63, p. 438.

37. Lindert, cited in note 14, pp. 385–6.

38. E. Biagini, *Liberty, Retrenchment and Reform: Popular Liberalism in the Age of Gladstone 1860–80* (Cambridge: Cambridge University Press, 1992); J. Prest, *Liberty and Locality: Parliament, Permissive Legislation, and Ratepayers'*

Democracies in the Mid-Nineteenth Century (Oxford: Oxford University Press, 1990); Hennock, cited in note 35.

39. Kellett, cited in note 32.

40. P. Curtin, *Death by Migration: Europe's Encounter with the Tropical World in the Nineteenth Century* (Cambridge: Cambridge University Press, 1989); R. Shlomowitz, *Mortality and Migration in the Modern World* (Aldershot: Variorum, 1996); R. Haines, R. Shlomowitz and L. Brennan, 'Maritime mortality revisited', *International Journal of Maritime History* 7 (1996): 133–72; S.R. Johansson, 'Death and the doctors: elites, mortality and medicine in Britain from 1500 to 1800', unpublished paper, April 1997.

41. A.C. Pigou, *The Economics of Welfare* (London: Macmillan, 1920).

42. J.A. Hassan, 'The growth and impact of the British water industry in the nineteenth century', *Economic History Review* 38 (1985): 531–47, esp. pp. 535–6.

43. Ibid.

44. S. Szreter, 'The importance of social intervention in Britain's mortality decline c. 1850–1914: a re-interpretation of the role of public health', *Social History of Medicine* 1 (1988): 1–37, pp. 25–6.

45. The most detailed and illuminating account of the origins and influence of the civic gospel is found in E.P. Hennock, *Fit and Proper Persons: Ideal and Reality in Nineteenth-Century Urban Government* (Montreal: McGill-Queens University Press, 1973), which examines its provenance among the dissenting congregations of the Birmingham social elite and its influence in the city of Leeds.

46. A. Briggs, *Victorian Cities* (Berkeley: University of California Press, 1965), p. 206.

47. This is a principal thesis of Hennock, cited in note 45. See also Briggs, cited in note 46, pp. 219–20.

48. Szreter, *Fertility, Class and Gender*, cited in note 1, Ch. 4, section 2.

49. Boyd Hilton has dubbed the earlier era 'the age of atonement', distinguishing it from the subsequent period of much more confident, incarnational religion and missionary zeal on the part of the upper and middle classes, earnestly endeavouring to bring the light of 'civilisation' to the poor and ignorant, both at home and abroad. B. Hilton, *The Age of Atonement: the Influence of Evangelicalism on Social and Economic Thought 1785–1865* (Oxford: Oxford University Press, 1988).

50. C.T. Harvie, *The Lights of Liberalism: University Liberals and the Challenge of Democracy 1860–86* (London: Allen Lane, 1976); C.D. Cashdollar, *The Transformation of Theology, 1830–1890: Positivism and Protestant Thought in Britain and America* (Princeton: Princeton University Press, 1989).

51. The history of change both in formal municipal voting qualifications and in the actual practices found in different towns is extraordinarily complex throughout the nineteenth century. A standard introductory text is B. Keith-Lucas, *The English Local Government Franchise: a Short History* (Oxford: Oxford University Press, 1952), Ch. III. I believe that H.P. Hennock's otherwise excellent, pioneering research in this area tended to discount too much the significance of change in the municipal electorate during the late 1860s and 1870s and placed too much emphasis, instead, on expansion of

the municipal electorate in the 1850s: Hennock, cited in note 35, esp. pp. 221, 224. The most recent research has concluded that the sequence of developments between 1867 and 1883 renders this the key period in the expansion of the urban municipal electorate to incorporate a dominant section of the working class: J. Davis and D. Tanner, 'The borough franchise after 1867', *Historical Research* 69 (1996): 306–27.

52. P.J. Waller, *Town, City and Nation* (Oxford: Oxford University Press, 1983), pp. 297–8; D. Read, *The Age of Urban Democracy: England 1868–1914* (Rev. edn, London: Longman, 1994), pp. 266–7.

53. H. Fraser, 'Municipal socialism and social policy', in Morris and Rodger, cited in note 32, pp. 258–80.

54. Szreter, cited in note 44, p. 25. During a period of minimal inflation these figures represent a real sevenfold increase in expenditure.

55. R. Millward and S. Sheard, 'The urban fiscal problem, 1870–1914: Government expenditure and finance in England and Wales', *Economic History Review* 48 (1995): 501–35.

56. J.F. Wilson, S. Sheard, and R. Millward, 'Trends in local authority loan expenditure in England and Wales 1870–1914', University of Manchester Working Papers in Economic and Social History No. 22 (1993), pp. 6–8.

57. R. Millward and S. Sheard, 'Government expenditure on social overheads and the infrastructure in England and Wales, 1870–1914', University of Manchester Working Papers in Economic and Social History No. 23 (1993), p. 9. These are trading profits after subtraction of loan charges, which can be calculated for these years, 1903–5.

58. McKeown, cited in note 5.

59. The principal comparative evidence in favour of public health expenditure and measures was assembled in S.H. Preston, *Mortality Patterns in National Populations: with Special Reference to Causes of Death* (New York: Academic Press, 1976).

60. The revisionist reworking of McKeown's historical epidemiological data for nineteenth-century Britain was published in Szreter, cited in note 44, pp. 5–17; see also S. Guha, 'The importance of social intervention in England's mortality decline: the evidence reviewed', *Social History of Medicine* 7 (1994): 89–113; S. Szreter, 'Mortality in England in the eighteenth and the nineteenth centuries: a reply to Sumit Guha', *Social History of Medicine* 7 (1994): 269–82; and S.R. Johansson, 'Food for thought: rhetoric and reality in modern mortality history', *Historical Methods* 27 (1994): 101–25.

61. C.A. Nathanson, 'Disease prevention as social change: toward a theory of public health', *Population and Development Review* 22 (1996): 609–37.

62. C. Hamlin, 'Muddling in Bumbledon: on the enormity of large sanitary improvements in four British towns, 1855–1885', *Victorian Studies* 32 (1988/89): 55–83; C. Hamlin, *A Science of Impurity: Water Analysis in Nineteenth-Century Britain* (Berkeley: University of California Press, 1990).

63. W.F. Bynum, 'Darwin and the doctors: Evolution, diathesis, and germs in nineteenth-century Britain', *Gesnerus* 40 (1983): 43–53.

64. Nathanson, cited in note 61, p. 631, note 2.

65. M. Mann, *The Sources of Social Power*, Vol. 2 (Cambridge: Cambridge University Press, 1993), Ch. 3.

66. On the concept of brokers, see H.R. Wolf, 'Aspects of group relations in a complex society: Mexico', in T. Shanin (ed.), *Peasants and Peasant Society* (Harmondsworth: Penguin Books, 1971), pp. 50–68.

67. Szreter, cited in note 44; on the GRO's public health role, see Szreter, cited in note 36.

68. J. Powles and N. Day, 'The East Europeans dying before their time', *European Brief* 2 (1995): 50–1. See also the papers from the session on 'Mortality Reversals and Their Causes in the Former USSR and Eastern Europe', by V.M. Shkolnikov, F. Meslé, V. Hertrich, *et al.*, in IUSSP, *International Population Conference, Beijing 1997*, Vol. 2 (Liège, 1997), pp. 473–579.

69. On the importance of the principle of universality in social security and welfare entitlements in promoting social inclusionism, avoiding social deprivations, and enhancing citizenship, see R.M. Titmuss, *Commitment to Welfare* (London: W. Pickering, 1968).

70. J. Chen, T.C. Campbell, J. Li and R. Peto, *Diet, Lifestyle and Mortality in China: a Study of the Characteristics of 65 Chinese Counties* (Oxford: Oxford University Press, 1990), pp. 102–3. See also the papers from the session on 'Mortality Trends in China', by Z. Weimin, X. Li, J. Banister, *et al.*, in IUSSP, *International Population Conference, Beijing 1997*, Vol. 3 (Liège, 1997), pp. 1325–69.

71. J. Drèze and A. Sen, *Hunger and Public Action* (Oxford: Oxford University Press, 1989), pp. 11–2.

72. On these issues in Britain, see for instance A. Offer, *Property and Politics 1870–1914: Landownership, Law, Ideology, and Urban Development in England* (Cambridge: Cambridge University Press, 1981); and M.A. Crowther and B.M. White, 'Medicine, property and the law in Britain 1800–1914', *Historical Journal* 31(1988): 853–70.

73. For the original work on entitlements, see A. Sen, *Poverty and Famines: an Essay on Entitlement and Deprivation* (Oxford: Oxford University Press, 1981); and for a summary of entitlements and capabilities, see Drèze and Sen, cited in note 71, pp. 9–19.

74. See references cited in note 3.

75. R. Dorfman, 'Review article: Economic development from the beginning to Rostow', *Journal of Economic Literature* 29 (1991): 573–91, p. 573.

76. W. Hutton, *The State We're In* (London: Cape, 1995), Ch. 10.

77. N.F.R. Crafts, 'The golden age of economic growth in Western Europe, 1950–1973', *Economic History Review* 48 (1995): 429–47, p. 434. For reviews of new growth theory, see the special issues of two journals devoted to this subject: *Oxford Review of Economic Policy* 8, no. 4 (1992) and *Journal of Economic Perspectives* 8, no. 1 (1994). More generally, see M. Abramovitz, *Thinking About Growth: and Other Essays on Economic Growth and Welfare* (Cambridge: Cambridge University Press, 1989).

78. J.S. Coleman, *Foundations of Social Theory* (Cambridge, MA: Belknap Press of Harvard University Press, 1990), Ch. 12. Social capital should not be confused with Pierre Bourdieu's notion of cultural capital (more or less corresponding to an individual's success in the educational system), though it is certainly related to it; see P. Bourdieu, 'Cultural reproduction and social reproduction', in R. Brown (ed.), *Knowledge, Education and Cultural Change* (London: Tavistock, 1973), pp. 71–112. Social capital is the property of a

social group and its institutions, not of an individual. Coleman distinguishes social capital from the related concepts of economic capital (productive plant and finance) and human capital (which is not dissimilar to Bourdieu's cultural capital, being the aptitudes, skills, and training possessed by an individual worker). Social capital is lodged neither in individuals, as their capacities, nor in the physical implements of production. It inheres in the pattern of relationships between persons: how they are able to communicate with each other. It is therefore constituted in the institutions, associations, and communities of society and the economy.

79. On social capital and both civic participation and economic performance, see in particular R.D. Putnam, *Making Democracy Work: Civic Traditions in Modern Italy* (Princeton: Princeton University Press, 1994). On social capital and health, see R.G. Wilkinson, 'Health inequalities: relative or absolute material standards?' *British Medical Journal* 314, no. 7080, 22 February 1997 (online publication); and R.G. Wilkinson, *Unhealthy Societies: the Afflictions of Inequality* (London: Routledge, 1996).

80. M. Granovetter, 'Economic action, social structure, and embeddedness', *American Journal of Sociology* 91 (1985): 481–510; P. Evans, *Embedded Autonomy: States and Industrial Transformation* (Princeton: Princeton University Press, 1995).

81. See the excellent special section of *World Development* 24, no. 6 (June 1996): 1033–132, introduced with a helpful review of other relevant work by P. Evans. This presents five empirical studies contributed by W.F. Lam (Taiwan), P. Heller (Kerala), E. Ostrom (Brazil and Nigeria), J. Fox (Mexico), and M. Burawoy (Russia and China).

6
Disease and International Development

Andrew T. Price-Smith

Over the centuries, there has been considerable debate concerning the sources of industrialization and the nature of the development of economies and societies. The most prominent explanations have been modernization theory and dependency theory. However, previous theories of development have generally overlooked a significant biological parameter that lies at the core of international development, specifically, the burden of infectious disease on the productivity and the consolidation of human capital in a given population. Following the lead of Robert Fogel, I argue that the mastery of high morbidity and mortality rates in a given population has been a central driver of state prosperity and economic strength throughout recorded history. Similarly, I argue that the continuing and unchecked proliferation of emerging and re-emerging infectious disease represents a considerable threat to the economic development, stability and prosperity of states throughout the world.

Let us perform a mental exercise at this point. Picture a Mercator projection map of the globe and note the global distribution of wealth between states. Wealth is generally located in the temperate regions of the world, with the exception of the Gulf Oil States. Societies in these temperate regions tend to be highly industrialized relative to those countries in the tropics. Even extremely cold countries, such as Canada and the Scandinavian nations, are exceptionally prosperous. I argue that there is a biological foundation for development, and that this bioeconomic axiom holds both across time and globally across diverse human societies.[1]

Pathogens have historically impeded the economic and social development of many societies, particularly those that lie within the tropical regions of the world. This chapter argues that the proliferation of

infectious disease can compromise the economic and social development of countries, and that the onerous burden of disease in tropical
regions may partially explain the vast economic development differential between societies in the tropics and their richer counterparts in the
temperate zones.

Over the span of centuries, historians and economists have specu-
lated that infectious disease has played a significant (if enigmatic) role
in the rise and fall of societies and empires. Fogel argued that much of
England's prosperity, if not the Industrial Revolution itself, resulted
from the conquest of high morbidity and mortality in Britain during
the late eighteenth and early nineteenth centuries.[2] This conquest of
mortality and morbidity was largely the result of significant advances
in public health and in the increasingly equitable distribution of food.
Conversely, William McNeill noted that the arrival of the Black Death
(bubonic/pneumonic plague) in Europe during the fourteenth century
had significant and pervasive negative economic and social effects on
the European societies of the time, generating widespread economic
and political instability throughout the continent.

> The buoyancy and self-confidence, so characteristic of the thirteenth
> century ... gave way to a more troubled age. Acute social tensions
> between economic classes and intimate acquaintance with sudden
> death assumed far greater importance for almost everyone than had
> been true previously. The economic impact of the Black Death was
> enormous. ... In highly developed regions like northern Italy and
> Flanders, harsh collisions between social classes manifested them-
> selves as the boom times of the thirteenth century faded into the
> past. The plague, by disrupting wage and price patterns sharply, exac-
> erbated these conflicts. ... Employers died as well as labourers. ...[3]

In *The Health of Nations*, the data show a pronounced negative association between the burden of disease on a society and that society's
ability to increase basal productivity and prosperity.[4] It is imperative
that we understand exactly how these causal processes function within
states. Only if we trace these pathways will we be able to develop and
evaluate policies that can mitigate the negative impact of infectious
disease on national economic development. Given that infectious
disease exerts a negative impact on state economic productivity and
development in myriad ways, the optimal means to analyse the general
economic effect of Emerging and Re-emerging Infectious Diseases
(ERIDs) is to examine their impact at the three standard levels of

economic analysis: microeconomic (individuals, households, firms), sectoral and macroeconomic.

Microeconomic analysis

Microeconomics deals with the economic behaviour of individual decision-making units in a free-market enterprise system, analysing consumer spending and saving patterns, the maximization of profits by firms, and the pricing of resources and products. Thus, microeconomics is the study of individual components of an economy, such as firms, households and prices of goods and services. Process-tracing techniques, which involve a qualitative examination of the probable relations between variables, allow us to demonstrate how ERIDs can erode household productivity. These maps will help to illuminate the 'break-points' in the causal chain so that effective policy can be formulated to mitigate the negative effects of poor health on productivity.

Within the household unit, disease undermines prosperity and generates significant shifts in family spending and saving behaviour. Households are defined as one or more individuals who represent both a consumption unit and a production unit.[5] Given their endowments of land, other wealth, and the time of their members, households engage in satisficing when they make production, consumption and savings decisions. At the micro level, increased disease incidence and lethality exert a significant negative effect on the household by debilitating and killing productive members, which in turn generates shifts in savings and consumption patterns and results in supply and demand-induced shocks that destabilize the household as an economic (and social) unit.

It is necessary to distinguish between directly and indirectly affected households. Directly affected households are those in which a member of the family unit is ill or has died from an infectious disease. Indirectly affected households are those that directly assist affected households by caring for orphans, assisting with funeral expenses and generating additional labour inputs. Ainsworth and Over argue that ERID-related adult mortality and morbidity will tend to affect macroeconomic aggregates such as wages and savings, and so everyone in an affected society will be influenced by the resurgence of infectious disease.[6]

Depending on their virulence and transmissibility, pathogens reduce the number of income-generating members of the household, lower household income, and alter patterns of consumption and savings. At the household level, pecuniary or direct costs that result from disease-induced illness, consist of personal health care expenditures, costs of prevention, diagnosis, treatment of illness and costs of death (which involves expenditures for funerals, mourning ceremonies and coffins). Increasing medical costs and higher funeral expenses will diminish general current expenditures, including those dedicated to savings. Households with infected members may try to increase savings rates in anticipation of paying onerous funeral costs in the near future.[7] These direct costs of death can be particularly burdensome on the poorer segments of society. For example, in southern Zambia, coffins cost from $66 to $200. The family of the deceased also pays for the food, lodging and transport of mourners. In Kinshasa, the funeral of a paediatric AIDS victim costs a family an average of $320, or the equivalent of 11 months' income.[8]

Other direct costs of ERIDs include nonpersonal costs for educational campaigns, biomedical research and blood screening. Arguably, the single most onerous health care costs for ERID patients are inpatient costs incurred during hospitalization. Annual inpatient costs reflect the treatment received (drugs, lab procedures, surgery, etc.), the duration of hospitalization and the frequency of episodes of hospitalization required in a year.[9] In their study of the economic affect of AIDS in Thailand, Myers *et al.*, found that the annual cost of AIDS treatment was approximately $1000 or 25 000 Baht per case, resulting in the loss of over 50 per cent of the average annual household income.[10] Similarly onerous treatment costs are also reported in sub-Saharan Africa: in Tanzania, the average cost of each adult AIDS patient over the duration of the patient's illness is roughly 50 000 T Sh, and for children, the corresponding figure is 34 000 T Sh. Given that per capita income in Tanzania was roughly 12 500 T Sh in 1988, it is obvious that these AIDS-related health care costs will become a tremendous burden on the household as the epidemic worsens.[11]

ERID-induced adult deaths can force vulnerable households into poverty. Even in countries such as Tanzania, where the government bears much of the burden of health costs, HIV-affected rural households in 1991 spent $60 (roughly the equivalent of annual rural income per capita) on treatment and funerals. Poonawala and Cantor observed similarly deleterious effects from ERIDs on household savings and productivity. They estimated that AIDS hospitalization in Zaire costs on average four months' wages for the average worker, while a funeral costs 11 months' wages.[12] For impoverished families, the reduced per capita income, taken with the needs of a chronically ill patient, tends to result in substandard diets and increasing levels of labour-substitution; this results in reduced school attendance for the children of affected households and lowered standards of living.[13]

Indirect or non-pecuniary costs result from the lost value of market and non-market output due to increased morbidity or mortality resulting from illness. Other ERID-induced indirect costs to the household consist of negative outcomes such as loss of remittances from labour, diminished agricultural inputs, diminished export and food crop production, reduced participation in labour-intensive and nonfood crop production, diminished household assets and increased levels of malnutrition within family members.[14] Nonpecuniary costs also include the weight that infected individuals, their families and friends, and other members of society place on the misery and mortality of affected persons, and changes in behaviour to avoid contracting or transmitting ERIDs.[15]

The combined direct and indirect costs of a lethal pathogen such as HIV/AIDS can have significant long-term detrimental effects on the annual net income of the household. Ainsworth and Over have determined that in severely affected states, roughly 75 per cent of annual household revenue may be lost as a result of HIV/AIDS infection.[16] The UN estimates that, 'the indirect costs of AIDS range from $890 to $2663 in Zaire and from $2425 to $5903 in ... Tanzania, which indicates that indirect costs represent roughly 95 per cent of the total costs associated with an AIDS infection'.[17]

The enormous economic burden of disease is in part a function of the synergistic interaction between various pathogens within both individual hosts and societies at large. For example, sexually transmitted diseases (herpes, gonorrhea, etc.) often create access points for HIV to enter and weaken the immune system, whereupon pathogens such as tuberculosis then kill the host. Of course, due to extensive data collection problems, it is extremely difficult to estimate co-infection rates throughout the developing world. Thus, most of the economic analyses to date have focused on the effects of a single pathogen upon a given population. It should be noted that HIV/AIDS has received the lion's share of this recent attention based on its lethality and rapidly increasing global prevalence rates. Despite the focus on HIV, other diseases including malaria, tuberculosis, leprosy and river blindness also generate negative micro- and macroeconomic outcomes. One example of how disease-induced morbidity affects individual productivity is found in the effects of leprosy.

A study of lepers in urban Tamil Nadu, India, estimates that the elimination of deformity would more than triple the expected annual earnings of those with jobs. The prevention of deformity in all of India's 645 000 lepers would have added an estimated $130 million to the country's 1985 GDP. This amount is the equivalent of almost 10 per cent of all the official development assistance received by India in 1985. Yet leprosy accounted for only a small proportion of the country's disease burden, less than 1 per cent in 1990.[18]

Infectious diseases in general, and HIV in particular, tend to generate economic 'shocks' to household savings and consumption patterns. Morbidity and mortality resulting from infection erodes the economic capacity of households as it reduces the time and labour available from members of the household, impairs the supply of education and health of the family unit, and, through inheritance customs, reduces the stock of land, housing and live-stock available to the household. Households adjust to these initial shocks over time by attempting to rationally re-distribute their limited human and financial capital in order to over-come the burden of disease, and change their behaviour concerning production, expenditure, savings and investment.[19] Non-infected indi-viduals may spend an increased amount of time caring for the debilitated, additional time working to make up for the lost productiv-ity of the sick, and less time in school. To pay for medical care, they may also deplete their savings, sell assets, borrow from others, or diminish other investments. In many developing nations, affected families may have to sell assets such as land and livestock in order to maintain economic subsistence levels. Indeed, according to World Bank figures, ill-health is the cause of 24 per cent of land transactions in Kenya.[20]

Despite the overwhelming (and largely justified) concern regarding the negative economic effects of HIV/AIDS, other diseases, such as malaria, represent resurgent impediments to development. While gen-erally less lethal than HIV/AIDS,[21] malaria frequently debilitates the populations of tropical societies, particularly during the peak months of the rainy growing seasons.

Poorer households often bear a much greater economic burden from infectious diseases than do their wealthier counterparts, and thus infectious disease tends to reinforce income inequalities within soci-eties and exacerbate income disparities between classes. In their study of malaria's effect on household income in Malawi, Ettling *et al.* observed that 'very low income households carried a disproportionate share of the economic burden of malaria, with total direct and indirect cost of malaria among these households consuming 32 per cent of annual household income. ...' Conversely, malaria consumes only 4.2 per cent of the annual income of the Malawian elite household.[22] The implication is that while all Malawians suffer the deleterious economic drag from the *Plasmodium* spp. the economic burden of the disease falls mainly on the poor, exacerbating the income gap between the average worker and the upper classes and driving marginalized populations into deeper poverty.[23] Thus, one of the principal negative effects of infectious disease on societies is that it increases both perceived and real inequalities between the rich and poor, particularly in the case of diseases like malaria, tuberculosis and cholera that tend to affect marginalized populations. Predictably, the economic gains from improved health are comparatively greater for poorer families, who are usually most handicapped by illness and stand to gain significantly from the development of improved human capital in the form of fewer work days lost to illness, worker productivity, per capita income, improved education and nutrition, greater opportunity to obtain better-paying jobs, longer working lives, and the ability to use previously under-utilized natural resources.[24]

Emerging and re-emerging infectious diseases and their legacy of orphans

One effect of the HIV pandemic that is commonly overlooked is the enormous increase in the numbers of orphaned children. The direct and indirect economic costs of caring for orphaned children will impose additional financial burdens on afflicted societies.

Based on the recent findings of a USAID study of 23 countries in the developing world, J. Brian Atwood predicts that more than 34.7 million children will have lost one or both parents to HIV by 2000, with the figure increasing to 41.6 million in 2010.[25] No figures are yet available for global estimates of the likely number of HIV orphans. Aside from the immense human suffering involved, such great numbers of orphaned children will create immense financial and social strains on heavily afflicted societies.

This means that for those sub-Saharan African countries that now exhibit general population HIV seroprevalence rates of 10 per cent or greater, we can expect the number of AIDS orphans in those societies to grow exponentially within the decade. In certain societies such as Zimbabwe, Zambia and Botswana (which now have HIV infection levels in excess of 30 per cent of the general adult population), one might reasonably expect that the rapid increase in orphans might generate increasing socioeconomic disruption over the long term.

The proliferation of infectious disease threatens the economic welfare of the family unit in all societies. However, process-tracing techniques suggest that ERID poses a relatively greater threat to poorer, marginalized families, particularly those in the developing world and in societies that rely on privately funded health-care systems. One of the most significant problems associated with the proliferation of pathogens is the strong possibility that it will exacerbate economic disparities between upper and lower economic strata within a given society. This may in turn contribute to perceptions of deprivation on the part of the marginalized. We shall pursue this point (and its attendant social and political ramifications) further at the end of the chapter.

Households are not the only actors at the microeconomic level which are negatively affected by the proliferation of infectious disease. Individual firms, which have endowments of land, buildings, equipment and a trained workforce, are also subject to the negative effects of disease. These firms operate in an environment that includes market prices, levels of morbidity and mortality in the community, infrastructure, climate, rainfall and government policies. The proliferation of disease will likely affect individual firms in several negative ways: increased sick leave and absenteeism, diminished productivity, increased worker turnover, the loss of highly skilled managers, greater training costs and larger expenditures on health and death benefits.[26] The World Bank argues that in severely affected states, the work force will become younger, and lack adequate training. For example, Tanzania and Uganda are already witnessing greater AIDS-induced absenteeism and declining productivity. The majority of macroeconomic models predict that adult AIDS-related deaths will greatly slow the rate of per capita economic growth as compared to a non-AIDS scenario.[27]

Extensive work has been done on the relationship between investment in human capital and the positive downstream effects on labour productivity.[28] ERIDs (notably HIV/AIDS) exert a negative impact on firms through the reduction of the local labour supply (particularly skilled workers), which will over time generate wage increases and cut the profit margins of firms. Reduced labour supply and productivity combined with increasing wages will undermine the productivity and profit-margins of firms in affected regions. For this reason, multinational firms may choose not to invest in areas where disease endemicity is particularly high. Thus, the proliferation of ERID (particularly HIV) generates disincentives over time to invest capital within severely affected societies. In extreme cases, exceptionally high rates of ERID infection in local populations may spur capital flight from affected regions to safer havens that have lower levels of endemic disease and hence are more productive.

Sectoral analysis

In the broadest sense, infectious diseases have a negative impact at the sectoral level of the economy, adversely affecting a host of economic mechanisms and generally undermining productivity throughout society. In the formal sector, the proliferation of infectious disease threatens the expansion of industry and the private sector, both of which exhibit a deep reliance on skilled workers, entrepreneurs and managers. In his 1997 address to the World Economic Forum at Davos, Sir Richard Sykes stated that the (HIV/AIDS) epidemic is already generating a negative effect on the global workforce, markets and overall business climate. Sykes cited studies done in southern and eastern Africa by the African Medical and Research Foundation (AMREF) for AIDSCAP, which concluded that the HIV/AIDS epidemic generates significant negative economic outcomes: the loss of skilled personnel; the need for greater resources to hire and maintain replacement workers; an increase in labour turnover and absenteeism; and a reduction in productivity.[29] Reductions in labour-supply resulting from increased mortality will also impose shocks to industry. Callisto Madavo notes that in a representative sample of 20 Zambian firms, worker mortality increased from 500 to 800 per cent between 1987 and 1992, largely as a direct result of HIV/AIDS.[30]

Further examples of the negative impact of HIV on skilled personnel include the loss of many of the senior managers of Barclay's Bank of Zambia to AIDS, while in Malawi nearly 30 per cent of all schoolteachers are HIV positive.[31] These highly skilled workers represent significant investments in human capital on the part of their employers and home states, and it will be very expensive and time-consuming to replace them. Indeed, African elites have generally been severely affected by HIV/AIDS. For example, in the former Zaire, 'among the [largely male] employees at a Kinshasa textile mill, managers had a higher infection rate than foremen, who in turn had a higher rate than workers'.[32]

Because HIV is so prevalent throughout African elites it is likely to have significant negative effects on senior management structures within firms, undercutting the reservoir of human capital within firms, sectors and macroeconomies. Peter Piot of UNAIDS argues that HIV/AIDS costs companies operating in Kenya roughly 4 per cent of annual profits, and that as a direct result of the HIV epidemic Kenya's GDP will be 15 per cent less than it would have been (in a non-AIDS scenario) by the year 2005.[33]

Besides the economic shocks to firms, resulting from pathogen-induced shortages in labour supply, Hancock and Cuddington agree that disease will undermine the economic productivity of nations as they exert general and profound negative effects on the overall size and quality of the labour force.[34] ERIDs (particularly HIV/AIDS) will affect individual sectors through both demand- and supply-side shocks. One example of supply-side shock occurs when a company which is dependent on an ERID-infected labour pool manufactures products for export. While international demand for the product is not affected by the local AIDS epidemic, the firm's labour supply and productivity are diminished, increasing costs and thus narrowing the company's profit margin.[35] Conversely, a healthy and stable work force enables employers to reduce the expense of allocating slack into their production schedules, permits greater investment in staff training that consolidates human capital, and provides employers with the benefits of specialization.[36] Cohen argues that labour costs will rise as productivity declines because of increasing morbidity and absenteeism: additional training costs will also result from greater labour turnover. Firm expenditures on health and other social programmes will also grow, such that the public and private outlays of firms will rise as a proportion of aggregate expenditure. Thus, the savings available to firms used for financing capital expenditures is diminished.[37]

Other effects of disease-induced morbidity and mortality on firms include reduced functional capacity in that workers may not be able to do their former jobs. Labour-substitution practices may result as other workers may be required to assume the former responsibilities of ill coworkers.[38] In their 1992 study of the microeconomic effects of AIDS on Thailand, Myers, Obremsky and Viravaidya concluded that the AIDS epidemic would have a significant negative effect on the performance of the Thai economy. In addition to greater health care costs and foregone income, HIV would likely result in a shortage of skilled labour, increased absenteeism, and significant training/re-training costs.[39]

Health

The global resurgence of disease will hurt the health care sector in affected nations through both supply- and demand-side shocks. As greater numbers of the population become infected and develop illness, the demand for medical care will soar, and the associated costs will drain national accounts where governments are the major providers of medical care.[40] Similarly, the increasing prevalence of infection will also debilitate and kill those medical professionals who must minister to the needs of the general population. Some diseases, particularly HIV, have the ability to generate significant supply-side shocks within the health sector, as the societal stock of medical personnel are infected, debilitated and die. Additionally, the HIV pandemic will generate much greater health care costs, as states need to employ greater numbers of healthcare staff. As well, the burdens of medical insurance, disability payments and life insurance premiums will add to the societal burden of healthcare costs.[41] Such health sector costs are by no means limited to the developing world, and are doubtless more costly (in absolute terms) to the economies of the developed world. For example, nosocomial (hospital-acquired) infections result in the deaths of over 20 000 Americans per year, and cost the US economy $5–10 billion annually.[42]

In absolute terms, disease is likely to have a much greater negative effect on the health care sector throughout the states of the developing world. For example, the World Bank estimates that the downstream costs of treating all current cases of AIDS cases in Tanzania will consume approximately 40.6 per cent of the public health budget and nearly 25 per cent of combined public and private spending. Similarly, the expense of treating current AIDS cases in Rwanda will absorb an astonishing 60 to 65.5 per cent of the public health budget.[43] What this means is that either far less money will be available to treat other health problems (i.e. malaria, tuberculosis, onchocerciasis, heart disease), or that money that would have gone into more productive sectors such as infrastructure or education will have to be diverted to cover national health expenditures. In many cases, the health care system will be completely overwhelmed by the strains imposed by high rates of infection. According to the UN 'the direct costs (drug costs, doctors' fees, hospitalization care, food, etc.) of treating AIDS patients are enormous and greatly surpass available resources in Africa. For instance, it has been estimated that the direct cost of treating one AIDS patient in Zaire ranges from a low of US $132 to $1585; in Tanzania, from $104 to $631. But the annual national budgets per capita for all health care were less than $5'.[44]

Additionally, developing countries are generally unable to afford expensive medications required for the treatment and care of their AIDS patients. The drug AZT, for instance, was estimated to cost $20 000 (US) per patient per annum in 1994. Given the low health care funding available on a per capita basis throughout most of the developing world, it is easy to see how ERIDs will drain government coffers, putting the expensive protease-inhibiting multi-drug cocktails of Western medicine out of reach for the majority of the world's inhabitants. Furthermore, hopes for the development of effective and inexpensive vaccines for the prevention of HIV and medications for the treatment of AIDS patients have been unsuccessful, further constraining countries unable to afford the costs needed for the treatment of its AIDS patients.[45] In Thailand, Viravaidya *et al.* estimated AIDS health care costs at between $658 and $1016 per year per infected person. Given that the national average GDP per capita was roughly $1270 in 1991, AIDS-related costs will drain household savings, and the government is forced to intervene when the family's resources are exhausted. The macro level cost of AIDS to the Thai economy include lost future earnings of $22 000 per death and ten-year aggregate costs of between $7.3 and $8.7 billion.[46]

The case of India is instructive in that surging HIV prevalence levels threaten to overwhelm the Indian health budget. If the HIV epidemic follows its current trend of proliferation throughout Indian society, by the year 2010 the government will have to spend about one-third more on health care than in a hypothetical non-AIDS scenario. This will necessitate an onerous $2.5 billion increase in the health care budget.[47] Such increases in the health budget are negative for most countries as the revenue must come from other government portfolios, (for example, education, housing, infrastructure) and the provision of other basic human services. Nelson Mandela has also recently voiced his concern that AIDS will drain the coffers of the South African government: 'It is anticipated that if current trends continue then AIDS will cost South Africa one per cent of our GDP by the year 2005; and that up to three quarters of our health budget will be consumed by direct health costs relating to HIV/AIDS. Even creative low cost alternatives to hospital care will leave us with a significant impact on our health care budget.'[48] Moreover, diseases such as AIDS, malaria and tuberculosis will combine synergistically to accelerate the fiscal drain from competing sectors of government expenditure. Thus, the proliferation of disease (HIV in particular) constitutes a very real fiscal problem for governments across the globe, and particularly those in the developing world.

This will likely result in increasing government deficits, greater debt, and generally undermine the ability of the government to provide for the basic needs of the population.

Agriculture

A major consequence of the improvement in rural health such as seems to have taken place in England in the century after 1650 was a notable increase in the efficiency of agricultural labour. Healthy people work better – and more regularly; and, as is obvious, losses to agricultural production resulting from inability to do necessary work at the right time of the year disappear in proportion as labourers cease to suffer from debilitating fevers and similar afflictions which tend to crest during the growing season. As health improved, fewer workers could therefore feed larger numbers of city folk. William McNeill[49]

The global spread of disease will also have a significant impact on the labour-intensive agricultural sector in affected regions. The UNDP notes that countries that bear the economic brunt of the HIV pandemic tend to be those that are most reliant on agriculture.[50] Diseases such as malaria, dengue, onchocerciasis, schistosomiasis and HIV have the greatest ability to undercut the productivity of affected agricultural workforces. Thus, the negative consequences of HIV on the agricultural sector will be substantial throughout developing societies.[51] The impact of disease proliferation on agricultural systems is also likely to be varied and complex depending on crop type, cash remittances, degree of labour-intensive cultivation practices and size of holding. In sub-Saharan Africa, the absolute number of individuals infected with HIV is likely to be higher in rural than in urban areas, because the majority of the population continues to live in rural areas. Furthermore, the age groups most seriously affected by the AIDS epidemic are those that are the most productive in the labour-intensive agricultural sector.[52]

Of course, agriculture is a core sector of many developing economies, particularly in Africa, Asia and Latin America. Agriculture contributes a large share of GDP and for many countries it contributes the majority share of the value of exported products through cash crops. Increasing disease prevalence rates will similarly afflict the agricultural sector with supply- and demand-induced shocks. For example, as pathogens debilitate and kill off the work force, the semi-skilled labour supply for this sector will be reduced, necessitating either labour substitution strategies within households/firms or the drawing of workers from other sectors. This problem of semi-skilled labour shortages tends to get particularly acute in the rainy season when vector-borne pathogens (for example, malaria, dengue) attain the highest prevalence within populations. However, given the facts that most developing societies possess an abundant labour-supply, and that labourers can be retrained to work in the agricultural sector rather quickly, we should not be overly concerned about supply-side shocks in this sector. The only obvious concern would arise in the case that an entire region, such as southern Africa,[53] suffered a rapid demographic implosion due to high prevalence of HIV in the 15–45 year segment of its population distributions. With HIV rates in the area ranging from 15–26 per cent of the total population, this remains a distinct possibility in the coming decade. Of course, imported labour from Central Africa would eventually be used to offset the demographic decline, but such massive adjustment would require some time to enact.

Demand-side shocks may also compromise sectoral productivity. Those citizens that succumb to diseases are also consumers of agricultural products; in seriously afflicted societies, domestic demand for these crops will therefore grow more slowly. If smallholders shift from the production of export to subsistence crops as a response to disease-induced shocks, export revenues will also suffer over the long term.[54] Barnett and Blaikie argue that:

> Those farming systems that are situated in the semi-arid tropics ... will be most vulnerable to labour loss as a result of AIDS ... the farming systems of southern and eastern Africa in Tanzania, Zimbabwe, Kenya, Botswana and Zambia seem particularly vulnerable, since seropositivity rates have already reached high levels in some rural areas of those countries. In all cases there will probably be implications for foreign-exchange earnings and urban food supplies.[55]

In her analysis of the Ugandan agricultural sector, Jill Armstrong found that the majority of production is concentrated within 'smallholder' farms and tends to be exceptionally labour-intensive. She concurs that HIV/AIDS will compromise key farm production parameters such as labour availability and productivity and it will also limit investment in capital equipment to improve output. Thus, HIV/AIDS will reduce the amount of available disposable income that can be used to acquire agricultural inputs (for example, occasional extra labour, new seeds or plants, fertilizer, pesticides or oxen power).[56]

Armstrong concludes that as a result of increasing ERID infection 'labor costs can be expected to increase, reflected in both market wage rates and the shadow wage rate implicit in family farm operations. This, in turn, could lead to a reversal in migration from urban areas or increased migration from other regions with surplus labour'.[57] Disease has a number of other possible effects on smallholder agricultural production: (a) the working day may be extended; (b) land under cultivation may decline; (c) cash crops may be substituted for by less labour-intensive subsistence crops; and (d) planting and weeding may be delayed leading to poor harvests and the loss of an agricultural season.[58]

Furthermore, human tendencies towards risk-aversion will also result in reduced agricultural productivity under certain circumstances, particularly when vector-borne pathogens are factored into the equation.[59] As a result of these vector-borne diseases, in many regions of the developing world, risk-averse farmers often forego higher output in exchange for diminished income volatility. For example, farmers in malarious regions of Paraguay frequently choose to produce crops that can be grown outside the malaria season, but which are of relatively lower value.[60] Thus the desire to avoid infection may result in sub-optimal economic outcomes for smallholder agricultural producers.

Under certain conditions, health investments can dramatically increase the productivity of land. For example, the reduction of malaria prevalence in Sri Lanka from 1947–77, increased national income by 9 per cent in 1977. The cumulative cost of disease-containment was $52 million, compared with a cumulative gain of $7.6 billion in national income over the same time period. This results in an impressive cost–benefit ratio of $140 gain per dollar originally invested in containment. During the exercise, regions that had been previously rendered hostile by vector-borne disease became increasingly settled as migrants moved in, generating increased output.[61]

ERIDs such as parasitic nematode worms can also have significant negative effects on the agricultural sector. In Nigeria, dracunculiasis (guinea worm disease) contributed to significant morbidity in over 2.5 million Nigerians during 1987. Cost–benefit analyses revealed that the disease was the chief impediment to increasing rice production in Nigeria, with the net effect of the disease being a reduction in rice production by $50 million in foregone revenue. Modelling suggested that the benefits of a worm control programme would exceed its costs after only four years.[62] The WHO is currently involved in a dracunculiasis control programme within selected regions of Africa, and the fruits of disease control are growing increasingly apparent. For example, reductions in dracunculiasis prevalence within targeted regions have resulted in a roughly 40 per cent increase in food production in those regions. The land under cultivation by farmers in these areas has increased by 25 per cent, and school absenteeism has declined from the level of 60 per cent to 13 per cent in certain regions.[63]

Thus, the proliferation of disease threatens 'food security' (i.e. the ability of the state to provide adequate nutritive resources for its population). This may in turn lead to increasing marginalization, famine and deprivation that will certainly contribute to increasing poverty and human misery. As HIV, tuberculosis, and vector-borne diseases spread across the globe, they have the potential to burden national economies that rely on labour-intensive agriculture to ensure both the sustenance of their own population and to generate exports in order to increase national revenue. The proliferation of disease threatens urban food supplies and foreign exchange earnings in a number of developing nations, particularly in sub-Saharan Africa, South and South-East Asia, and Latin America.

Education/training

One peculiar characteristic of the global AIDS pandemic is that unlike many other ERIDs (i.e. malaria) HIV does not spare the elite. HIV prevalence rates in high-income, urban, and well-educated African men are as high (or frequently higher) as rates in low-income and rural men. Since the elites have greater levels of consumption and investment and accrue higher wages, any disease affecting this group relatively more than other diseases is likely to have a greater impact per case.[64] Thus, decisions to make long-term societal investments in education are risky in Africa, as these investments in human capital are lost to HIV/AIDS with increasing frequency.[65] Cuddington argues that premature HIV-induced mortality will continue to erode national stocks of experienced workers, depleting existing reservoirs of human capital and limiting national output.

> [A]s AIDS becomes more prevalent, the perceived costs and benefits from undertaking new investments in human capital will change. Total expenditure will shift toward health care and away from schooling. To the extent that AIDS reduces expected lifetime, the incentives for individual workers or their employers to invest in education and training will also be reduced. Shifts in the relative wages of skilled and unskilled workers caused by differences in the

prevalence of AIDS among various skill groups might also affect decisions to invest in human capital.[66]

Infectious disease levels exhibit a significant negative correlation with the percentage of the eligible population of a state that is enrolled in secondary school.[67] The cases presented below demonstrate that outbreaks and/or rising levels of disease can prevent children from attending school, or from doing well if they do attend school. As the prevalence of infectious disease continues to grow, the costs and benefits from current investments in human capital are likely to shift. As a result, reduced spending on education will be the consequence of increasing national expenditures on health care to counter the effects of ERID.[68] Given that infectious diseases (particularly HIV/AIDS) tend to reduce life expectancy, the incentives for labourers or their employers to invest in training and education will diminish correspondingly. This results from the logic that there is little point in investing scarce resources in the education of someone who may be permanently debilitated by illness and therefore not likely to live to use the skills acquired through education. Furthermore, ERIDs may limit the efficacy of investing in human capital as poor health tends to undermine to capacity of children to learn and acquire skills. Dasgupta has observed that people who have been prone to illness and malnutrition in their youth, tend to have learning disabilities and reduced cognitive function which is directly related to their poor health status.[69] The World Bank has found that healthier and well-fed children do much better in school, and enrol with greater frequency than do their deprived counterparts. A recent study on Jamaican children infected with whipworm showed that those debilitated by nematode infection scored 15 per cent lower before treatment than healthy children in the same school. Following treatment, the previously-ill children were retested and achieved scores significantly closer to those of the healthy control group.[70]

Ainsworth, Over and Cuddington expect the HIV pandemic to produce demand and supply shocks resulting in negative outcomes within the education sector. They argue that AIDS will reduce the demand for education relative to an AIDS-free scenario for a number of reasons: reduced cohort size of those entering school, declining enrolment rates due to the fact that affected households may find school fees too burdensome or because children may be needed as labourers or caregivers.[71] USAID figures show that HIV/AIDS in Tanzania will reduce the number of children attending primary school by 22 per cent and the number of children in secondary school by 14 per cent from the level that could be expected without HIV/AIDS.[72] Supply-side shocks include depletion of the number of teachers available (due to increasing morbidity and mortality), increased teacher training and turnover costs, and reductions in the efficiency of the education system.[73] According to the World Bank, '(B)y 2010, Tanzania will have lost 14 460 teachers to AIDS. By 2020, some 27 000 teachers will have died. Training replacement teachers for the year 2020 will cost about $37.8 million (in 1991 dollars) in recurrent costs.'[74] Ultimately, these disruptions of the education sector will have a significant negative effect on the downstream formation and consolidation of human capital in severely-affected societies. Over time, as a result of these disruptions, the quality of the labour force will be significantly degraded, impairing long-term prospects for national growth. Demand-induced shocks to the education sector resulting from disease will also have a significant negative effect on the downstream formation of human capital overall.

Mining

As I have argued in the preceding pages, infectious diseases have a particularly negative economic impact on those sectors associated with labour-intensive modes of production. Mining is therefore among the most vulnerable of these sectors to the increasing global proliferation of ERID. Mining also tends to make a significant contribution to the economic output of many nations, particularly those in the developing world where resource extraction generates significant employment and revenues from export that can be used to offset foreign debt. For example, the copper industry in Zambia, which depends on young workers for its labour-intensive operations, accounts for almost 25 per cent of the country's Gross National Product, and 90 per cent of the country's export earnings.[75] The United Nations estimates that approximately 60 per cent of the copper industry's labour force will be HIV-infected by year 2000. This AIDS-induced morbidity and mortality will impair individual productivity and increase man-hours lost to illness. In addition, AIDS will generate increased expenditures resulting from benefits for ill employees and their dependents, death benefits, and the need to train new employees. The combination of these pressures will undermine industry profits and have a significant negative effect on Zambia's downstream prosperity, particularly if global copper prices recover from their current low level.[76]

The mining sector in Namibia accounts for approximately 12 per cent of GDP and for some 3.5 per cent of national employment. Thus, mining is a major contributor to national output and generates more than 50 per cent of total national export revenues. The industry will have to cope with the direct costs associated with the epidemic, namely absenteeism, health costs for employees and dependents, retraining costs and additional recruitment costs. But the greatest costs of the epidemic will result from the loss of skilled managerial and supervisory workers. This erosion of national reserves of human capacity will be difficult, costly and time-consuming to replace.[77]

Tourism

Increasing levels of infectious disease may also disrupt tourism in severely affected regions with the attendant reduction in revenue from foreign sources. Many countries in the developing world extract significant economic benefit from their tourism industries, particularly countries in the Caribbean basin and Oceania. The proliferation of diseases such as malaria, dengue, cholera and HIV may have serious and long-term negative impacts on the tourism sector for many nations, particularly those in the tropics. States that depend on revenues from tourism for employment and foreign exchange are vulnerable to the myriad negative effects of disease through the reduction of labour supply, changing domestic demand priorities as ERID reduces income, and demand shifts as tourists visit more benign destinations.[78]

In their study of the effect of AIDS on the Thai economy, Myers *et al.* concluded that, 'Thailand's $5 billion tourism industry may already be feeling the effects of AIDS. Tourist arrivals are down for a variety of reasons, with the fear of AIDS certain to be a significant factor in the future.'[79] Aside from attrition processes such as the HIV/AIDS pandemic, outbreak events such as the sudden re-emergence of ebola in Zaire, plague in India, and cholera in Peru generate extreme levels of fear derived from the human tendency of risk-aversion, and thus tourists avoid affected regions during the outbreak period. For example, the outbreak of cholera (the El Tor strain) in Peru during 1991 had a significant immediate effect on tourism revenues within that country. Kimball and Davis estimate that during the outbreak tourism revenues declined between 60 to 70 per cent in the first quarter of 1991 as compared to the first quarter of 1990.[80] Given that the fear of contagion can drive down tourism and deplete sectoral earnings, many afflicted states have an initial incentive not to report an outbreak, or to downplay its seriousness.

Macroeconomic analysis

The current resurgence in infectious disease promises increasing poverty and economic destabilization for severely affected countries. At the microeconomic level, we have noted the adverse impact of disease on economic well-being within individual families and firms, on the general quality of the labour force, on human capital formation and maintenance and on various sectors of the economy. It is logical to conclude that these microeconomic effects will generate, through multiplier effects, significant negative macroeconomic outcomes. Direct costs to the economy may be enormous, and indirect costs will include lost output due to increasing mortality and (to a lesser extent) ERID-induced morbidity.

The four factors of production are capital, land, technology and labour. Ainsworth argues that 'if the first three of these [factors] grow at a constant rate the slower growth in labour caused by the epidemic will ... slow the growth of output'.[81] ERIDs act synergistically, however, to exert negative effects on capital (both human capital and foreign investment) and land (diminishing access due to endemic infestation). This negative synergy should result in significant limits on national economic growth, and may result in growing poverty and national economic decline (particularly within the developing world). In their study of the effects of HIV on the Cameroonian economy, Kambou, Devarajan and Over argue that the worst economic effects of HIV manifest themselves when significant infection levels are prevalent in skilled urban workforces, and predict that HIV will result in a 2.2 per cent drag on the annual national GDP growth rate in Cameroon. They posit that the growth rates of saving and investment will decline rapidly, undercutting the GDP growth rate. This contraction of real output growth will accompany the simultaneous erosion of macroeconomic competitiveness in international markets. These effects have already been demonstrated in the declining growth rates of exports and increasing current account problems.[82]

Thus, ERID impedes the investment of foreign capital, erodes human capital resources (limiting the endogenous supply of social and technical ingenuity within a given state), and renders infested land and its natural resources economically useless. ERID may also affect technology as disease-induced mortality may reduce the pool of skilled individuals such as scientists and doctors who would otherwise have contributed to endogenous technological innovation.

Foreign investment

High rates of infectious disease prevalence in a given state will generate a disincentive for foreign capital owners to invest in states with high endemic ERID rates. High disease rates tend to correlate with diminished state productivity, and such countries may be less able to attract exogenous capital in order to improve infrastructure and stimulate economic reforms. States with higher pathogen prevalence levels are, therefore, less productive and prosperous. Thus, soaring disease rates in much of the developing world will diminish the probability of increasing foreign investment and undermine the ability of severely affected nations to generate economic growth.

As Fogel had suggested, declining disease rates over time increase the productivity of a given state. It is important to note the centrality of human capital in the economic equation of state prosperity and understand the significant role that public health plays in the generation and preservation of that valuable human capital. Thus, we may conclude that as public health improves, so does societal economic productivity. Conversely, as HIV, tuberculosis, malaria and other ERIDs continue to proliferate, we can conclude that this will undermine the economic productivity of severely affected states such as those in sub-Saharan Africa.

Savings

Infectious disease will also affect savings patterns at the macroeconomic level to produce negative outcomes. In Cuddington's analysis of the effect of AIDS on the Tanzanian economy, he predicts that one of the outcomes of the epidemic is a negative domestic saving effect. According to Cuddington, infectious diseases such as onchocerciasis, HIV and malaria will affect savings patterns in several ways. First, the immediate effect of increased medical expenditures will diminish saving as well as non-health current expenditures to a certain extent. Second, infectious diseases may negatively alter savings patterns through their pernicious effects on the life expectancy, age structure, healthiness and growth rate of the population. The attributes of national health delivery systems will determine whether the negative savings effect burdens the private or the public sector. Cuddington argues that the decline in domestic savings will generate a corresponding reduction in the formation of capital, and if the savings decline is significant it will produce a correspondingly large negative effect on per capita income over the long term.[83]

In developing countries, available savings and their use will significantly affect the growth rate of GNP. There are reasons to expect that the effects of HIV and the general proliferation of disease will be to reduce total national savings, resulting in reduced investment, diminished productive employment, lower per capita incomes, a drag on GNP growth rate, and in all likelihood a lower level of GNP.[84] Cohen concludes that disease-induced declines in national savings, resulting from domestic and exogenous sources, will generate a decline in the rate of investment, precipitating a fall in the GNP growth rate. Ultimately, expenditures on current output will likely grow, resulting in fewer savings to generate capital formation. As domestic savings decline, less investment is likely. Thus, exogenously supplied savings will decline in volume and will diminish relative to the growing needs induced by disease. Furthermore, it is probable that domestic savings will also decline as most productive sectors will be affected by ERID (notably by HIV). Additionally, declining foreign savings as a result of declining net long-term capital inflow will compromise national savings reservoirs over time.[85]

Trade

At the systems level, trade goods from ERID-affected areas may be subject to international embargo. This has been the keystone of the continuing discordance between the United Kingdom and its European partners, as British beef and beef by-products have been banned by the rest of the European Community due to the fear of contamination by the BSE agent that causes a lethal new variant of Creutzfeldt–Jakob disease (V-CJD) in humans. This trade embargo has seriously strained Britain's relationship with Brussels, to the extent that the then Prime Minister, John Major, once declared 'diplomatic war' on the rest of the European Union in an attempt to disrupt the agenda of European unification.[86] The economic damage to Britain has yet to be accurately measured but estimates run from a bare minimum of $8.4 billion (US) to upwards of $48 billion (US).[87]

Similarly, the re-emergence of cholera in Peru from 1991–96 had significant effects on trade and national prosperity. The epidemic generated over 600 000 cases and 4500 deaths in Peru and spread rapidly throughout equatorial South America. As a result of the epidemic, Peru experienced trade-related costs due to cancelled orders for exports of foodstuffs, including fresh fruit and seafood. These export costs, including deterioration in prices of export goods, delayed sales, cancelled orders, and increased inspection costs, resulted in the loss of $700 million in export revenue for 1991 alone.[88]

The Indian city of Surat saw an outbreak of plague in September 1994, resulting in mass panic and the rapid out-migration of peoples from the affected region. Because of the nature of the contagion, the pestilence generated a global epidemic of fear. Despite the fact that only 56 people perished as a result of the contagion, the economic damage to India resulting from foregone export revenues was significant. Specifically, many Indian goods were the subject of international embargo for the duration of the epidemic, ranging from foodstuffs to fabric and diamonds. Costs of the epidemic to India range from $1.3 to $1.7 billion, a significant sum given the persistent frailty of the Indian economy.[89]

It is important to differentiate between *outbreak events* and *attrition processes* when we evaluate the potential for ERID to increasingly disrupt trade. Attrition processes are highly unlikely to generate the significant levels of affect (fear) that may lead to an international boycott of a given country's exports. Conversely, outbreak events tend to generate high levels of fear, which when coupled with the generalized human tendency to risk-aversion, result in extreme (and often inappropriate) measures, such as trade restrictions on Indian diamonds. Once the hysteria of an outbreak event dissipates, normal trade patterns will likely resume. Attrition processes, on the other hand, are likely to have greater negative long-term effects on trade, as every factory worker felled by contagion fails to produce marketable products indefinitely into the future, depending upon the nature of the good in question.

National costs

Malaria

According to recent USAID estimates, more than 85 per cent of global malaria cases occur in sub-Saharan Africa where the disease is responsible for approximately 2.5 million deaths per year. The negative economic impact of malaria on the region is substantial and increasing: for example, the direct economic cost of malaria in Africa for 1987 was $800 million; it rose to $1.7 billion by 1995; and it is projected to reach $3.5 billion by the year 2000. Moreover, USAID estimates that health care costs for malaria on an out-patient basis account for approximately 40 per cent of current national public health expenditures in sub-Saharan Africa.[90] USAID predicts that the region can expect a 7–20 per cent annual increase in the burden of malaria-induced mortality and morbidity in the coming decade.[91] As Shepard, Ettling, Brinkmann and Sauerborn pointed out in 1991, the direct and indirect costs of disease are often greater than the amount of economic aid provided to afflicted regions by international donor agencies:

> (I)n 1987 the cost of malaria in sub-Saharan Africa was about $791 million per year. This figure is projected to rise to $1684 million by 1995. By comparison, the entire health assistance to Africa of a major bilateral donor, the U.S. Agency for International Development, was only $52 million for all conditions.[92]

Ettling and Shepard's study of malaria's economic cost to Rwanda demonstrated that malaria's drag on the national GDP rose from 1 per cent in 1989 to an estimated 2.4 per cent in 1995, a 140 per cent increase over 5 years.[93] Recent studies by the World Health Organization in Burkina Faso, Chad, Congo and Rwanda, show that the cost of an average case of malaria in sub-Saharan Africa is equivalent to about 12 days of productive output. The total cost for the area in 1995 was projected at $1684 million or 1 per cent of GDP (having risen from $791 million or 0.6 per cent of the GDP in 1987).[94] This represents an increase in costs to the regional GDP of 66.7 per cent from 1987 to 1995. Extrapolating conservatively from the trendline, malaria alone will exert a drag of 1.67 per cent on the regional GDP by 2003, and possibly as high as 4.64 per cent by 2012.

Of course, one must consider the fact that the impact of malaria differs from state to state; South Africa has a relatively minor malaria problem, for example, compared to the tropical states in the Great Lakes region of Central Africa. Shepard estimates that malaria incidence in Rwanda increased an average of 21 per cent every year through the 1980s (an eightfold increase since 1979), while malaria incidence in Togo increased by a relatively modest 10.4 per cent/annum over the same time period. Furthermore, malarial resistance to quinine increased from 0 to 30 per cent for the whole of Africa, and rose to an astonishing level of 66 per cent in Rwanda over the same time period. Regional resistance to another powerful anti-malarial agent (the drug fansidar) is estimated at 34 per cent.[95] Unfortunately, malaria is not confined to the African continent and its spread bodes ill for other tropical regions, particularly South Asia. In a detailed study, V.P. Sharma concludes that malaria generates an annual economic loss of anywhere between US $0.5 to $1 billion annually to the Indian economy.[96] As malaria spreads throughout South and South-East Asia, Oceania and Latin America, we should expect to see mounting damage to the economies of those affected regions.

HIV/AIDS

> We have every reason to assume that the epidemic in South-East Asia will soon be just as widespread as it is in Africa. And that East Africa's experience – a slow down of its economy – will be replicated in Eastern Europe and the developing countries of Asia and Latin America.
>
> Peter Piot, Director UNAIDS[97]

The significance of the economic costs resulting from the HIV pandemic are now becoming clearer, draining government coffers and markets in both the developing and developed world. Hellinger notes the burdensome costs imposed by HIV infection on the American health care budget. He estimates that the lifetime cost of treating a person with HIV from the time of infection until death is approximately $119 000.[98] Hanveldt *et al.* compared the societal impact of HIV/AIDS with other selected causes of male mortality to determine the indirect costs of lost future production in Canada. Over the period 1987–91, the HIV/AIDS epidemic resulted in the loss of $2.11 billion (US) to the Canadian economy.

> Assuming a 2 per cent annual growth in earnings and a 3 per cent annual real discount rate. ... Deaths due to HIV/AIDS accounted for 2.11 billion in 1990 US$. Future production loss due to HIV/AIDS more than doubled during the period from 1987 to 1991, from 0.27 to 0.60 billion 1990 US$. Our findings demonstrated HIV/AIDS mortality is already having a dramatic impact on future wealth production in Canada. If the past trend continues, the production lost in 1994 should exceed 0.86 billion 1990 US$ and will account for more than 10 per cent of the total annual loss for men aged 25–64 years.[99]

In 1993, D.C. Lambert estimated the costs of AIDS-related deaths in France. He concludes that the annual cost of AIDS-induced mortality in France is between 10 and 12 billion ($US) in 1989 and between 18 and 20 billion in 1992. Based on the trendline of the epidemic, he argues that the costs of HIV to the French economy will reach between $32.4 and $36 billion for 1995.[100] Furthermore, Newton *et al.* examined the past and potential impact of HIV/AIDS in 19 English-speaking nations of the Caribbean, and estimated that the total annual costs of the epidemic will approach $US 500 million per annum (in constant 1989 US$) or 2 per cent of GDP in the low scenario, and will exceed $US 1200 million per annum or 5 per cent of GDP in the high scenario.[101]

Bloom *et al.* conducted a study to estimate the significant negative impact of HIV on the Human Development Index. The researchers used a sample of 56 countries over the 1980–92 period, and concluded that HIV resulted in the global loss of 1.3 years of human development progress per country. Some countries in particular have borne an enormous toll: Zambia has lost ten years of development, Tanzania has lost 8 years, and Malawi and Zimbabwe have lost approximately 5 years.[102] It should be noted that the pandemic has greatly increased in seroprevalence levels since the 1980–92 era, and thus the negative developmental impacts will likely be significantly greater than Bloom's original figures.

Recent studies by USAID conclude that AIDS will infect 25 per cent of Kenya's population by 2005, and reduce Kenya's GDP by 10 per cent.[103] Cuddington argues that HIV/AIDS may reduce Tanzanian GDP in the year 2010 by 15–25 per cent in relation to a counter-factual non-AIDS scenario.[104] Julia Dayton concurs, noting that the presence of AIDS in Tanzania will likely reduce the average real growth rate in the 1985–2010 period by between 15 and 28 per cent, from 2.9 to 4.0 per cent per annum. Over a 25 year period, this decreases potential output by between (1980) Tsh 15 billion to Tsh 25 billion. The net impact of HIV on growth of potential Tanzanian GDP per capita is estimated at a reduction of 12 per cent (vs a counter-factual non-HIV scenario).[105]

Piot has warned that several of the most promising emerging markets, particularly China, India and Thailand, are likely to replicate the experience of sub-Saharan Africa in a few years, something that would be a disaster for the global economy.[106] Myers *et al.* predict that the negative macroeconomic effects of HIV/AIDS in Thailand will continue to slow the rate of economic growth:

> The total annual health care costs plus the value of lost income is projected to grow from $100 million in 1991 to $2.2 billion by 2000 in the high scenario and from $97 million to $1.8 billion in the low scenario. Over a ten year period, $8.7 billion will be lost due to AIDS illness and death in the high case and $7.3 billion in the low case. These annual costs, both direct and indirect, equal about 16–18 times the per capita GDP.[107]

A recent study, commissioned by the UNDP's Regional Bureau for Asia and the Pacific, has examined the detrimental effect of the HIV/AIDS pandemic on development and concludes that the HIV pandemic will cost Thailand approximately nine years of human development, while denying Myanmar (Burma) five years of developmental progress between 1992 and 2005. India, which will soon be the HIV/AIDS capital of Asia, will forego one year of development progress by 2005, with the loss accelerating thereafter.[108]

Piot warns that by the year 2000, the world economic impact of AIDS could be as high as equivalent to 4 per cent of the GDP of the United States or the entire economy of India.[109] In the 1994 version of the UNDP's Human Development Report, the cumulative direct and indirect costs of HIV/AIDS throughout the 1980s have been estimated at $240 billion. The report states: 'The social and psychological costs of the epidemic for individuals, families, communities and nations are also huge – but inestimable.' The report goes on to predict that 'The global cost – direct and indirect – of HIV and AIDS by 2000 could be as high as $500 billion a year – equivalent to more than 2 per cent of global GDP.'[110]

Based on the balance of evidence, we can reasonably conclude that the global proliferation of ERID will impose a general drag on the productivity and prosperity of seriously affected states. Under extreme conditions of endemic pathogen infection within the national population pool (i.e. most countries in sub-Saharan Africa), disease has the potential to destabilize economies and push entire regions into economic decline. Unfortunately, social scientists currently have no idea where the threshold of collapse may lie, after which the system may rapidly slide into a negative economic spiral dynamic.[111] Available models are based upon the anecdotal experience of historians and their observations of the effects that various forms of pestilence had upon local populations at distant points in time. Given the rapid and significant changes in population density, urbanization, migration, environmental decay and travel times in the twentieth century, we have no clear idea of the levels at which pathogen seroprevalence in local populations may push societies across a poorly demarcated threshold into such a negative economic spiral.

Given the evidence presented above, it is reasonable to speculate that one of the principal barriers to the development of pathogen-laden tropical areas is the economic burden that ERID inflicts on those societies. If we extrapolate from Fogel's arguments it becomes apparent that one reason for the significant gap between the developed states of temperate regions and the generally underdeveloped tropical states is the intensity of infectious disease in tropical regions.[112] Such arguments are taken as obvious within the medical community, but have yet to be recognized by the community of scholars of international development in the social sciences.

The strong association between health and prosperity is certainly evident in sub-Saharan Africa, which is the area of highest ERID prevalence in the world, and, not surprisingly, the poorest region of the world as well, despite the presence of significant natural resources. Besides having the highest prevalence of endemic regional pathogens, sub-Saharan Africa is also host to the most virulent sub-epidemic of the AIDS pandemic. Now that the HIV pandemic is thoroughly entrenched in Africa, we should be concerned about the economic instability that the epidemic will bring in its wake as it spreads through both South and South-East Asia and Eastern Europe. The UNDP has predicted that economic losses resulting from AIDS could soon exceed total foreign aid to seriously affected states.[113] Based on the experience of sub-Saharan Africa, and given the data we now have, it seems reasonable to predict that as ERID continues to proliferate on a global scale, we will see increasing poverty and economic polarization between social classes within societies.

Ultimately, the global proliferation of ERID poses a significant long-term threat to the economic capacity of states, as ERID-induced economic shocks force a contraction of the frontier of national production possibilities and threaten the development prospects of many societies. Indeed, ERID is already undermining hard-won economic and social gains throughout the developing world, particularly in the tropical regions of the globe. The available evidence suggests that the negative effects of infectious disease on economic productivity are, unfortunately, likely to be greatest in the developing world (due to initially low state capacity, geographical endemicity and lower endogenous adaptation capacity). ERID constitutes a significant long-term threat to the economic stability of states and possibly entire regions, particularly those within the tropical zones of the planet.

Notes

1. The geographical distribution of industrialized and developing nations, and its possible relation to disease prevalence, was discussed with Daniel Deudney during a conversation in Toronto on 18 November 1997.

2. See Robert W. Fogel, 'The Conquest of High Mortality and Hunger in Europe and America: Timing and Mechanisms' in David Landes, Patrice Higgonet, and Henry Rosovsky, eds, *Favorites of Fortune: Technology, Growth and Economic Development Since the Industrial Revolution* (Cambridge, MA: Harvard University Press, 1991). Also see Fogel's 'Nutrition and the Decline in Mortality Since 1700: Some preliminary Findings in Long-Term Factors in American Economic Growth' in Stanley L. Engerman and Robert E. Gallman, eds, *Conference on Research in Income and Wealth* (Vol. 41. Chicago, IL: University of Chicago Press, 1986); and *Economic Growth, Population Theory, and Physiology: the Bearing of Long-Term Processes in the Making of Economic Policy*, Working Paper no. 4638 (Cambridge, MA: National Bureau of Economic Research, April 1994).

3. William McNeill, *Plagues and Peoples*, p. 162.

4. Price-Smith, *Health of Nations*, 1999, Ch. 3.

5. See Desmond Cohen, *Socio-Economic Causes and Consequences of the HIV Epidemic in Southern Africa: a Case Study of Namibia* (UNDP HIV and Development Programme. Issues Paper #31, available at http://www.undp.org:80/hiv/issues/English/issue31.htm), pp. 10–18.

6. Martha Ainsworth, and A. Mead Over, 'The Economic Impact of AIDS on Africa' in Max Essex *et al.*, eds, *AIDS in Africa* (New York: Raven Press, 1994), p. 564.

7. See John Cuddington, 'Modeling the Macroeconomic Effects of AIDS, with an Application to Tanzania', *World Bank Economic Review*, Vol. 7, No. 2 (May 1993), p. 175.

8. Op. cit., p. 565.

9. Myers, Charles, Stasia Obremsky and Mechai Viravaidya, *The Economic Impact of AIDS on Thailand. Working Paper No. 4* (Boston: Harvard School of Public Health, 1992), p. 9.

10. Ibid., p. 8.

11. World Bank, *The Macroeconomic Effects of AIDS: Development Brief Number 17, July 1993*, available at http://www.worldbank.org/html/dec/Publications/Briefs/DB17.html (March 8, 1997), p. 1.

12. See S. Poonawala, and R. Cantor, *Children Orphaned by AIDS: a Call for Action for NGOs and Donors* (Washington, DC: National Council for International Health, 1991).

13. *AIDS and the Demography of Africa* (Department for Economic and Social Information and Policy Analysis, United Nations, New York, 1994), p. 3.

14. Ainsworth and Over, 'The Economic Impact of AIDS on Africa', p. 565.

15. For an excellent discussion of pecuniary and non-pecuniary costs associated with ERIDs, see David E. Bloom, and Geoffrey Carliner, 'The Economic Impact of AIDS in the United States', *Science*, Vol. 239, p. 604.

16. Kimberly A. Hamilton, *Global HIV/AIDS: a Strategy for U.S. Leadership* (Washington, DC: Center for Strategic and International Studies, 1994), p. 5.

17. *AIDS and the Demography of Africa* (Department for Economic and Social Information and Policy Analysis, United Nations, 1994), p. 4.

18. *World Development Report 1993: Investing in Health* (New York: Oxford University Press, 1993), p. 18.

19. For additional information on these re-adjustment processes, see Ainsworth and Over, 'The Economic Impact of AIDS on Africa', p. 564.
20. *The World Health Report 1996: Fighting Disease Fostering Development* (Geneva: World Health Organization, 1996), p. 7.
21. With the obvious exception of the highly lethal *P. falciparum* malaria.
22. D. Ettling, D.A. McFarland, L.J. Schultz and L. Chitsulo, 'Economic Impact of Malaria in Malawian Households', *Tropical Medicine and Parasitology*, Vol. 45, No. 1 (March 1994), p. 74.
23. See R. Barlow, *The Economic Effects of Malaria Eradication* (Ann Arbor: University of Michigan, 1967); M. Gomes, 'Economic and Demographic Research on Malaria: a Review of the Evidence', *Social Science and Medicine*, Vol. 37, No. 9 (November 1993), pp. 1093–108; R. Sauerborn *et al.*, 'Estimating the Direct and Indirect Costs of Malaria in a Rural District of Burkina Faso', *Tropical Medicine and Parasitology*, Vol. 42 (1991), pp. 219–23; R.E. Castilla and D.O. Sawyer, 'Malaria Rates and Fate: a Socioeconomic Study of Malaria in Brazil', *Social Science and Medicine*, Vol. 37, No. 9, November 1993, pp. 1137–45; D. Sawyer, 'Economic and Social Consequences of Malaria in New Colonization Projects in Brazil', *Social Science and Medicine*, Vol. 37, No. 9 (November 1993), pp. 1131–6.; E.T. Nur, 'The Impact of Malaria on Labour Use and Efficiency in the Sudan', *Social Science and Medicine*, Vol. 37, No. 9 (November 1993), pp. 1115–19; N.K. Kere *et al.*, 'The Economic Impact of *Plasmodium falciparum* Malaria on Education Investment: a Pacific Island Case Study', *Southeast Asian Journal of Tropical Medicine and Public Health*, Vol. 24, No. 4 (December 1993), pp. 659–63; A. Mills. 'The Household Costs of Malaria in Nepal', *Tropical Medicine and Parasitology*, Vol. 44, No. 1 (March 1993), pp. 9–13; W.K. Asenso-Okyere, 'Socioeconomic Factors in Malaria Control', *World Health Forum*, Vol. 15, No. 3 (1994), pp. 265–8; B.M. Popkin, 'A Household Framework for Examining the Social and Economic Consequences of Tropical Diseases', *Social Sciences and Medicine*, Vol. 16, No. 5 (1982), pp. 533–43.
24. *World Development Report 1993: Investing in Health*, p. 17.
25. J. Brian Atwood, *Speech at USAID Conference on Infectious Disease*, Washington DC, 17 December 1997, available at http://www.info.usaid. gov/press/spe_test/speeches/spch560.htm, p. 1.
26. Ainsworth and Over, 'The Economic Impact of AIDS on Africa', p. 566.
27. *Better Health in Africa: Experience and Lessons Learned* (Washington, DC: World Bank, 1994), p. 27.
28. See T.W. Schultz, 'Investment in Human Capital', *American Economic Review*, Vol. 51 (1961), pp. 1–17; T.W. Schultz, *Investing in People: the Economics of Population Quality* (Berkeley: University of California Press, 1981); G.S. Becker, K.M. Murphy and R. Tamura 'Human Capital, Fertility, and Economic Growth', *Journal of Political Economy*, Vol. 98 (1990), pp. S12–S37; N.L. Stokey, 'Human Capital, Product Quality, and Growth', *Quarterly Journal of Economics*, Vol. 105 (1991), pp. 587–616; and Dasgupta, 1993, Ch. 16.
29. Sir Richard Sykes, *Private and Public Partnerships in the Fight Against HIV/AIDS*, address to the World Economic Forum 1997 Annual Meeting, Davos, available at http://www.us.unaids.org/highband/speeches/sykes, 30 January–4 February.

30. Callisto Madavo, *AIDS, Development, and the Vital Role of Government*, speech, available at http://worldbank.org/aids-econ/madavo.htm, p. 2.
31. Dr Piot is currently the head of UNAIDS in Geneva.
32. *World Development Report 1993: Investing in Health* (New York: Oxford University Press, 1993), p. 20.
33. Peter Piot, *Business in a World of HIV/AIDS*. Statement at World Economic Forum, 3 February 1997, Davos. Available at http://www.us.unaids.org/highband/speeches/davspc.html, p. 3.
34. John T. Cuddington, and John D. Hancock, 'Assessing the Impact of AIDS on the Growth Path of the Malawian Economy', *Journal of Development Economics*, Vol. 43 (1994), p. 364.
35. Ainsworth and Over, 'The Economic Impact of AIDS on Africa', p. 567.
36. *World Development Report 1993: Investing in Health*, p. 18.
37. Desmond Cohen, *The Economic Impact of the HIV Epidemic: Issues Paper #2*, UNDP HIV and Development Programme (New York: UNDP, 1998). Available at http://www.undp. org:80/hiv/issues2e.htm, p. 6.
38. *AIDS in Uganda: Impacts and Responses* (Washington, DC: World Bank, 1994), p. 4.
39. Myers, Obremsky and Viravaidya, *The Economic Impact of AIDS on Thailand*, p. 15.
40. Ainsworth and Over, 'The Economic Impact of AIDS on Africa', p. 568.
41. Sir Richard Sykes, *Private and Public Partnerships in the Fight Against HIV/AIDS*, p. 3.
42. Joshua Lederberg *et al.*, *Emerging Infections*, p. 58.
43. See *World Health Report 1996: Fighting Disease Fostering Development* (Geneva: World Health Organization, 1996), p. 7; Ainsworth and Over, 'The Economic Impact of AIDS on Africa', p. 569.
44. *AIDS and the Demography of Africa*, Department for Economic and Social Information and Policy Analysis, United Nations, p. 3.
45. See Chin, J. 'The Epidemiology and Projected Mortality of AIDS' in Richard G. Feacham and Dean T. Jamison, eds, *Diseases and Mortality in Sub-Saharan Africa* (New York: Oxford University Press, 1994); *AIDS and the Demography of Africa*, Department for Economic and Social Information and Policy Analysis, United Nations, p. 4.
46. See Mechai Viravaidya, Stasia A. Obremsky and Charles Myers, 'The Economic Impact of AIDS on Thailand' in David Bloom and E. Lyons, eds, *Economic Implications of AIDS in Asia* (New Delhi: UNDP, 1993); Kimberly A. Hamilton, *Global HIV/AIDS: a Strategy for U.S. Leadership* (Washington, DC: Center for Strategic and International Studies, 1994), p. 20.
47. Lyn Squire, 'Confronting AIDS' in *Finance and Development* (March 1988), p. 17.
48. Nelson Mandela, *AIDS: Facing up to the Global Threat*, p. 3.
49. William McNeill, *Plagues and Peoples*, p. 220.
50. See *The Implications of HIV/AIDS for Rural Development Policy and Programming: Focus on Sub-Saharan Africa*, UNDP HIV and Development Programme, Study Paper #6. Available at http://www/undp.org:80/hiv/Study /SP6/sp6chap1&2. htm, p. 3.
51. See James Sender and S. Smith, *Poverty, Class and Gender in Rural Africa: a Tanzanian Case Study* (London: Routledge, 1990), and S. Devereux. and

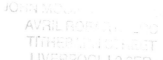

G. Eele, *Monitoring the Social and Economic Impact of AIDS in East and Central Africa* (Food Studies Group, Oxford University, Report Commissioned for UNDP, September 1991).

52.   *AIDS and the Demography of Africa*, p. 4.

53.   Southern Africa may be understood in this case to incorporate Botswana, Zambia, Zimbabwe, Namibia and South Africa.

54.   Ainsworth and Over, 'The Economic Impact of AIDS on Africa', p. 570.

55.   Tony Barnett, and Piers Blaikie, 'The Impact of AIDS on Farming Systems' in *AIDS in Africa: Its Present and Future Impact* (London: Guilford Press, 1992), p. 151.

56.   *AIDS and the Demography of Africa*, p. 4.

57.   Jill Armstrong, *Uganda's AIDS Crisis: Its Implications for Development* (Washington, DC: World Bank, 1994), p. 4.

58.   *The Socio-Economic Impact of HIV and AIDS on Rural Families in Uganda: an Emphasis on Youth: Study Paper #2* (UNDP HIV and Development Programme), available at http://www/undp. org:80/hiv/Study/sp2Echap2. htm, pp. 15–16.

59.   For example, aerial vector-borne diseases such as malaria, dengue, yellow fever, and various strains of encephalitis have significant negative effects on agricultural productivity throughout the tropical regions of the planet.

60.   *World Development Report 1993: Investing in Health*, p. 18. Such crops include cheap staples such as maize, wheat and potatoes.

61.   Ibid., p. 18.

62.   World Bank. *Better Health in Africa: Experience and Lessons Learned* (Washington, DC: World Bank, 1994), p. 25.

63.   *World Health Report 1996: Fighting Disease Fostering Development* (Geneva: World Health Organization, 1996), p. 45.

64.   Ainsworth and Over, 'The Economic Impact of AIDS on Africa', p. 561.

65.   Gerald Helleiner recently noted that of the 20 agro-economists that his group had recently trained in Africa, 10 had died of HIV/AIDS within the last year. Author's conversation with Dr Helleiner, 18 December 1998.

66.   John Cuddington, 'Modeling the Macroeconomic Effects of AIDS, with an Application to Tanzania', *World Bank Economic Review*, Vol. 7, No. 2 (May 1993), p. 176.

67.   See Andrew T. Price-Smith, *The Health of Nations: Infectious Disease and its Effects on State Capacity, Prosperity and Stability*, Doctoral Dissertation, Department of Political Science, University of Toronto, July 1999.

68.   Ibid., p. 175.

69.   For an extensive review of this argument see Partha S. Dasgupta, *An Inquiry into Well-Being and Destitution*.

70.   *World Development Report 1993: Investing in Health*, p. 18.

71.   John Cuddington, 'Modeling the Macroeconomic Effects of AIDS, with an Application to Tanzania', p. 175.

72.   See USAID at http://www.info.usaid.gov/press/spe_test/speeches/spch560. htm, p. 2.

73.   Ainsworth and Over, 'The Economic Impact of AIDS on Africa', p. 571.

74.   World Bank, *Tanzania: AIDS assessment and planning study, no. 9825-TA* (Population and Human Resources Division, Southern Africa Department, Washington, DC: World Bank, 1992).

75. See B. Nkowane, 'The Direct and Indirect Cost of HIV Infection in Developing Countries: the Cases of Zaire and Tanzania' in Alan F. Fleming *et al.*, eds, *The Global Impact of AIDS* (New York: Alan Liss, 1988); and Desmond Cohen, *The Economic Impact of the HIV Epidemic: Issues Paper #2*, p. 11.

76. *AIDS and the Demography of Africa*, p. 4.

77. Desmond Cohen, *Socio-Economic Causes and Consequences of the HIV Epidemic in Southern Africa: a Case Study of Namibia, Issues Paper #31* (UNDP HIV and Development Programme), available at http://www.undp.org:80/hiv/issues/ English/issue31.htm, p. 16.

78. See Desmond Cohen, *The Economic Impact of the HIV Epidemic: Issues Paper #2* (New York: UNDP HIV and Development Programme), available at http://www.undp.org:80/hiv/issues2e.htm, p. 11.

79. Myers, Obremsky and Viravaidya, p. 15.

80. See Ann-Marie Kimball and Robert Davis, *The Economics of Emerging Infections in the Asia Pacific: what do we know and what do we need to know?* Paper presented at CIS/CIH Conference on the Social and Economic Impact of Emerging and Re-emerging Infectious Diseases, 30 October 1997, University of Toronto, Toronto, Canada. Published by Program on Health and Global Affairs/CIS and available on line at http://www.utoronto.ca/cis/pgha.html, p. 7.

81. Ibid., p. 578.

82. See G. Kambou, S. Devarajan and M. Over, 'The Economic Impact of the AIDS Crisis in Sub-Saharan Africa: Simulations with a Computable General Equilibrium Model', *Journal of African Economies*, Vol. 1, No. 1 (1992).

83. John Cuddington, 'Modeling the Macroeconomic Effects of AIDS, with an Application to Tanzania', p. 175.

84. See Desmond Cohen, *The Economic Impact of the HIV Epidemic: Issues Paper #2*, p. 4.

85. Ibid., p. 4.

86. Madelaine Drohan, 'Major Thwarts EU to Protest Beef Ban', *Globe and Mail*, 23 May 1996.

87. Economist. 'Mad Cows and Englishmen', reprinted in *Globe and Mail*, 25 March 1996, p. A15.

88. See Kimball and Davis, p. 7.

89. Ibid., p. 8.

90. See USAID Factsheets, available at http://www.info.usaid.gov/pop_health/child_sur/malaria.htm.

91. J. Brian Atwood, *Combatting Malaria*, available at http://www.info.usaid.gov/press/spe_test/speeches/spch556.htm, p. 1.

92. See Donald S. Shepard *et al.*, 'The Economic Cost of Malaria in Africa', *Tropical Medicine and Parasitology*, Vol. 42 (1991), pp. 119–203.

93. Mary B Ettling, and D.S. Shepard, 'Economic Cost of Malaria in Rwanda', *Tropical Medicine and Parasitology*, Vol. 42 (1991), p. 214.

94. World Health Organization, *A Global Strategy for Malaria Control* (Geneva: WHO, 1994), pp. 1–7.

95. Uwe Brinkmann and A. Brinkmann, 'Malaria and Health in Africa: the Present Situation and Epidemiological Trends', *Tropical Medicine and Parasitology* (Vol. 42, 1991), p. 204.

96. V.P. Sharma, 'Malaria: Cost to India and Future Trends', *Southeast Asian Journal of Tropical Medicine and Public Health*, Vol. 27, No. 1, pp. 4–14.

97. Peter Piot, *Business in a World of HIV/AIDS*, statement at World Economic Forum, 3 February 1997 Davos, available at http://www.us.unaids.org/highband/speeches/davspc.html, p. 3.

98. Disaggregated, the estimated costs of individual care from HIV infection until the development of AIDS is $50 000 while the estimated costs from AIDS development until death is approximately $69 000. F J. Hellinger, 'The Lifetime Cost of Treating a Person with HIV', *JAMA*, Vol. 270, No. 4 (28 July 1993), p. 74.

99. R.A. Hanvelt *et al.*, 'Indirect Costs of HIV/AIDS Mortality in Canada', *AIDS*, Vol. 8, No. 10 (October 1994), pp. F7–11.

100. D.C. Lambert, 'Prospects of the Cost of AIDS-Related Death in France: 1970–2020' (French), *Cahiers de Sociologie et de Demographie Medicales*, Vol. 33, No. 3 (Jul–Sep 1993), pp. 249–87.

101. E.A. Newton *et al.*, 'Modeling the HIV/AIDS Epidemic in the English-speaking Caribbean', *Bulletin of the Pan American Health Organization*, Vol. 28, No. 3 (Sep. 1994), pp. 239–49.

102. See David Bloom *et al.*, 1996. Cited in Desmond Cohen, *Socio-Economic Causes and Consequences of the HIV Epidemic in Southern Africa: a Case Study of Namibia, Issues Paper #31*, p. 12.

103. 'Kenya faces 10 per cent drop in GDP as result of AIDS, US study finds', *Independent Online*, http://www.inc.co.za/online/news/politics/africa/ afdigest.html, 25/07/97.

104. World Bank, *The Macroeconomic Effects of AIDS: Development Brief Number 17, July 1993*, available at http://www.worldbank.org/html/dec/Publications/Briefs/DB17.html, p. 1.

105. Julia Dayton, *World Bank HIV/AIDS Interventions: Ex-Ante and Ex-Post Evaluation, World Bank Discussion Paper #389* (Washington, DC: World Bank, 1 June 1998), p. 30.

106. *UNAIDS Director Calls Upon Business Leaders to Initiate Aggressive Efforts Against AIDS* (UNAIDS, 3 February 1997). Available at http://www.us.unaids.org/highband/press/davospr.html, p. 2.

107. See Myers, Obremsky and Viravaidya, p. 8.

108. 'AIDS Leading Threat to Public Health', *HINDU ONLINE*, available at http://www.webpage.com/hindu/950916/18/1516c.html.

109. Peter Piot, *Business in a World of HIV/AIDS*, p. 3.

110. United Nations Development Programme, *Human Development Report 1994* (New York: Oxford University Press, 1994), p. 28.

111. As with many natural systems, the level of inputs into a system may cross boundaries at which the entire system suddenly and chaotically shifts, gradually establishing a new equilibrium that may be irreversible. This argument follows on Thomas F. Homer-Dixon's concept of 'threshold' dynamics as detailed in Thomas F. Homer-Dixon, 'On the Threshold: Environmental Changes as Causes of Acute Conflict', pp. 43–83.

112. See Fogel, 'The Conquest of High Mortality and Hunger in Europe and America: Timing and Mechanisms'.

113. UNAIDS, *UNAIDS Director Delivers Opening Plenary at U.S. AIDS Research Conference*, press release, 22 January 1997, available at http://www.us.unaids.org/highband/press/retpren.html, p. 2.

7
The Map is not the Territory: Reconceiving Human Security

Jim Whitman

However broad their scope, theories of world politics are abstractions from the richness and complexity of life. Of course, theorizing necessitates boundaries which define and limit what is deemed pertinent and within which coherent understanding and explanatory power can be developed and defended. This generally holds, however difficult it might sometimes be to clearly distinguish the border between, say, international relations and international political economy; or between economics and economic sociology.[1]

Theories are refined, strengthened expanded – and challenged – by empirical evidence. They are also open to challenge on part-empirical/conceptual grounds. So, in common with others, theories of world politics can be judged on their comprehensiveness, their ability to predict the trajectory of variables within their bounds, and by their inclusion of features or actors thought by some to be salient rather than peripheral. Within academic circles, the re-evaluation of classic texts and established theories, while sometimes appearing to be rather arcane, helps to drive research agendas. More pragmatically, but to an extent difficult to determine, theories of international relations are thought to provide some framework for practitioners.[2] Whatever the utility of such theories for those who shape and execute public policy, James Rosenau and Mary Durfee point out that 'the alternatives to seeking comprehension are too noxious to contemplate, ranging as they do from resorting to simplistic and ideological interpretations to being propelled by forces we can neither discern nor influence'.[3]

Our delineation and separation of aspects of social and political life are necessary abstractions, then, but our actual engagement with the world is rarely so tidy. For example, the insights of cognitive psychology place decisions of historical moment in a light which reveals the

151

underlying human frailties of high politics.[4] Similarly, might we search the familiar world for the 'rational actor' of economic theory.

Theories are tentative and their boundaries permeable. Specific challenges can be accommodated, rejected or form part of the substance of exchange between disciplines – a rich source of creative thinking and intellectual growth. But what is of fascination in the last decade of world politics is not so much the meaning to be had from theoretical refinements and painstaking research into minor anomalies, but the sheer scale, variety and pace of change and the formidable strain this places on our capacities, formal and informal, to fashion a satisfactory picture of the world. Consider for example the apparent 'epidemic of epidemics' (including but not limited to HIV/AIDS);[5] a single investment company generating a crisis within the world political economy by exposing itself to US$900 billion of debt; that natural disasters (including environmental degradation) now generate more refugees than war and conflict;[6] the diminution of planetary biodiversity;[7] and the implications of global warming and ozone layer depletion.

Against well-established theories, especially in the field of international relations, the simple but searching question, 'of what is this an instance?'[8] now often appears uncomfortably oblique. This applies particularly to Realist theories, with their assertion of the predominance of state power. Realists might well counter that the turbulence of world politics renders considerations of state power all the more important;[9] and that in any event, the impacts of non-state actors and global dynamics hardly diminish the significance of matters more directly within the orbit of state competence: war in the Balkans and elsewhere; nuclear rivalry between India and Pakistan; and the development of chemical and biological weapons by states such as North Korea, Libya and Syria.[10] Yet ours is a world in which the pervasiveness and practical import of the larger forces of world politics and the direct impact of the planet's changing natural systems have come to be matters of urgent concern for governments, even as their capacity to summon and exert the requisite authority is diminished. The inability of states to control global flows of capital is a familiar case in point;[11] and there is abundant evidence that the potential of a variety of human groups to bring about large-scale, often devastating environmental change is running well ahead of our capacity to frame effective regimes and international institutions in response. In view of the likely human consequences of current trends, what Richard Falk describes as the 'realist mindset' which 'forecloses the political imagination' begins to look disturbingly reductionist.[12] This is not to overlook the insights and refinements which have been brought to bear on the rigidities of Realism. However:

> It took long enough for neorealism to come to terms with economic variables ... [but] ... even neorealism is intellectually incapable of embracing questions of ecological interdependence. Realism makes positivist claims to objective knowledge and explicitly excludes values not associated with national interest. It would not admit that universalist values of the type associated with the preservation of the biosphere can have political relevance in a world of selfish and competing states.[13]

One need not subscribe to the Gaia hypothesis[14] to recognize that the indifference of the natural world to 'political relevance' is still more profound. Yet despite a growing body of literature on the environment, globalization, governance, sub-state actors and other aspects of world politics, our conceptions of order, security and political possibility remain doggedly hierarchical and state-centric. What gives an environmental crisis its political character is its relationship to existing configurations of power and interest. It is not surprising then that the most important and influential theoretical work on environmental matters within the discipline of International Relations is concentrated on environmental problem-solving[15] and since states are the largest and most concerted form of political agency, the paradigms are largely undisturbed.

The contention here is not that the study of international politics is conceptually deficient, but that its predominance as part of our larger thinking about world politics, particularly when expressed in exclusivist terms, is misplaced. Necessary though it is to abstract notions of state power from other, large-scale dynamics, particularly those of the natural world, the latter are not (or are at least no longer) a 'given' or even a precondition, but are an active element in the security and progress of states and the state system. In this regard, the 'anarchy' of Realist theory (that is, the lack of any sovereign authority over states), is a condition masquerading as an arena – essentially, one devoid of anything other than discrete states in competition with one another. However, the observable world is one in which a variety of actors and dynamics exist in complex, tensioned relationships. The relegation of these relationships to a level of relative unimportance in theoretical terms can all too easily be carried across to a dismissal of their functional significance. The defence of theory at the expense of our broader comprehension of the workings of the world is not merely an abstraction of international politics from natural phenomena, but also from a good deal of world history and contemporary developments of considerable consequence for states and peoples alike.[16,17]

The international and the global

The usefulness of theories of the international system is in their explanatory power. Challenging new developments that a theory cannot be extended to encompass become part of the larger context in which the theory continues to have some purchase – albeit sometimes reduced. For example, much of the established body of theorizing about the world economy has not been invalidated by the growing force of transnational, electronic currency exchange and the mobility of capital, even if its explanatory reach has shortened. Yet as Susan Strange noted, the new analytical approaches which these and other developments invite are typically regarded as '... deeply subversive of the exclusivity of the 'disciplines' and sub-disciplines of social science'.[18] However, siting theories of state power and international order within a larger, dynamic context is not to divest them of their meaning and integrity, but to ensure it. Fixed and impermeable boundaries between abstraction and context are not possible; and the defence of disciplinary turf against innovative, multi-disciplinary perspectives is hardly a substitute for outward-looking, intellectual engagement.

But which context? Toward the end of his classic study devoted to how order is maintained in the state system, Hedley Bull maintained that

> World order, or order within the great society of all mankind, is not only wider than international order or order among states, but also more fundamental and primordial than it, and morally prior to it. The system of states has constantly to be assessed in relation to the goal of world order.[19]

This purposeful contextualization should be extended further: theories of international relations must be assessed not only in relation to a goal, but also in respect of the human condition as shaped by environmental conditions and a globalizing humanity acting – and in turn, being acted upon – the ecosystems of which we are a part. The dynamic interactions between human and natural systems are also 'more fundamental and primordial' than international order.

The recognition of a global arena is more than making a logical assumption explicit; it also makes clear the nature and extent of what international relations theories are abstracted from.

The viability and duration of societies and states rests upon a sustaining ecosystem – a truism rooted in biological necessity, but also a fact of contemporary international politics, as we work to build regimes to deal with matters as considerable as global warming and the loss of biodiversity.[20] As aspects of the biosphere lose their resilience in the face of a variety of human pressures, the sense in which the world is becoming a single, shared arena of human activity is an historic change in the human situation – and by extension, the situation of states. (Consider the shift from the shared understanding that 'the seas belong to no one' to 'the seas belong to everyone.') And as the fundamentals of human existence – air, water, land and soil quality, non-renewable resources, oceans – become ever more stressed, the world can also stand as a single political arena. What is most compelling about global atmosphere politics is not the scientific and political contention, but that the issues are global in character as well as in extent – a striking instance of international politics in a global arena.

There remain distinct levels of analysis and clear 'actor realms' and few would claim to foresee a future in which states are not powerful actors. Even so, the rich literature on globalization and the evidence of a vast array of contemporary developments[21] (not least in economics and communications) has made the 'hard shell' of states beloved of some Realists into something more like a semi-permeable membrane. It follows that arguments about whether our world is definitively state-centric or a multi-centric are essentially sterile contests over theoretical predominance. Rather than debates around a contrived polarization, we might more meaningfully engage the question, 'What would a satisfactory theory of world politics be a theory of?'[22]

Human security

While theories of international politics remain central to our comprehension of many of the most important socio-political actors and dynamics, it is no longer the case that 'international security' and 'human security' are effectively indistinguishable. The most immediate sense in which 'human security' has come to have political meaning is through a common human fate arising from an encompassing threat. The Cold War did much to bring this about, in the form of possible ecocide through nuclear war. Less dramatically, but no less profoundly, global environmental crises have brought new meaning to the phrase, 'the human condition'. In addition, one of the many outcomes of globalization is the extent to which identity and allegiance are no longer so closely bound to territory and sovereignty. Finally, the development of a global culture of human rights brings an important normative element to perceptions of order and security.

As a concern with the security of peoples begins to impinge on the better established concern with state security and international order, a range of new perspectives on levels of analysis, significant actors, structure/agency and hitherto overlooked dynamics begin to emerge. R.J.B. Walker's 1988 depiction has gained considerable force in subsequent years:

> there has been a broadening of the subject of security to include people in general, indeed life on earth, rather than just citizens of states. The concept of national security incorporates a specific resolution of the competing claims of people as people and people as citizens. It gives absolute priority to the latter. Under modern conditions, the pursuit of the security of citizens of states renders everyone more and more insecure as people. Furthermore, the emergence of new structures of inclusion and exclusion – not the spatial or territorial divisions between states but the complex social, cultural, economic and political divisions between peoples who can or cannot participate effectively in contemporary global processes – renders one-third of humanity radically unable to secure the minimum conditions for survival.[23]

Walker's 'modern conditions' are not confined to the structural injustices which effectively disenfranchise such a large portion of humanity from a minimum standard of living.

One of the interests of emerging and resurgent infectious diseases is that an examination of the socio-political forces driving and responding to them reveals the security of states and the security of peoples in a complex of causation and response which makes clear that the global arena is not a static backdrop to inter-state actions.[24] Pathogens and high politics; individual behaviours and pandemics; community health and state viability; viral traffic and globalization – the relationships between the microbial and the international defy rigid demarcations of 'high' and 'low'. This is not to suggest that the viability of International Relations theories is thereby undermined, but that in a world which has global characteristics as well as international structures, their explanatory compass is useful but not sufficient for comprehending the full range of forces now shaping human life.

Although any number of phenomena can be characterized as comprising or operating within a global sphere – from new communications technologies to the culture of human rights – it is the planetary biosphere that reveals the most profound and dynamic links between international politics and global processes.[25] Although the international politics of the environment are highly visible intersections of human and natural systems, the substance of these interactions is much deeper than crisis response and belated management and control regimes might lead us to believe. The susceptibility of human societies to the uncertainties of nature, from the microbial to the climatic, is well-recorded and by no means the stuff of pre-modern times, or confined to under-developed regions. The natural world also comprises more than 6 billion human beings capable of bringing about considerable change to the earth's biosphere both cumulatively and synergistically. Although the discovery of a hole in the ozone layer came as a shock, it is not yet clear that we have absorbed the underlying meaning of this and other environmental threats: that the resilience of the earth's life support systems are ever more subject to the pressures of population growth and the attendant repercussions of industrialization, resource depletion, consumerism and the generation of wastes. The point here is that planetary-scale changes are not the outcome of intention and planning – quite the reverse; moreover, the international politics of environmental protection are frequently set in train by an accumulation of local, often diffuse actions (the use of CFCs; over-fishing; long-term and/or widely spaced species loss leading to a crisis of biodiversity).

Calculations of human security naturally turn on immediate and recurring matters, as is clear in regions prone to earthquakes, typhoons or droughts. However, the sense in which 'human security' pertains to humanity as much as to individual societies, is not merely an expression of solidarity, but a reflection of the variety of global dynamics that are swiftly eliminating isolation of every kind. A few examples will suffice. In a six-month period in 1918–19, the influenza pandemic killed at least 21 million people. At that time, the fastest means of travel between continents was by ship. Today, the number of people making international journeys by air increases by 11 million per year, on top of an increase of 7 per cent per year for the last four decades.[26] Enhanced means of transport has also ensured that thousands of 'exotic' species are now moving through the world trading system, posing a variety of threats to biodiversity, agriculture, fishing and human health in many parts of the world.[27] And the implications of the release of genetically-modified organisms into the environment – both legal and illegal – are incalculable.[28]

Because interdependence and causation are a much more intricate web than can be captured in any hierarchical schema, human security has many dimensions. For this reason, coming to an understanding of an encompassing (as opposed to national or regional) human security necessitates a recognition of the limitations of our abstractions in the face of a globalizing humanity now capable of altering the conditions of its continued existence.[29]

Emerging and resurgent infectious diseases

At the microbial level, globalization has long been a reality, while epidemics, pandemics and the biological consequences of human expansion and conquest are central to world history.[30] New or hitherto unrecorded diseases are not in themselves surprising, given our less than comprehensive knowledge of the microbial world and ecology more generally. However, their number and aetiology, together with a disturbing pattern of resurgent diseases in areas where they were thought to have been 'conquered' not only pose threats to particular human societies, but also point to a grave fissure in the relationship between human and natural systems. This is easier to appreciate in reverse: the advance of global warming has considerable implications for human health, in matters ranging from extreme weather events to the altered conditions of disease vector ecology.[31] (The advance of malarial mosquitoes into formerly temperate zones has been recorded.) The political 'drivers' for the unprecedented, encompassing condition of global warming are an intricate complex of relatively small acts and omissions – a cumulative 'politics of the environment' sited locally and nationally, but global in their effect. In the first instance, the appropriate political responses to the consequences are from within the realm of international politics; likewise, there are a variety of state and international organizations to deal with epidemics.[32] Important as they are, however, initiatives at this level are often belated and nearly always reactive, while the intensification of challenges to human-ecological equilibrium continue apace – with disease outbreaks of disturbing character and extent now widely regarded as critical indicators of 'a world out of balance'.[33]

International efforts at disease surveillance and control are not inconsiderable,[34] but they can only monitor the most visible outcomes of the considerable changes being brought about by human activity and the opportunistic advances by disease organisms in changed and changing circumstances. Any of those developments – rapid urbanization, the toxic legacy of industrialized farming, degraded ecosystems, the pace of plant and animal extinction – can re-configure the suscepti-bilities of humans to disease organisms. Political inertia as well as polit-ical initiative are closely bound up not only with the socio-political consequences of diseases, but also with their emergence and persist-ence. This is not merely a matter of crumbling infrastructures and strained social services such as can now be witnessed in Russia. It is also a matter of microbial ecologies and human ecologies in ever-closer, sometimes unprecedented communion. Recent patterns of infectious diseases make plain to everyone what has long been familiar to epidemiologists: that pathogens do not respect nationality, class or gender divides – nor in many cases, species boundaries.[35] From the per-spective of 'high' politics, the distant consequences of violent conflict in developing countries or the formal ordering of international trade may be of little importance – as when a dispossessed social group clears land for subsistence farming and thereby comes into routine contact with a new zoonotic pool. These were the circumstances under which Bolivian hemorrhagic fever emerged;[36] and the possibilities, which extend to varieties of lethality and communicability, are incalculable.

Of existing patterns of disease and epidemic, the eradication of smallpox in the 1970s stands as a rebuke to narrow self-interest and the manner in which rich world/poor world cleavages persist in the prioritization of disease control and treatment.[37] Those most con-cerned with international order will readily engage the implications of globalization for state viability and the coherence of the international system. But beneath the marvel and the anxiety over the pace of change we are all enduring, we need to grasp that one of the conse-quences of globalization is a kind of desegregation – of the political and the environmental; of high and low; and political order and life-system stability and predictability.

What then is the place of International Relations theory in a world which more resembles a web than a hierarchy; in which states are as easily acted upon as act; in which causal relations are linear largely only in intent; and in which 'human security' is less a normative vari-able than a condition of practical politics?

Conclusion

Above all, let us regard theories as tools for comprehension, not a sub-stitute. Our larger understanding of the dynamics of the world is immeasurably enriched by the painstaking work of theorists of every intellectual disposition; likewise, our theoretical abstractions are not private fictions but the discovery, articulation and dissemination of important facets of socio-political life. A recognition that the uses of theory are sometimes lost to rather inward-looking academic debates probably lies at the heart of Ken Booth's call for a 'revolution in the ontology, epistemology and agenda of the discipline'.[38] A further, important assertion was made by Susan Strange, who wrote that, '... our times no longer allow us the comfort of separatist specialisation in the social sciences, and that, however difficult, the attempt has to be made at synthesis and blending, imperfect as we know the results are bound to be'.[39] This call for a breaking down of barriers (not disciplinary boundaries) should not be read as an interest in a social sciences 'unified field theory', but as intellectual need shaping new disciplinary approaches and scholarly communication.

Because we need a deeper and more sophisticated understanding of the profoundly inter-connected and dynamic links between human activity and environmental constraints – and in particular, the interaction of human and natural systems – we need to start from a more generous conception of the basis of human security. Those with a view to revolution might consider embracing of ecology as a social science. One of the virtues of bringing ecology within the realms of social science is that it has as its operating principle the essential unity of knowledge and the comprehension of whole systems.[40] Is it likely to be any more 'awkward' – or any less productive – than human geography, which also depends on the information and insights from many disciplines?

The map is not the territory: the use of any individual theory depends on a recognition of its limitations as well as on a validation of its substance. Our work as theorists is all the more meaningful for being part of the larger endeavour of all disciplines to conceive – and reconceive – human security.

Notes

1. As it was for Schumpeter. See Neil J. Smelser and Richard Swedberg, 'The Sociological Perspective on the Economy', in Neil J. Smelser and Richard Swedberg (eds), *The Handbook of Economic Sociology* (Princeton: Princeton University Press, 1994), p. 13.
2. Christopher Hill and Pamela Beshoff (eds), *The Two Worlds of International Relations: Academics, Practitioners and the Trade in Ideas* (London: Routledge, 1994).

3. James N. Rosenau and Mary Durfee, *Thinking Theory Thoroughly: Coherent Approaches to an Incoherent World* (Boulder: Westview Press, 1997), p. 1.
4. Jonathan M. Roberts, *Decision-Making During International Crises* (London: Macmillan, 1988); Yaacov Y.I. Vertzberger, *The World in Their Minds: Information Processing, Cognition, and Perception in Foreign Policy Decisionmaking* (Stanford: Stanford University Press, 1990).
5. Jonathan Mann and Daniel Tarantola (eds), *AIDS in the World II* (Oxford: Oxford University Press, 1996); *The World Health Report 1996* (Geneva: World Health Organisation, 1996); Laurie Garrett, *The Coming Plague: Newly Emerging Diseases in a World Out of Balance* (New York: Farrar, Straus and Giroux, 1994).
6. International Federation of Red Cross and Red Crescent Societies, *World Disasters Report 1999* (Key information reproduced at: http://www.ifrc.org/pubs/wdr/keyfacts.htm.)
7. Edward O. Wilson, *The Diversity of Life* (London: Penguin Books, 1992), Ch. 12.
8. James N. Rosenau and Mary Durfee, op. cit., p. 3.
9. A phrase made familiar by James Rosenau in *Turbulence in World Politics: a Theory of Change and Continuity* (New York: Harvester/Wheatsheaf, 1990).
10. See Avigdor Haselkorn, *The Continuing Storm: Iraq, Poisonous Weapons and Deterrence* (New Haven: Yale University Press, 1999).
11. Susan Strange, *The Retreat of the State: the Diffusion of Power in the World Political Economy* (Cambridge: Cambridge University Press, 1996).
12. Richard Falk, *On Humane Governance: Toward a New Global Politics* (Cambridge: Polity Press, 1995), p. 37.
13. John Volger, 'Introduction: The Environment in International Relations: Legacies and Contentions', in John Volger and Mark F. Imber, *The Environment and International Relations* (London: Routledge, 1996), pp. 6–7.
14. James Lovelock, *Gaia: a New Look at Life on Earth* (Oxford: Oxford University Press, 1979).
15. David G. Victor, Kal Raustiala and Eugene Skolnikoff (eds), *The Implementation and Effectiveness of International Environmental Commitments: Theory and Practice* (Cambridge, MA: MIT Press, 1998); Volker Ritterberger (ed.), *Regime Theory and International Relations* (Oxford: Clarendon Press, 1993).
16. See William H. McNeill, *Plagues and Peoples* (London: Penguin Books, 1976); Alfred W. Crosby, *Ecological Imperialism: the Biological expansion of Europe, 900–1900* (Cambridge: Cambridge University Press, 1986); Stephen Boyden, *Western Civilization from a Biological Perspective* (Oxford: Clarendon Press, 1987).
17. Laurie Garrett, op. cit.; Jonathan Mann and Daniel Tarantola (eds), op. cit.; Bernard Roizman (ed.), *Infectious Diseases in an Age of Change: the Impact of Human Ecology and Behaviour on Disease Transmission* (Washington, DC: National Academy Press, 1995).
18. Susan Strange, op. cit., pp. xiv–xv.
19. Hedley Bull, *The Anarchical Society: a Study of Order in World Politics* (London: Macmillan, 1977), p. 319.

20. David G. Victor, Kal Raustiala and Eugene Skolnikoff (eds), op. cit.; Tim O'Riordan and Jill Jäger (eds), *Politics of Climate Change: a European Perspective* (London: Routledge, 1996); Timothy M. Swanson, *The International Regulation of Extinction* (London: Macmillan, 1994).

21. An excellent, wide-ranging overview is James Rosenau, *Along the Domestic-Foreign Frontier: Exploring Governance in a Turbulent World* (Cambridge: Cambridge University Press, 1997).

22. Compare with the following: 'The academic study of international relations is often presented as being founded on the fundamental difference between domestic 'society' and international 'anarchy'. Yet one of the most striking features of European thought before 1914 was just how few theorists actually accepted such a dichotomy'. Andrew Hurrell, 'International Society and the Study of Regimes: a Reflective Approach', in Volker Ritterberger (ed.), op. cit., p. 50.

23. R.J.B. Walker, *One World, Many Worlds: Struggles for a Just World Peace* (London: Zed Books, 1998), p. 121.

24. Jim Whitman, 'Political Processes and Infectious Diseases', in Jim Whitman (ed.), *The Politics of Emerging and Resurgent Infectious Diseases* (London: Macmillan, 2000), pp. 1–14.

25. Ian Bradbury, *The Biosphere* (London: Belhaven Press, 1991); for an excellent overview of dynamic systems from a sustainability perspective, Hartmut Bossel, *Earth at a Crossroads: Paths to a Sustainable Future* (Cambridge: Cambridge University Press, 1998); see also Geoffrey Vickers, *Human Systems Are Different* (London: Harper & Row, 1983).

26. Henryk Handszuh and Sommerset R. Waters, 'Travel and Tourism Patterns', in Herbert L. DuPont and Robert Steffen, *Textbook of Travel Medicine and Health* (Hamilton, ON: B.C. Decker, Inc., 1997), p. 20.

27. Chris Bright, *Life Out of Bounds: Bio-Invasions in a Borderless World* (London: Earthscan, 1999).

28. J.R.S. Fincham and J.R. Ravetz, *Genetically Modified Organisms: Benefits and Risks* (Milton Keynes: Open University Press), 1991.

29. A.J. McMichael, *Planetary Overload: Global Environmental Change and the Health of the Human Species* (Cambridge: Cambridge University Press, 1994); Barbara Sundberg Baudot and William Moonmaw, *People and Their Planet: Searching for Balance* (London: Macmillan, 1999).

30. Joshua Lederberg, 'Medical Science, Infectious Disease, and the Unity of Mankind', *Journal of the American Medical Association*, Vol. 260, No. 5 (5 August 1988), pp. 684–5; Alfred W. Crosby, op. cit.; William H. McNeill, *The Human Condition: an Ecological and Historical View* (Princeton: Princeton University Press, 1992).

31. A.J. McMichael, A. Haines, R. Slooff and S. Kovats (eds), *Climate Change and Human Health: an Assessment Prepared by a Task Group on behalf of the World Health Organisation, the World Meteorological Organisation and the United Nations Environment Programme* (Geneva: World Health Organisation, 1996).

32. Milton I. Roemer, *National Health Systems of the World* (Oxford: Oxford University Press, 1993); Javed Siddiqi, *World Health and World Politics: the World Health Organization and the UN System* (London: Hurst & Company, 1995); Leon Gordenker, Roger A. Coate, Christer Jönsson and Peter

Söderholm, *International Cooperation in Response to AIDS* (London: Pinter, 1995).

33. Laurie Garrett, op. cit.
34. Report of the National Science and Technology Council Committee on International Science, Engineering, and Technology Working group on Emerging and Re-Emerging Infectious Diseases, 'Infectious Disease – a Global Threat' (Washington, DC: September 1995).
35. Note recent reports on pig and avian viruses infecting humans. 'Malaysia kills pigs as virus jumps to humans', *The Guardian* (30 March 1999); Pete Davies, 'The Plague in Waiting', *Guardian Weekend*, 7 August 1999.
36. Laurie Garrett, op. cit., p. 27.
37. UK NGO AIDS Consortium, Report of the Workshop Series, 'Access to HIV Treatments in Developing Countries': Interim Report (4 November–2 December, 1997).
38. Ken Booth, 'Dare Not to Know: International Relations Theory Versus the Future', in Ken Booth and Steve Smith, *International Relations Theory Today* (Cambridge: Polity Press, 1995), p. 330.
39. Susan Strange, op. cit., p. xvi.
40. Edward Goldsmith, *The Way: an Ecological World-View* (Athens: The University of Georgia Press, 1998).

8
Ghosts of Kigali: Infectious Disease and Global Stability at the Turn of the Century

Andrew T. Price-Smith

> Beyond the enormous suffering of individuals and families, South Africans are beginning to understand the cost (of HIV/AIDS) in every sphere of society, observing with growing dismay its impact on the efforts of our new democracy to achieve the goals of reconstruction and development.
>
> Nelson Mandela, 1997[1]

As the spectre of the Cold War recedes into the past, international relations and national security analysts have begun to embrace concepts of human security and preventive defence, arguing that factors such as environmental degradation, resource scarcity and overpopulation represent significant threats to global security. But another threat looms large on the horizon, namely the proliferation of emerging and re-emerging infections on a global scale. Indeed, the HIV pandemic is entrenched in sub-Saharan Africa,[2] and is accelerating through Eastern Europe, South Asia and East Asia. Other widening pandemics include old scourges such as tuberculosis, malaria, cholera and dengue. New threats have also emerged in the form of Hanta, Ebola, *Legionella*, and such antibiotic resistant organisms as vancomycin-resistant enterococci and methycillin-resistant *Staphylococcus aureus*.

International relations theory

Arguably, the primary raison d'être of International Relations theory is to construct models that will assist in averting the premature loss of human life and productivity as a result of war. Indeed, as Thomas Hobbes claimed, it is the central function of the state to guarantee the physical safety of its citizens from both internal and external forms of predation.[3] However, traditional concepts of security have traditionally ignored the greatest source of human misery and mortality, the microbial penumbra that surrounds our species. I argue here that it is time to consider the additional form of ecological predation wherein the physical security and prosperity of a state's populace is directly threatened by the global phenomena of emerging and re-emerging infectious disease.[4]

Emerging and re-emerging infectious diseases are significant obstacles to the political stability and economic development of seriously affected societies. Thus, the global resurgence of infectious disease presents a direct and significant long-term threat to international governance and prosperity.[5] Over the broad span of human history, infectious disease has consistently accounted for the greatest proportion of human morbidity and mortality, easily surpassing war as the foremost threat to human life and prosperity. Historians have long argued that infectious disease has had a profound impact on the evolution and at times the dissolution of societal structures, governments and empires.[6] Indeed, Robert Fogel argues that much of England's prosperity, if not the Industrial Revolution itself, resulted from the conquest of high morbidity and mortality in Britain during the late eighteenth and early nineteenth centuries.[7] This was largely because of significant advances in public health and in the increasingly equitable distribution of food. However, even in the era of modern medicine, states annually suffer much greater mortality and morbidity from infectious disease than from casualties incurred during inter- and intrastate military conflict.

According to the World Bank, of the 49 971 000 deaths recorded in 1990, infectious disease claimed 16 690 000 lives or 34.4 per cent of deaths, while war killed 322 000 (0.64 per cent of total deaths) a ratio of 52:1.[8] These statistics demonstrate the relative destruction wrought by disease when compared to deaths from military actions, and in terms of a ratio, the deaths resulting from infectious disease compared to war are a significant 52:1 in this year. From the standpoint of human security, then, disease is a relatively greater threat to human well-being than war, and yet the subject remains poorly understood within the general policy community.

According to statistics gathered by the Harvard-based Global AIDS Policy Coalition, approximately 22 million people were infected with HIV/AIDS, and 4.7 million new infections occurred globally during 1995. Of these new infections, 2.5 million occurred in South-East Asia and 1.9 million in sub-Saharan Africa while the industrialized world accounted for approximately 170 000 new HIV cases.[9] The pace of the HIV/AIDS pandemic is accelerating, with a total of 33.4 million people now infected, 5.8 million new HIV infections annually, and 2.5 million HIV-induced deaths in 1998.[10] Thus the global pace of infection has increased by 24 per cent over 1995 levels. The HIV pandemic now rivals (in terms of the absolute magnitude of mortality) the greatest plagues of history, including the Black Death of Middle Ages Europe and the Influenza Pandemic of 1918, both of which killed over 20 million people. As of 1999, the HIV pandemic had resulted in the infection of 47 million and was responsible for the deaths of 14 million people, and the contagion is spreading rapidly throughout South and South-East Asia, Eastern Europe and Latin America.[11]

The heart of the HIV pandemic lies in sub-Saharan Africa where many states are now reporting HIV seroprevalence levels in excess of 10 per cent. Indeed, South Africa, Kenya, Uganda, Zambia, Namibia, Swaziland, Botswana and Zimbabwe all have seroprevalence levels ranging from 10 to 36 per cent of the population.[12] Botswana, for example, has seen national HIV seroprevalence rates rise from 10 per cent in 1992 to 25.1 per cent in 1997, an increase of 250 per cent over five years.[13] South Africa has seen total HIV infection levels rise from 1.4 million in 1995 to over 3 million in 1998.[14] This represents an increase of HIV seroprevalence in the South African population of over 200 per cent over a period of three years. Some regions within these states have even higher infection levels, HIV prevalence in KwaZulu-Natal (South Africa) has now reached the level of 30 per cent,[15] and Francistown in Botswana reports that 43 per cent of its citizens are infected.[16] Certain towns along the South African–Zimbabwe border boast astonishing rates of approximately 70 per cent HIV seroprevalence.[17]

The pandemic is expanding into Eastern Europe at an ever-increasing pace. Former Russian Minister of Health, Tatyana Dmitriyeva, has predicted that over 1 million Russians will be infected with HIV by the year 2000.[18] Ukraine has also seen HIV incidence soar from a modest 44 cases in 1994 to an astonishing 110 000 cases as of mid-1998.[19] India is also seeing the epidemic spread throughout its vast population at a rapacious pace. Five years ago, HIV was practically unheard of in India; now almost 1 per cent of all pregnant women tested throughout the country are HIV positive.[20] Disturbingly, by 1997, the epidemic was already firmly entrenched in regions of India such as Nagaland along the Burmese border (7.8 per cent HIV seroprevalence), and nearby Manipur (over 10 per cent HIV seroprevalence).[21] Indeed, with the exception of the developed world, and certain states such as Uganda and Thailand (which have seen some reduction in the rate of new infections), the HIV pandemic continues to expand at a rapid pace.

Tuberculosis (TB) has been making a steady comeback as a global scourge, and WHO declared the TB pandemic a global crisis in 1993. WHO estimates that '8.9 million people developed tuberculosis in 1995, bringing the global total of sufferers to about 22 million, of whom about 3 million will have died in the same space of time'.[22] Furthermore, in the absence of increased effectiveness and availability of tuberculosis control measures, over 30 million tuberculosis deaths and more than 90 million new TB infections are forecast to occur by the turn of the century.[23] Tuberculosis is making inroads into the industrialized nations, particularly Canada and the United States, where it infects disadvantaged urban and incarcerated populations and then spreads throughout society. The incidence of tuberculosis in the United States is climbing rapidly. For example, in the US, reported cases of TB had declined from 84 300 in 1953 to 22 200 in 1984, a drop of approximately 4 per cent per annum. However, from 1985 to 1993, the number of cases increased by a cumulative 14 per cent, and the pace of increase continues to accelerate.[24] Similarly, Zimbabwe has reported massive increases in TB incidence, from 5000 cases in 1986 to 35 000 cases in 1997.[25] Feschbach notes that the incidence of tuberculosis in Russia is increasing rapidly, and based on estimates provided by the Russian Ministry of the Interior, he predicts that tuberculosis will result in the deaths of 1.75 million Russians per year by 2000.[26]

Malaria continues its relentless expansion into former regions of endemicity. For example, in 1989, malaria claimed 100 lives in Zimbabwe while debilitating many thousands; by 1997, malaria was responsible for the deaths of 2800 in that country, an astonishing rate of increase for a disease that was once thought to be controlled.[27] Indeed, the best available estimates project that malaria currently claims 5000 lives every day in Africa, approximately 1.8 million deaths a year.[28] Global estimates put the total annual death rate from malaria at upwards of 2.7 million and note that malaria debilitates as many as 500 million people every year.[29] Ellen Shell claims that global incidence of malaria has increased by approximately 400 per cent over the 1992–97 period, and notes that the disease has re-emerged in North America from urban centres in California to Michigan, to New York City and Toronto.[30]

Meanwhile, familiar pathogens continue to exact their toll on humanity with relentless vigour. For example, acute lower respiratory infections slay nearly 4 million children annually, while diarrhoeal diseases such as adenovirus and rotavirus kill nearly 3 million infants every year. Viral hepatitis is another global scourge as a minimum of 350 million people are chronic carriers of the hepatitis B virus, and an additional 100 million harbour the hepatitis C virus. The World Health Organization projects that at least 25 per cent of these carriers will die due to related liver disease.[31] To make matters worse, many of the ten million new cases of cancer diagnosed in 1995 were caused by viruses, bacteria and parasites. WHO calculates that 15 per cent of all new cancer cases (1.5 million) are the result of exposure to infectious agents, and this percentage of ERID-induced cancer mortality is estimated to increase as our knowledge of both infectious disease and cancer advances. New evidence is linking many other supposedly chronic or genetic diseases such as heart disease and multiple sclerosis to common infectious agents (chlamydia and herpes, respectively) which promote long-term disease processes within human hosts.[32] If certain conditions such as cancer, heart disease and MS are in fact pathogen-induced, then the global burden of disease may be far greater than we previously thought.

While it is relatively easy to see that disease is a central agent of misery throughout the developing world, it is not often apparent that infection-induced mortality has been on the rise in the developed world as well. For example, the United States – with its enormous levels of state capacity – has seen steadily increasing mortality from infectious disease over the last two decades, ranging from 15 360 deaths in 1979 to 77 128 ERID-induced deaths in 1995,[33] a significant increase of 502 per cent over that time period.

Interdisciplinary models that combine the natural and social sciences require a fundamental reconceptualization of standard definitions of national interest and security. Constricting definitions that focus exclusively on the relative military capability of states are increasingly sterile in the face of the many global challenges of the post-Cold War world. Threats to human welfare such as global environmental degradation, resource scarcity and infectious disease, present policy-makers with difficult policy dilemmas. Novel global collective action problems are exceptionally difficult to resolve given the primacy of national sovereignty in an arena of international anarchy. In articulating the complex linkages between increasing disease prevalence and state capacity, some light can be shed on the association between the prevalence of infectious disease and growing poverty and political destabilization in regions such as sub-Saharan Africa.

To begin with a specific definition: emerging and re-emerging infectious diseases (ERIDs) are pathogen-induced human illnesses which have increased in incidence, lethality, transmissibility and/or have expanded their geographical range since 1973. Re-emerging diseases are those pathogen-induced human illnesses that were previously controlled or were declining in range and/or incidence, but are now expanding – and not just in range and incidence, but also in drug-resistance, and increasing transmissibility and/or lethality. Pathogens are defined as viral, bacterial, parasitic or proteinic organisms or agents that live in a parasitic and debilitating relationship with their human host.

Pathogenic microbes exist independently throughout the Earth's biosphere with the vast majority of them present in the zoonotic pool and outside of human ecology. In a very real way these pathogens are independent variables and are exogenous to the state because they are global phenomena (existing at the system level). They may cross over from the zoonotic reservoir into the human ecology at any time according to the principles of chaos.[34] A classic example of such zoonotic transfer is *Plasmoduim falciparum* malaria, which seems to have crossed over from various avian species to humans at some time within the last 5000 years. Because of the recent nature of the crossover, *p. falciparum* is far deadlier to humans than its cousin *p. vivax*, which has had a much longer time to adjust to its human hosts.

After pathogenic agents enter the human ecology (and become endogenized within human societies), their effects are magnified by intervening variables called 'disease amplifiers' (DAs). Examples of potent DAs are phenomena such as environmental degradation, warfare, climate change, the misuse of antibiotics, changes in the speed of human transportation technologies, famine, natural disasters and global trade.[35] These DAs generate changes in viral traffic that result in ERIDs. Thus ERIDs are a product of the synergy between the independent variable (pathogens) and the disease amplifiers.

States and societies may at this point use adaptive resources to mitigate the effects of ERIDs on state capacity. The state's ability to adapt is limited by several factors. First, the initial level of state capacity will determine the scale of adaptive resources that can be mobilized to deal with the ERID problem. States with higher initial capacity will therefore have greater technical, financial and social resources to adapt to crises. State adaptation will also be affected by exogenous inputs of capital and social and technical ingenuity, courtesy of international organizations such as the World Health Organization, United Nations

Children's Fund and NGOs such as the International Committee of the Red Cross. It may also be compromised by certain outcomes generated by intervening variables, such as war, famine and ecological destruction. Exogenous inputs (EIs) take the form of capital, technology and ingenuity into the state from external sources such as IOs, NGOs, and direct foreign aid supplied by donor countries. Exogenous inputs, such as direct foreign capital infusions, also directly affect the resources available to the state to respond to crises and, therefore, augment the efficacy of adaptation responses.

There is a logically positive association between state capacity (SC) and state adaptation because greater initial capacity means that there are more human, economic, and technical resources within the state to mobilize to deal with various crises. The lower the initial value of SC, the fewer the resources that can be mobilized to offset the crisis. This relationship operates in a reciprocal spiral: greater initial capacity leads to greater adaptive ability, which should in turn reduce the ERID-induced loss to SC. Thus states that have lower SC when ERIDs afflict them generally suffer much greater SC losses than states with high initial SC. The only means by which states with lower SC can ameliorate the effects of ERID is through exogenous inputs which give them greater resources to mobilize and advance tactical knowledge to deal with the crisis.[36]

Intra-state effects of ERID

A brief explanation of the effects of disease on SC, in the domains of economics and governance, is in order at this point. The destructive effects of ERIDs reverberate throughout all levels of the economy, from households and firms, to sectors such as resource extraction, agriculture, insurance and banking. When infected workers are debilitated or killed, the productivity of the workforce is reduced, particularly in labour-intensive sectors such as agriculture or mining.[37] Infectious disease imposes additional costs on the household (loss of revenue, loss of savings, and labour substitution), particularly affecting those units in the lower economic strata of society, such that income inequalities between the lower and upper classes are exacerbated. ERIDs also change expenditure patterns in the household, as money is increasingly spent on medication instead of food, clothing, shelter, and so on. Thus, ERIDs generate economic shocks to the household, changing savings and consumption patterns, eroding aggregate household wealth, and making significant labour substitution necessary. Rising levels of infectious disease also decrease incentives to invest in child education, as children spend more time working to support debilitated or bereaved family members. As well, there is little incentive to allocate resources to educate a child if that child is likely to die of some infection in the near future.[38]

Thus, the negative effects of disease in the domain of economic productivity include decreases in worker productivity, labour shortages and increased absenteeism, higher costs imposed on household units (particularly on the poor), reductions in per capita income, reduced savings, capital flight, reductions in national GDP and increases in income inequalities within a society which may in turn generate increased governance problems. ERID also impedes the settlement of marginal regions and the development of natural resources, negatively affects tourism and results in the embargoing of infected goods. A prime example of this occurred when the European Union banned all beef-related products from Britain in 1997, from foodstuffs to soaps to cosmetics, for fear of contamination with the BSE agent that causes Creutzfeldt–Jakob disease in humans. All told, increasing disease prevalence poses a serious threat to the economic health of societies across the globe.

In the domain of governance, high levels of ERID incidence undermine the capacity of political leaders and their respective bureaucracies to govern effectively as the infection of government personnel results in the debilitation and death of skilled administrators who oversee the day-to-day operations of governance. For example, AIDS has resulted in a significant winnowing of educated and skilled workers in government, industry and education in Tanzania. The destructive impact of ERID-induced mortality in capital-intensive institutions generates institutional fragility that will undermine the stability of nascent democratic societies. As the burden of disease increases on the population of a state, the resulting poverty and physical destruction visited on the populace will over time erode governmental legitimacy. Therefore, ERID-induced poverty, morbidity and mortality, migration, and psychological stresses wear upon the economic and social fabric of society. This may contribute to repression and the collapse of democracy as a weakening state seeks to maintain order while the government's legitimacy erodes and as governmental institutions become increasingly fragile.[39] This poses problems for the advocates of democratization and development and the US strategy of 'engagement and enlargement' which places a premium on establishing and strengthening democratic regimes on a global level. Furthermore, the presence of ERIDs in military populations jeopardizes military readiness, international co-operation, national security and the ability of a state to preserve its territorial integrity. At the intra-state level, ERIDs reduce force strength through the death or debilitation of military personnel, deplete the supply of healthy recruits and generate costs that limit military budgets, all of which impairs a state's capacity to defend itself against a potential aggressor and limits a state's ability to project power for peacekeeping or coercive measures.

The adaptive capability of states depends on their current and future supply of technical and social ingenuity, on their domestic reservoirs of capacity, and on the contribution that outside actors make in the form of capital, goods and technical assistance. Homer-Dixon's concept of ingenuity is a partial factor in the ability of states to adapt to crises. While the ingenuity model that he has constructed deals with the issue of economic development in a climate of resource scarcity and environmental degradation, the concept of ingenuity is useful in determining the capacity of a state to adapt in the face of significant challenges. Homer-Dixon argues that 'resource scarcity can simultaneously increase the requirement and impede the supply (of ingenuity), producing an "ingenuity gap" that may have critical consequences for adaptation and, in turn, social stability'.[40] Similarly, the negative economic and social effects as a result of ERID, can also increase the requirement for ingenuity while limiting its supply.[41] The lesson to be drawn from the ingenuity argument is that the longer we wait to address the problem of infectious disease the greater the costs of generating the levels of ingenuity that will be required to resolve the problem.

Because of low initial levels of state capacity and ingenuity in the developing world, the global proliferation of infectious disease presents the greatest threat to the least developed societies. This has given rise to a disturbing tendency on the part of some Western scholars, policy-makers and the media to see ERID as a threat only to the populations in those societies. But hubris and denial are shortsighted and bound to lead to significant downstream losses for developed societies as well. The natural world is, of course, infinitely complex and interdependent, and as the human species continues to alter the global environment it will produce corresponding responses from that environment, such as the continuing emergence of human pathogens. As we have seen from the emergence of AIDS, hepatitis, drug-resistant tuberculosis, and 'flesh eating disease', the developed world remains vulnerable to the ravages of infection.[42]

ERID's negative effect on state capacity at the unit level produces related pernicious outcomes at the systems level. Within the domain of economics, as ERID produces a significant drag on the economies of affected countries, we may see chronic regional underdevelopment, which may in turn exert a net drag on global trade and impair global prosperity. In all likelihood, due to the nature of spiral dynamics inherent in the relationship between ERID and state capacity, countries with low initial levels of SC will suffer greater losses over time from increasing prevalence of infectious disease within their populations. Due to this negative spiral effect, ERID's negative influence on the economic development of states may exacerbate the economic divide between North and South. Furthermore, the negative effects of infectious disease are not confined to the developing world. At the systems level, trade goods from ERID-affected regions may be subject to international embargo (for example, BSE in British beef, and influenza-infected chickens in Hong Kong). As infectious agents continue to emerge and re-emerge, and as agricultural crops and animal stocks become increasingly infested, we should expect that presumably infected trade goods from affected states will be embargoed, tourism to affected regions may decline, and economic damage to affected states will likely intensify.

One conclusion we can draw from the emergence of v-CJD, Ebola, HIV, and plague is that people are extremely risk-averse when it comes to the emergence of new pathogens, and that emergence tends to generate paranoia, hysteria and xenophobia that may manifest itself in the foreign policy of a state, impairing rational decision-making. The recent epidemic of pneumonic plague (*Yersinia pestis*) in western India during the latter part of 1994 gives an idea of how the psychological effects of infectious disease (in the form of *outbreak events*) may affect both SC and an afflicted state's relations with its neighbours. The very rumour of plague in Surat prompted the frenetic exodus of over 300 000 refugees from the city who could have carried the pestilence with them to Bombay, Calcutta and as far as New Delhi.[43] Out of fear, Pakistan, Bangladesh, Nepal and China rapidly closed their borders to both trade and travel from India, with some going so far as to restrict mail from the affected state: India had become an instant international pariah. As the plague spread, concern mounted and international travel to, and trade with, India became increasingly restricted. On 22 September 1994, the Bombay stock exchange plunged and soon thereafter many countries began to restrict imports from India, placing impounded goods in quarantine or turning them back altogether at the border.[44]

As the crisis deepened, the Indian army was called in to enforce a quarantine on the affected area in western India, and doctors who had fled Surat were forced back to work under threat of legal prosecution by the government. In the aftermath of the epidemic that killed 56 people, the Indian government was notified by the CDC in Atlanta that the *Yersinia pestis* bacillus was an unknown and presumably new strain. This information was interpreted by Indian authorities as 'unusual', and they promptly accused rebel militants (Ultras) of procuring the bacillus from a pathogen-manufacturing facility in Almaty, Kazakhstan with the object of manufacturing an epidemic in India. This paranoia on the part of Indian officials resulted in the transference of the inquest of the epidemic from public health authorities to the Department of Defence.[45] Beyond the acrimony that the plague fostered between India and its Islamic neighbours, the economic toll of the plague has been estimated at a minimum of $1 billion in lost revenue from exports and tourism.[46] While the loss of $1 billion may seem trivial, to a developing state like India it represents a serious blow to the economy with negative repercussions throughout numerous sectors.

As we can see in the Surat event and the current BSE scare in Europe, infectious disease and the irrational behaviour that it generates may worsen relationships between states, and/or cultures.[47] For example, the recent panic in Britain over bovine spongiform encephalopathy (BSE) or 'Mad Cow Disease' has resulted in the embargo of many beef-derived British products, and dictated the cull of a significant proportion of the UK's beef stocks. The BSE scare has frightened the British population as scientists talk about the possibility that thousands of Britons are infected with a new variant of Creutzfeldt–Jakob disease (human BSE), and the UK's European partners have summarily banned the import of British beef in violation of EC trade law.[48]

Increasing levels of ERID correlate with a decline in the state capacity of affected countries. As State Capacity declines, coupled with an increase in pathogen-induced deprivation and increasing demands upon the state, we may observe an attendant increase in the incidence of chronic sub-state violence and state failure. State failure frequently produces chaos in affected regions, as neighbouring states seal their borders to prevent the massive influx of ERID-infected refugee populations. Adjacent states may also seek to fill the power vacuum, and seize valued territory from the collapsing state, prompting other proximate states to do the same, exacerbating regional security dilemmas. As ERID incidence and lethality increase, deprivation will mount and SC will decline, generating increasing levels of stress and demands upon government structures and undermining its legitimacy. Thus, disease-induced stresses may combine with other environmental, demographic and economic stressors to generate riots, rebellions and insurgencies. As ERID prevalence increases and the geographical range of pathogens expands, the number of failing states may rise, necessitating increased humanitarian intervention by UN security forces to maintain order in affected regions. As we have seen from its experiences in Central and West Africa, the UN is unlikely to have a lasting effect in restoring order to areas where ERID incidence and lethality remains high.

Conclusions

The global resurgence of infectious disease has significant implications for state survival, stability and prosperity, and ramifications for inter-state relations as well. The premature death and debilitation of a significant proportion of a state's population erodes worker productiv-ity and undermines state prosperity, induces high levels of psychologi-cal stress in the populace, fosters internal migration and emigration, threatens the state's ability both to defend itself and to project force, generates institutional fragility and undermines the legitimacy of authority structures, thus impairing the state's ability to govern effect-ively. While disease acts as a stressor on state capacity, it simultaneously generates poverty and misery within the population of the state which may result in deprivation conflicts, widespread insurrection and gover-nance problems.[49] At the global level, ERID-induced poverty generates a drag on both regional development and global prosperity. Disease-induced poverty and instability may exacerbate migration from the biologically onerous regions of the South to the prosperous and rela-tively benign regions of the North. Furthermore, as ERID-induced shortcomings in the realms of governance and defence impair state survival, the international community may be called on to intervene and restore order in affected states.

It is likely that plagues have contributed to the collapse of gover-nance over the broad span of history: they hampered the Athenian war effort during the Peloponnesian War, contributed to the demise of Byzantine Rome and to the destruction of the feudal order in Europe, and were the primal force in the annihilation of the pre-Colombian societies in the Americas after their first contacts with Europeans.[50] This dynamic is not relegated to the annals of history but continues to affect state capacity in the modern era. Because of the negative associ-ation between infectious disease and state capacity, the global proliferation of emerging and re-emerging diseases (particularly HIV, tuberculosis and malaria) is a threat to international economic development and global governance. This allows us to draw several preliminary conclusions. First, the growing destabilization of sub-Saharan Africa is at least partly due to the exceptionally high ERID levels in the region, particularly that of HIV/AIDS and malaria. Indeed, the extreme governance problems in the Democratic Republic of the Congo, Rwanda, Uganda and Burundi may be related to increasing ERID stresses on state capacity.

Based on the experience of sub-Saharan Africa, we can project that the continuing and rapid spread of HIV and other ERIDs in Eastern Europe, South Asia and East Asia will erode state capacity in those regions as well, generating widespread poverty and political instability in seriously affected nations. In particular, the proliferation of infectious diseases such as HIV and tuberculosis threatens the economic well-being and political stability of several key states in the world, notably Russia, Ukraine, India, South Africa, Thailand and perhaps China. To promote global stability and prosperity, significant resources must be allocated to reinforcing public health infrastructures within these countries and public health must be made a central component of foreign development assistance packages.

Global phenomena such as infectious diseases frequently act in concert with other global collective action problems such as environmental degradation, resource scarcity and overpopulation, to strain state capacity. This synergy between stressors of state capacity will increasingly destabilize seriously affected states and in some cases entire regions (such as sub-Saharan Africa). We must foster increased communication and cooperation between the global policy and medical communities and provide increased resources for surveillance, containment and co-operative policy measures to check the global proliferation of emerging and re-emerging diseases. Above all, we must bring the gravity of these issues to the attention of the heads of all governments, as the greatest requirement for stemming the global tide of infection is political will.

Tangible actions that governments should take include the establishment of a global disease surveillance system, incorporating the successful civil-society model of the ProMED network that currently monitors disease outbreaks. Governments should also undertake the collection of 'health intelligence' such that we can monitor the progression of diseases through the populations of states that either cannot provide accurate statistics on disease prevalence, or refuse to for political reasons.[51] Policy-makers must also take action to reduce the pace of global environmental degradation, curb the abuse of anti-microbial medications within their societies, and provide increased funding for research to develop vaccines and other anti-microbial agents.

Although the World Health Organization has been the principal actor engaged in tracking disease emergence and proliferation, the WHO faces several problems in dealing with these issues. Although funding is increasingly diverted within the WHO to infectious surveillance, treatment and control, these programmes are generally underfunded and understaffed and have proven generally to be less than effective in fighting the re-emergence of ERID on many different fronts. Thus, greater resources must be given to WHO to increase its capacity, and these funds should be specifically targeted to deal with the greatest current ERID threats (HIV, tuberculosis and malaria). The United States and Japan are currently developing a policy framework for greater cooperation in checking the spread of disease within and between their own territories. Furthermore, the G7 states are exploring the means by which they might collaborate to reduce the threat of emerging diseases to their populations. While these efforts have produced few concrete results in the form of multilateral anti-contagion regimes, they are a step in the right direction. Given the will, policy-makers can enact the required redistribution of fiscal resources, ingenuity and technology to stem the rising tide of disease and promote global prosperity and stability.

Notes

1. Nelson Mandela. *AIDS: Facing Up to the Global Threat*. Address to the World Economic Forum. Davos, 3 February 1997. (http://www.us.unaids.org/high-band/speeches/mandela.html) p. 2. off-web 20/04/97.
2. It is increasingly disturbing to note the exceptionally high HIV infection rates throughout sub-Saharan Africa. Indeed, in Zimbabwe and Botswana UNAIDS estimates that a minimum of 25 per cent of the total population is currently infected with HIV. See http://www.unaids.org/highband.
3. See Thomas Hobbes, *Leviathan*. C.B. Macpherson, ed. Harmondsworth: Penguin, 1968.
4. Until very recently the concept of microbial threats to human security had not been explored. Two recent works which begin to explore the threat are: Laurie Garret, 'The Return of Infectious Disease', *Foreign Affairs*. Jan/Feb 1996. pp. 66–79, and Dennis Pirages, *Ecological Security: Micro-Threats to Human Well-Being*, paper presented at the International Studies Association Annual Meeting, San Diego. April 1996.

5. The author originally makes this argument in Price-Smith, Andrew T., *Contagion and Chaos: Infectious Disease and its Effects on Global Security and Development*. CIS Working Paper 1998–1. Toronto: Centre for International Studies, University of Toronto. January 1998.

6. See McNeill, William H. *Plagues and Peoples*. Toronto: Doubleday, 1989; Crosby, Alfred W., *Ecological Imperialism: The Biological Expansion of Europe, 900–1900*. New York: Cambridge University Press, 1994; Crosby, Alfred W., *The Colombian Exchange: Biological and Cultural Consequences of 1492*. Westport: Greenwood, 1972.; Sheldon Watts, *Epidemics and History: Disease, Power, and Imperialism*. New Haven, CT: Yale University Press, 1997; Zinsser, Hans. *Rats, Lice, and History*. New York: Little, Brown, & Co., 1934.

7. See Robert W. Fogel, 'The Conquest of High Mortality and Hunger in Europe and America: Timing and Mechanisms' in David Landes, Patrice Higgonet and Henry Rosovsky, eds, *Favorites of Fortune: Technology, Growth and Economic Development Since the Industrial Revolution*. Cambridge, MA: Harvard University Press, 1991. Also see Fogel's 'Nutrition and the Decline in Mortality Since 1700: Some Preliminary Findings in Long-Term Factors in American Economic Growth', in Stanley L. Engerman and Robert E. Gallman, eds, *Conference on Research in Income and Wealth*, Vol. 41. Chicago, IL: University of Chicago Press, 1986, and *Economic Growth, Population Theory, and Physiology: the Bearing of Long-Term Processes in the Making of Economic Policy*, working paper no. 4638. Cambridge, MA: National Bureau of Economic Research, April 1994.

8. Statistics on the causes of global deaths in 1990 are derived from the World Bank's *World Development Report 1993: Investing in Health*. New York: Oxford University Press, 1993. pp. 224–5.

9. Global AIDS Policy Coalition. Johnathan Mann, ed. *Status and Trends of the HIV/AIDS Pandemic as of January 1996*: Cambridge, MA. Harvard School of Public Health, François-Xavier Bagnoud Center for Health and Human Rights. January 18, 1996. p. 2.

10. See UNAIDS. AIDS Epidemic Update: December 1998, pp. 2–3. Available at the following URL, http://www.unaids.org/highband/document/epdemio/wadr98e.pdf.

11. Ibid., p. 3.

12. Namibia and Swaziland currently report HIV seroprevalence levels in excess of 20 per cent, and Zimbabwe, Botswana have the dubious distinction of having infection levels of over 25 per cent of the total population. See the individual country annual seroprevalence statistics available at http://www.unaids.org/highband.

13. Lawrence K. Altman. 'Parts of Africa Showing HIV in 1 in 4 adults', *New York Times*, 24 June 1998. p. A1.

14. Suzanne Daly. 'A Post-Apartheid Agony: AIDS on the March', *New York Times*, 23 July 1998. p. A1.

15. Donald McNeil, Jr. 'AIDS Stalking Africa's Struggling Economies', *New York Times*, 15 November 1998. p. A1.

16. Op. cit., p. A1.

17. Andre Picard, 'UN Warns of Alarming Gap in Prevention of AIDS', *Globe and Mail*, 24 June 1998. p. B.4.

18. Murray Feschbach, 'Dead Souls', *Atlantic Monthly*, January 1999. p. 26.

19. 'HIV Rising in CIS Countries', *Globe and Mail*, 22 April 1998. p. A16.
20. Lawrence K. Altman, 'Dismaying Experts, HIV infections Soar', *New York Times*, 24 November 1998. p. F7.
21. John Stackhouse, 'Nagaland Choking in Grip of AIDS ...', *Globe and Mail*, 1 December 1997. p. A11.
22. *World Health Report 1996*, p. 27.
23. Ibid.
24. Ibid., p. 28.
25. Michael Specter, 'Doctors Powerless as AIDS rakes Africa', *New York Times*, 6 August 1998. p. A1.
26. Feschbach, p. 27.
27. Specter, p. A1.
28. Ellen Ruppel Shell, 'Resurgence of a Deadly Disease', *Atlantic Monthly*, August 1997. p. 47.
29. Ibid., p. 48.
30. Ibid., p. 45. Malaria's re-emergence as an endemically transmitted pathogen in Toronto, Canada has been verified by Kevin Kain of the Tropical Disease Unit, Toronto General Hospital. Comments made to the author 30 October 1998.
31. *World Health Report 1996*, p. 2.
32. Note the evidence compiled by Paul Ewald, cited in Judith Hooper, 'A New Germ Theory', *Atlantic Monthly*. February 1999. pp. 41–53.
33. See http://cdc.gov/nchswww/fastats for this data.
34. 1973 may be viewed as a turning point in the 'health transition'. Up until the early 1970s, advances in public health had contributed to the dramatic fall in infectious-disease induced morbidity and mortality on a global scale. Thus the prevalence of infectious disease had reached its nadir circa 1973. This year also saw the recognition of a new pathogen 'rotavirus', the first of many new pathogenic agents to emerge in the coming decades. Essentially, 1973 is the turning point in the health transition where the curve of infectious disease incidence stops declining and begins its ascension. See *Report of the NSTC Committee on International Science, Engineering, and Technology (CISET) Working Group on Emerging and Re-Emerging Infectious Diseases. Global Microbial Threats in the 1990s*. Washington, DC: White House, September 1995.
35. Stephen S. Morse, ed. *Emerging Viruses*. New York: Oxford University Press, 1993.
36. This methodology (and the use of surrogate measures of disease prevalence such as infant mortality and life expectancy) is presented in full in Price-Smith, Andrew T. *Wilson's Bridge: a Consilient Methodology for the Analysis of Complex Biological-Political Relationships*. CIS Working Paper 1998–8. Toronto: Centre for International Studies, University of Toronto. November 1998.
37. See Randall M. Packard. *White Plague, Black Labour: Tuberculosis and the Political Economy of Health and Disease in South Africa*. Berkeley: University of California Press, 1989.
38. These hypothetical causal relationships are empirically confirmed via diachronic national and global correlations in Andrew T. Price-Smith, *Statistical Evidence of a Negative Association between Infectious Disease and*

State Capacity: 1951–1991. CIS Working Paper 1999–1. Toronto: Centre for International Studies, University of Toronto.

39. This collapse of governance in the presence of rapidly declining population health has been anecdotally noted over the broad span of history by observers such as Thucydides, Galen, McNeill, Crosby, and Watts. For example see Thucydides, *The Peloponnesian War*. New York: Penguin, 1980. pp. 151–6.

40. Thomas F. Homer-Dixon. 'The Ingenuity Gap: Can Poor Countries Adapt to Resource Scarcity?' *Population and Development Review*, 21 (3) September 1995, p. 589.

41. The determinants of adaptation are (1) the change in the requirements for adaptation (i.e. how hard is the job?); and (2) can we supply the knowledge, adaptive strategies and technologies we need, when and where we require them, at the optimal time?

42. Note the significant penetration of developed societies by pathogens such as HIV, Hepatitis C and B, and our continuing vigilance against another lethal influenza pandemic.

43. 'The Old Enemy'. *Economist*. 1 October 1994. p. 40.

44. Hamish MacDonald. 'Surat's Revenge: India Counts the Mounting Costs of Poverty'. *Far Eastern Economic Review*. 13 October 1994. p. 76.

45. 'Were Ultras responsible for Surat Plague?' *The Hindustan Times*. 9 July 1995.

46. 'Was it the Plague?' *Economist*. 19 November 1994. pp. 38–40.

47. For an analysis of human reaction to, and aversion of, risk with the attendant irrational behavior that results, see Roger E. Kasperson *et al. The Social Amplification of Risk: a Conceptual Framework*. Center for Technology, Environment, and Development (CENTED), Clark University, Worcester, Massachusetts. 1989.

48. As of 23 March 1996 France, Italy, Germany and Belgium among others had banned UK beef imports. John Darnton. 'France and Belgium ban British Beef over Cow Disease'. *New York Times*. 22 March 1996. p. A4; David Wallen. 'European partners ban UK beef'. *Globe and Mail*. 22 March 1996. pp. A1, A10.

49. For further literature on deprivation-conflicts and state-failure see Jack Goldstone. *Revolution and Rebellion in the Early Modern Era*. Berkeley: University of California Press, 1991; Homer-Dixon, Thomas F. 'On the Threshold: Environmental Changes as Causes of Acute Conflict'. pp. 43–83 in Sean M. Lynn-Jones and Steven E. Miller, eds. *Global Dangers: Changing Dimensions of International Security*. Cambridge, MA: MIT Press, 1995; Thomas F. Homer-Dixon, 'Environmental Scarcities and Violent Conflict: Evidence from Cases'. pp. 144–82 in Sean M. Lynn-Jones and Steven E. Miller, eds. *Global Dangers: Changing Dimensions of International Security*. Cambridge, MA: MIT Press, 1995; Colin Kahl. 'Population Growth, Environmental Degradation, and State-Sponsored Violence; The case of Kenya, 1991–93'. International Security Vol. 23 (2), Fall 1998. pp. 80–119; Holsti, Kalevi J. *The State, War, and the State of War*. Cambridge: Cambridge University Press, 1996; Ted Gurr. *Why Men Rebel*, 1970; and Rice, Edward. *Wars of the Third Kind: Conflict in Underdeveloped Countries*. Berkeley: University of California Press, 1988.

50. This conclusion is based on the aforementioned negative empirical association between infectious disease and SC. The statistical evidence shows that the arguments of historians such as McNeill, Crosby, Zinsser, Watts and Oldstone (linking plagues with the collapse of empires and societies) are likely accurate. See Michael Oldstone. *Viruses, Plagues and History*. New York: Oxford University Press, 1998.
51. See Johnson and Snyder, Ch. 11.

Bibliography

Barber, C.V. *The Case Study of Indonesia*. Occasional Paper. Project on Environmental Scarcities, State Capacity, and Civil Violence. Cambridge: American Academy of Arts and Sciences and the University of Toronto, 1997.

Crosby, A.W. *Ecological Imperialism: the Biological Expansion of Europe, 900–1900*. New York: Cambridge University Press, 1994.

Crosby, A.W. *The Colombian Exchange: Biological and Cultural Consequences of 1492*. Westport: Greenwood, 1972.

Economy, E. *The Case Study of China – Reforms and Resources: the Implications for State Capacity in the PRC*. Occasional Paper. Project on Environmental Scarcities, State Capacity, and Civil Violence. Cambridge: American Academy of Arts and Sciences and the University of Toronto, 1997.

Fogel, R.W. The Conquest of High Mortality and Hunger in Europe and America: Timing and Mechanisms, in D. Landes, P. Higgonet and H. Rosovsky (eds). *Favorites of Fortune: Technology, Growth and Economic Development Since the Industrial Revolution*. Cambridge, MA: Harvard University Press, 1991.

Fogel, R.W. Nutrition and the Decline in Mortality Since 1700: Some Preliminary Findings in Long-Term Factors in American Economic Growth, in Stanley L. Engerman and Robert E. Gallman (eds). *Conference on Research in Income and Wealth*, Vol. 41. Chicago, IL: University of Chicago Press, 1986.

Fogel, R.W. *Economic Growth, Population Theory, and Physiology: the Bearing of Long-Term Processes in the Making of Economic Policy*, working paper no. 4638. Cambridge, MA: National Bureau of Economic Research. April 1994.

Goldstone, J. *Revolution and Rebellion in the Early Modern Era*. Berkeley: University of California Press, 1991.

Holsti, K.J. *The State, War, and the State of War*. Cambridge: Cambridge University Press, 1996.

Gurr, T.R. *Why Men Rebel*. Princeton: Princeton University Press, 1970.

Homer-Dixon, T.F. On the Threshold: Environmental Changes as Causes of Acute Conflict, pp. 43–83, in S.M. Lynn-Jones and S.E. Miller (eds). *Global Dangers: Changing Dimensions of International Security*. Cambridge, MA: MIT Press, 1995.

Homer-Dixon, T.F. Environmental Scarcities and Violent Conflict: Evidence from Cases, pp. 144–82, in S.M. Lynn-Jones and S.E. Miller (eds). *Global Dangers: Changing Dimensions of International Security*. Cambridge, MA: MIT Press, 1995.

Homer-Dixon, T.F. The Ingenuity Gap: Can Poor Countries Adapt to Resource Scarcity? *Population and Development Review* 21 (3). September 1995.

Homer-Dixon, T.F. and V. Percival. *The Case Study of Bihar, India.* Occasional Paper. Project on Environmental Scarcities, State Capacity, and Civil Violence. Cambridge: American Academy of Arts and Sciences and the University of Toronto, 1997.

Kahl, C. Population Growth, Environmental Degradation, and State-Sponsored Violence; The case of Kenya, 1991–93, *International Security* 23 (2). Fall 1998. pp. 80–119.

McNeill, W.H. *Plagues and Peoples.* Toronto: Doubleday, 1989.

Morse, S.S. (ed.), *Emerging Viruses.* New York: Oxford University Press, 1993.

Packard, R.M. *White Plague, Black Labour: Tuberculosis and the Political Economy of Health and Disease in South Africa.* Berkeley: University of California Press, 1989.

Oldstone, M. *Viruses, Plagues and History.* New York: Oxford University Press, 1998.

Price-Smith, A.T. *Statistical Evidence of a Negative Association between Infectious Disease and State Capacity: 1951–1991.* CIS Working Paper 1999–1. Toronto: Centre for International Studies, University of Toronto, February 1999.

Price-Smith, A.T. *Wilson's Bridge: a Consilient Methodology for the Analysis of Complex Biological–Political Relationships.* CIS Working Paper 1998–8. Toronto: Centre for International Studies, University of Toronto, November 1998.

Price-Smith, A.T. *Contagion and Chaos: Infectious Disease and its Effects on Global Security and Development.* CIS Working Paper 1998–1. Toronto: Centre for International Studies, University of Toronto, January 1998.

Rice, E. *Wars of the Third Kind: Conflict in Underdeveloped Countries.* Berkeley: University of California Press, 1988.

Thucydides, *The Peloponnesian War.* New York: Penguin, 1980.

Watts, S. *Epidemics and History: Disease, Power, and Imperialism.* New Haven, CT: Yale University Press, 1997.

Zinsser, H. *Rats, Lice, and History.* New York: Little, Brown & Co., 1934.

World Development Report 1993: Investing in Health. New York: Oxford University Press, 1993. pp. 224–5.

Report of the NSTC Committee on International Science, Engineering, and Technology (CISET) Working Group on Emerging and Re-Emerging Infectious Diseases. Global Microbial Threats in the 1990s. Washington: DC, White House, September 1995.

9

The Return of Infectious Disease

Laurie Garrett

The post-antibiotic era

Since World War II, public health strategy has focused on the eradication of microbes. Using powerful medical weaponry developed during the postwar period – antibiotics, antimalarials and vaccines – political and scientific leaders in the United States and around the world pursued a military-style campaign to obliterate viral, bacterial and parasitic enemies. The goal was nothing less than pushing humanity through what was termed the 'health transition', leaving the age of infectious disease permanently behind. By the turn of the century, it was thought, most of the world's population would live long lives ended only by the 'chronics' – cancer, heart disease and Alzheimer's.

The optimism culminated in 1978 when the member states of the United Nations signed the 'Health for All, 2000' accord. The agreement set ambitious goals for the eradication of disease, predicting that even the poorest nations would undergo a health transition before the millennium, with life expectancies rising markedly. It was certainly reasonable in 1978 to take a rosy view of *Homo sapiens'* ancient struggle with the microbes; antibiotics, pesticides, chloroquine and other powerful antimicrobials, vaccines, and striking improvements in water treatment and food preparation technologies had provided what seemed an imposing armamentarium. The year before, the World Health Organization (WHO) had announced that the last known case of smallpox had been tracked down in Ethiopia and cured.

The grandiose optimism rested on two false assumptions: that microbes were biologically stationary targets and that diseases could be geographically sequestered. Each contributed to the smug sense of immunity from infectious diseases that characterized health professionals in North America and Europe.

Anything but stationary, microbes and the insects, rodents and other animals that transmit them are in a constant state of biological flux and evolution. Darwin noted that certain genetic mutations allow plants and animals to better adapt to environmental conditions and so produce more offspring; this process of natural selection, he argued, was the mechanism of evolution. Less than a decade after the US military first supplied penicillin to its field physicians in the Pacific theatre, geneticist Joshua Lederberg demonstrated that natural selection was operating in the bacterial world. Strains of staphylococcus and streptococcus that happened to carry genes for resistance to the drugs arose and flourished where drug-susceptible strains had been driven out. Use of antibiotics was selecting for ever-more-resistant bugs.

More recently, scientists have witnessed an alarming mechanism of microbial adaptation and change – one less dependent on random inherited genetic advantage. The genetic blueprints of some microbes contain DNA and RNA codes that command mutation under stress, offer escapes from antibiotics and other drugs, marshal collective behaviours conducive to group survival, and allow the microbes and their progeny to scour their environments for potentially useful genetic material. Such material is present in stable rings or pieces of DNA and RNA, known as plasmids and transposons, that move freely among microorganisms, even jumping between species of bacteria, fungi and parasites. Some plasmids carry the genes for resistance to five or more different families of antibiotics, or dozens of individual drugs. Others confer greater powers of infectivity, virulence, resistance to disinfectants or chlorine, even such subtly important characteristics as the ability to tolerate higher temperatures or more acidic conditions. Microbes have appeared that can grow on a bar of soap, swim unabashed in bleach, and ignore doses of penicillin logarithmically larger than those effective in 1950.

In the microbial soup, then, is a vast, constantly changing lending library of genetic material that offers humanity's minute predators myriad ways to outmanoeuvre the drug arsenal. And the arsenal, large as it might seem, is limited. In 1994, the Food and Drug Administration licensed only three new antimicrobial drugs, two of them for the treatment of AIDS and none an antibacterial. Research and development has ground to a near halt now that the easy approaches to killing viruses, bacteria, fungi and parasites – those that mimic the ways competing microbes kill one another in their endless tiny battles throughout the human gastrointestinal tract – have been exploited. Researchers have run out of ideas for countering many microbial scourges, and the lack of profitability has stifled the development of drugs to combat organisms that are currently found predominantly in poor countries. 'The pipeline is dry. We really have a global crisis', James Hughes, director of the National Center for Infectious Diseases at the Centers for Disease Control and Prevention (CDC) in Atlanta, said recently.

Diseases without borders

During the 1960s, 1970s and 1980s, the World Bank and the International Monetary Fund devised investment policies based on the assumption that economic modernization should come first and improved health would naturally follow. Today the World Bank recognizes that a nation in which more than 10 per cent of the working-age population is chronically ill cannot be expected to reach higher levels of development without investment in health infrastructure. Furthermore, the bank acknowledges that few societies spend health care dollars effectively for the poor, among whom the potential for the outbreak of infectious disease is greatest. Most of the achievements in infectious disease control have resulted from grand international efforts such as the expanded programme for childhood immunization mounted by the UN Children's Emergency Fund and WHO's smallpox eradication drive. At the local level, particularly in politically unstable poor countries, few genuine successes can be cited.

Geographic sequestration was crucial in all postwar health planning, but diseases can no longer be expected to remain in their country or region of origin. Even before commercial air travel, swine flu in 1918–19 managed to circumnavigate the planet five times in 18 months, killing 22 million people, 500 000 in the United States. How many more victims could a similarly lethal strain of influenza claim now, when some half a billion passengers will board airline flights?

Every day, one million people cross an international border. One million a week travel between the industrial and developing worlds. And as people move, unwanted microbial hitchhikers tag along. In the nineteenth century, most diseases and infections that travellers carried manifested themselves during the long sea voyages that were the primary means of covering great distances. Recognizing the symptoms, the authorities at ports of entry could quarantine contagious individuals or take other action. In the age of jet travel, however, a person incubating a disease such as Ebola can board a plane, travel 12 000 miles, pass unnoticed through customs and immigration, take a domestic carrier to a remote destination, and still not develop symptoms for several days, infecting many other people before his condition is noticeable.

Surveillance at airports has proved grossly inadequate and is often biologically irrational, given that incubation periods for many incurable contagious diseases may exceed 21 days. And when a recent traveller's symptoms become apparent, days or weeks after his journey, the task of identifying fellow passengers, locating them and bringing them to the authorities for medical examination is costly and sometimes impossible. The British and US governments both spent millions of dollars in 1976 trying to track down 522 people exposed during a flight from Sierra Leone to Washington, DC, to a Peace Corps volunteer infected with the Lassa virus, an organism that produces gruesome haemorrhagic disease in its victims. The US government eventually tracked down 505 passengers, scattered over 21 states; British Airways and the British government located 95, some of whom were also on the US list. None tested positive for the virus.

Towards the end of 1994, the New York City Department of Health and the US Immigration and Naturalization Service took step to prevent plague-infected passengers from India from disembarking at New York's John F. Kennedy International Airport. All airport and federal personnel who had direct contact with passengers were trained to recognize symptoms of *Yersinia pestis* infection. Potential plague carriers were, if possible, to be identified while still on the tarmac, so fellow passengers could be examined. Of ten putative carriers identified in New York, only two were discovered at the airport; the majority had long since entered the community. Fortunately, none of the ten proved to have plague. Health authorities came away with the lesson that airport-based screening is expensive and does not work.

Humanity is on the move worldwide, fleeing impoverishment, religious and ethnic intolerance, and high-intensity localized warfare that targets civilians. People are abandoning their homes for new destinations on an unprecedented scale, both in terms of absolute numbers and as a percentage of population. In 1994, according to the UN High Commissioner for Refugees and the Worldwatch Institute, at least 110 million people immigrated, another 30 million moved from rural to urban areas within their own country, and 23 million more were displaced by war or social unrest. This human mobility affords microbes greatly increased opportunities for movement.

The city as vector

Population expansion raises the statistical probability that pathogens will be transmitted, whether from person to person or vector – insect, rodent or other – to person. Human density is rising rapidly worldwide. Seven countries now have overall population densities exceeding 2000 people per square mile, and 43 have densities greater than 500 people per square mile. (The US average, by contrast, is 74.)

High density need not doom a nation to epidemics and unusual outbreaks of disease if sewage and water systems, housing and public health provisions are adequate. The Netherlands, for example, with 1180 people per square mile, ranks among the top 20 countries for good health and life expectancy. But the areas in which density is increasing most are not those capable of providing such infrastructural support. They are, rather, the poorest on earth. Even countries with low overall density may have cities that have become focuses for extraordinary overpopulation, from the point of view of public health. Some of these urban agglomerations have only one toilet for every 750 or more people.

Most people on the move around the world come to burgeoning metropolises like India's Surat (where pneumonic plague struck in 1994) and Zaire's Kikwit (site of the 1995 Ebola epidemic) that offer few fundamental amenities. These new centres of urbanization typically lack sewage systems, paved roads, housing, safe drinking water, medical facilities and schools adequate to serve even the most affluent residents. They are squalid sites of destitution where hundreds of thousands live much as they would in poor villages, yet so jammed together as to ensure astronomical transmission rates for airborne, waterborne, sexually transmitted and contact-transmission microbes.

But such centres are often only staging areas for the waves of impoverished people that are drawn there. The next stop is a megacity with a population of ten million or more. In the nineteenth century only two cities on earth – London and New York – even approached that size. Five years from now there will be 24 megacities, most in poor developing countries: São Paulo, Calcutta, Bombay, Istanbul, Bangkok, Tehran, Jakarta, Cairo, Mexico City, Karachi, and the like. There the woes of cities like Surat are magnified many times over. Yet even the developing world's megacities are way stations for those who most aggressively seek a better life. All paths ultimately lead these people – and the microbes they may carry – to the United States, Canada and Western Europe.

Urbanization and global migration propel radical changes in human behaviour as well as in the ecological relationship between microbes and humans. Almost invariably in large cities, sex industries arise and multiple-partner sex becomes more common, prompting rapid increases in sexually transmitted diseases. Black market access to antimicrobials is greater in urban centres, leading to overuse or outright misuse of the precious drugs and the emergence of resistant bacteria and parasites. Intravenous drug abusers' practice of sharing syringes is a ready vehicle for the transmission of microbes. Underfunded urban health facilities often become unhygienic centres for the dissemination of disease rather than its control.

The emblematic new disease

All these factors played out dramatically during the 1980s, allowing an obscure organism, HIV, to amplify and spread to the point that WHO estimates it has infected a cumulative total of 30 million people and has become endemic to every country in the world. Genetic studies of the human immunodeficiency virus that causes AIDS indicate that it is probably more than a century old, yet HIV infected perhaps less than .001 per cent of the world population until the mid-1970s. The virus population then surged because of sweeping social changes: African urbanization; American and European intravenous drug use and homosexual bathhouse activity; the Uganda–Tanzania war of 1977–79, in which rape was used as a tool of ethnic cleansing; and the growth of the American blood products industry and the international marketing of its contaminated goods. Government denial and societal prejudice everywhere in the world led to inappropriate public health interventions or plain inaction, further abetting HIV transmission and slowing research for treatment or a cure.

The estimated direct (medical) and indirect (loss of productive labour force and family-impact) costs of the disease are expected to top $500 billion by the year 2000, according to the Global AIDS Policy Coalition at Harvard University. The US Agency for International Development predicts that by then some 11 per cent of children under 15 in sub-Saharan Africa will be AIDS orphans, and that infant mortality will soar fivefold in some African and Asian nations, due to the loss of parental care among children orphaned by AIDS and its most common opportunistic infection, tuberculosis. The agency forecasts that life expectancy in the African and Asian nations hit hardest by AIDS will plummet to an astonishing low of 25 years by 2010.

Medical experts now recognize that any microbe, including ones previously unknown to science, can take similar advantage of conditions in human society, going from isolated cases, camouflaged by generally high levels of disease, to become a global threat. Furthermore, old organisms, aided by mankind's misuse of disinfectants and drugs, can take on new, more lethal forms.

A White House-appointed interagency working group on emerging and re-emerging infectious diseases estimates that at least 29 previously unknown diseases have appeared since 1973 and 20 well-known ones have re-emerged, often in new drug-resistant or deadlier forms. According to the group, total direct and indirect costs of infectious disease in the United States in 1993 were more than $120 billion; combined federal, state and municipal government expenditures that year for infectious disease control were only $74.2 million (neither figure includes AIDS, other sexually transmitted diseases or tuberculosis).

The real threat of biowarfare

The world was lucky in the September 1994 pneumonic plague epidemic in Surat. Independent studies in the United States, France and Russia revealed that the bacterial strain that caused the outbreak was unusually weak, and although the precise figures for plague cases and deaths remain a matter of debate, the numbers certainly fall below 200. Yet the epidemic vividly illustrated three crucial national security issues in disease emergence: human mobility, transparency and tensions between states up to and including the threat of biological warfare.

When word got out that an airborne disease was loose in the city, some 500 000 residents of Surat boarded trains and within 48 hours dispersed to every corner of the subcontinent. Had the microbe that caused the plague been a virus or drug-resistant bacterium, the world would have witnessed an immediate Asian pandemic. As it was, the epidemic sparked a global panic that cost the Indian economy a minimum of $2 billion in lost sales and losses on the Bombay stock market, predominantly the result of international boycotts of Indian goods and travellers.

As the number of countries banning trade with India mounted towards the end of the year, the Hindi-language press insisted that there was no plague, accusing Pakistan of a smear campaign aimed at bringing India's economy to its knees. After international scientific investigations concluded that *Yersinia pestis* had indeed been the culprit in this *bona fide* epidemic, attention turned to the bacteria's origin. By the following June, several Indian scientists claimed to have evidence that the bacteria in Surat had been genetically engineered for biowarfare purposes. Though no credible evidence exists to support it, and Indian government authorities vigorously deny such claims, the charge is almost impossible to disprove, particularly in a region rife with military and political tensions of long standing.

Even when allegations of biological warfare are not flying, it is often exceedingly difficult to obtain accurate information about outbreaks of disease, particularly from countries dependent on foreign investment or tourism or both. Transparency is a common problem; though there is usually no suggestion of covert action or malevolent intent, many countries are reluctant to disclose complete information about contagious illness. For example, nearly every country initially denied or covered up the presence of the HIV virus within its borders. Even now, at least ten nations known to be in the midst of HIV epidemics refuse to cooperate with WHO, deliberately obfuscating incidence reports or declining to provide any statistics. Similarly, Egypt denies the existence of cholera bacteria in the Nile's waters; Saudi Arabia has asked WHO not to warn that travellers to Mecca may be bitten by mosquitoes carrying viruses that cause the new, and particularly lethal, dengue haemorrhagic fever; few countries report the appearance of antibiotic-resistant strains of deadly bacteria; and in 1998 central authorities in Serbia rescinded an international epidemic alert when they learned that all the scientists WHO planned to send to the tense Kosovo region to halt a large outbreak of Crimean–Congo haemorrhagic fever were from the United States, a nation Serbia viewed with hostility.

The spectre of biological warfare having raised its head, Brad Roberts of the Centre for Strategic and International Studies is particularly concerned that the New Tier nations – developing states such as China, Iran and Iraq, that possess technological know-how but lack an organized civil society that might put some restraints on its use – might be tempted to employ bioweapons. The Federation of American Scientists has sought, so far in vain, a scientific solution to the acute weaknesses of verification and enforcement provisions in the 1972 Biological Weapons Convention, a convention which most of the world's nations have signed.

That treaty's flaws, and the very real possibility of bioweapons use, stand in sharp focus today. Iraq's threat in 1990–91 to use biological weapons in the Persian Gulf conflict found allied forces in the region virtually powerless to respond: the weapons' existence was not verified in a timely manner, the only available countermeasure was a vaccine against one type of organism, and protective gear and equipment failed to stand up to windblown sand. Last June the UN Security Council concluded that Iraqi stocks of bioweaponry might have been replenished after the Gulf War settlement.

More alarming were the actions of the Aum Shinrikyo cult in Japan in early 1995. In addition to releasing toxic sarin gas in the Tokyo subway on March 18, cult members were preparing vast quantities of *Clostridium difficile* bacterial spores for terrorist use. Though rarely fatal, clostridium infections often worsen as a result of improper antibiotic use, and long bouts of bloody diarrhoea can lead to dangerous colon inflammation. Clostridium was a good choice for biological terrorism: the spores can survive for months and may be spread with any aerosol device, and even slight exposure can make vulnerable people (particularly children and the elderly) sick enough to cost a crowded society like Japan hundreds of millions of dollars for hospitalizations and lost productivity.

The US Office of Technology Assessment has calculated what it would take to produce a spectacular terrorist bioweapon: 100 kilograms of a lethal sporulating organism such as anthrax spread over Washington, DC, by a crop duster, could cause well over two million deaths. Enough anthrax spores to kill five or six million people could be loaded into a taxi and pumped out from its exhaust as it meandered through a heavily populated city. Vulnerability to terrorist attacks, as well as to the natural emergence of disease, increase with population density.

A world at risk

A 1995 WHO survey of global capacity to identify and respond to threats from emerging disease reached troubling conclusions. Only six laboratories in the world, the study found, met security and safety standards that would make them suitable sites for research on the world's deadliest microbes, including those that cause Ebola, Marburg and Lassa fever. Local political instability threatens to compromise the security of the two labs in Russia, and budget cuts threaten to do the same to the two in the United States (the army's facility at Fort Detrick and the CDC in Atlanta) and the one in Britain. In another survey, WHO sent samples of hantaviruses (such as Sin Nombre, which caused the 1993 outbreak in New Mexico) and organisms that cause dengue, yellow fever, malaria and other diseases, to the world's 35 leading disease-monitoring facilities. Only one – the CDC – correctly identified all the organisms; most got fewer than half right.

Convinced that newly emerging diseases, whether natural or engineered, could endanger national security, the CDC requested $125 million from Congress in 1994 to bolster what it termed a grossly inadequate system of surveillance and response; it received $7.3 million. After two years of inquiry by a panel of experts, the Institute of Medicine, a division of the National Academy of Sciences, declared the situation a crisis.

Today's reality is best reflected in New York City's battle with tuberculosis. Control of the W-strain of the disease – which first appeared in the city in 1991–92, is resistant to every available drug, and kills half its victims – has already cost more than $1 billion. Despite such spending, there were 3000 TB cases in the city in 1994, some of which were the W-strain. According to the surgeon general's annual reports from the 1970s and 1980s, tuberculosis was supposed to be eradicated from the United States by 2000. During the Bush administration, the CDC told state authorities they could safely lower their fiscal commitments to TB control because victory was imminent. Now public health officials are fighting to get levels down to where they were in 1985 – a far cry from elimination. New York's crisis is a result of both immigration pressure (some cases originated overseas) and the collapse of the local public health infrastructure.

National preparedness has further eroded over the past five years in the face of budgetary constraints. Just as WHO cannot intercede in an epidemic unless it receives an invitation from the afflicted country, the CDC may not enter a US state with out a request from the state government. The US system rests on an increasingly shaky network of disease surveillance and response by states and territories. A 1992 survey for the CDC showed that 12 states had no one on staff to monitor microbial contamination of local food and water; 67 per cent of the states and territories had less than one employee monitoring the food and water of every one million residents. And only a handful of states were monitoring hospitals for the appearance of unusual or drug-resistant microbes.

State capacity rests on county and municipal public health, and there too weaknesses are acute. In October, dengue hemorrhagic fever, which had been creeping steadily northward from Brazil over the past eight years, with devastating results, struck in Texas. Most Texas counties had slashed their mosquito control budgets and were ill prepared to combat the aggressive Tiger mosquitoes from South-East Asia that carry the virus. In Los Angeles County that month, a $2 billion budget shortfall drove officials to close all but 10 of the 45 public health clinics and to attempt to sell four of the county's six public hospitals. Congress is contemplating enormous cuts in Medicare and Medicaid spending; the American Public Health Association predicts that this would result in a widespread increase in infectious disease.

Prescriptions for national health

Bolstering research capacity, enhancing disease surveillance capabilities, revitalizing sagging basic public health systems, rationing powerful drugs to avoid the emergence of drug-resistant organisms, and improving infection control practices at hospitals, are only stopgap measures. National security warrants bolder steps.

One priority is to find scientifically valid ways to use polymerase chain reaction (popularly known as DNA fingerprinting), field investigations, chemical and biological export records, and local legal instruments to track the development of new or re-emergent lethal organisms, whether naturally occurring or in the form of bioweapons. The effort should focus not only on microbes directly dangerous to humans but on those that could pose major threats to crops or livestock.

Most emerging diseases are first detected by health providers working at the primary-care level. Currently there is no system, even in the United States, whereby the providers can notify relevant authorities and be assured that their alarm will be investigated promptly. In much of the world, the notifiers' reward is penalties levied against them, primarily because states want to hush up the problem. But Internet access is improving worldwide, and a small investment would give physicians an electronic highway to international health authorities that bypassed government roadblocks and obfuscation.

Only three diseases – cholera, plague and yellow fever – are subject to international regulation, permitting UN and national authorities to interfere as necessary in the global traffic of goods and persons to stave off cross-border epidemics. The World Health Assembly, the legislative arm of WHO, recommended at its 1995 annual meeting in Geneva that the United Nations consider both expanding the list of regulated diseases and finding new ways to monitor the broad movement of disease. The Ebola outbreak in Kikwit demonstrated that a team of international scientists can be mobilized to swiftly contain a remote, localized epidemic caused by known non-airborne agents.

If a major epidemic were to imperil the United States, the Office of Emergency Preparedness and the National Disaster Medical System (part of the Department of Health and Human Services) would be at the helm. The office has 4200 private-sector doctors and nurses throughout the 50 states who are at its disposal and committed to rapid mobilization in case of emergency. The system is sound but should be bolstered. Participants should be supplied with protective suits, respirators, mobile containment laboratories and adequate local isolation facilities.

As for potential threats from biological weapons, the US Department of Energy has identified serious lapses in Russian and Ukrainian compliance with the Biological Weapons Convention. Large stockpiles of bioweapons are believed to remain, and employees of the Soviet programme for biological warfare are still on the state payroll. Arsenals are also thought to exist in other nations, although intelligence on this is weak. The location and destruction of such weapons is a critical priority. Meanwhile, scientists in the United States and Europe are identifying the genes in bacteria and viruses that code for virulence and modes of transmission. Better understanding of the genetic mechanisms will allow scientists to manipulate existing organisms, endowing them with dangerous capabilities. It would seem prudent for the United States and the international community to examine that potential now and consider options for the control of such research or its fruits.

To guard against the proliferation of blood-associated diseases, the blood and animal exports industries must be closely regulated, plasma donors must be screened for infections and an internationally acceptable watchdog agency must be designated to monitor reports of the appearance of new forms of such diseases. The export of research animals played a role in a serious incident in Germany in which vaccine workers were infected with the Marburg virus and in an Ebola scare in Virginia in which imported monkeys died from the disease.

Nobel laureate, Joshua Lederberg, of Rockefeller University, has characterized the solutions to the threat of disease emergence as multitudinous, largely straightforward and commonsensical, and international in scope; 'the bad news', he says, 'is they will cost money'.

Budgets, particularly for health care, are being cut at all levels of government. Dustin Hoffman made more money playing a disease control scientist in the movie *Outbreak* than the combined annual budgets for the US National Center for Infectious Diseases and the UN Programme on AIDS/HIV.

10
Microsecurity

Sara Glasgow and Dennis Pirages

Hardly a week goes by without new evidence of a growing microbial threat to human well-being. In the United States, thousands are killed and millions are sickened each year from food-borne illnesses caused by *E. coli, Salmonella* spp., cyclospora, and cryptosporidium.[1] Outbreaks of hepatitis A have become so common that it is now recommended that children be vaccinated against it in 17 US states.[2] Exotic diseases, such as West Nile fever, appear in parts of the country where they have never been seen before. Food shipments from abroad, often carrying various pathogens, are increasingly taxing the ability of the Food and Drug Administration to inspect them. Less than two per cent of the 2.7 million shipments of fruit, vegetables, seafood and processed foods shipped yearly ever get inspected.[3]

The situation is even grimmer in other parts of the world. A deadly AIDS epidemic grinds methodically around the world leaving millions of casualties in its wake. Extremely lethal diseases such as Ebola continue to emerge from tropical rain forests. Millions of chickens have been slaughtered as a preventive measure in Hong Kong in order to stop a deadly virus from spreading to human beings.[4] Similarly, nearly a million pigs have been culled in Malaysia to keep another fatal virus from decimating the human population.[5] And 'mad cow' disease continues to poison economic relations among members of the European Union. The war with infectious diseases, once thought to have been won, now seems to be escalating.

The causes of these new microbial challenges can be found by studying processes of coevolution and the growth of ecological interdependence. Biological populations of *Homo sapiens* (societies) historically have coevolved with other species and a wide variety of microorganisms within the ever-changing constraints of local ecosystems.

Ecological interdependence refers to the delicate networks of symbiotic relationships among these various organisms and between them and the sustaining physical environments. Rapid changes in these relationships can rebound to the detriment of human beings, other creatures, microorganisms or even the ecosystem itself. Thus, a mutation in a pathogenic microorganism, a rapid increase in a human population, or even a change in rainfall patterns, could destabilise an ecosystem with unfortunate consequences for all the creatures that share it.

For much of human history these coevolutionary processes have taken place in local and somewhat isolated ecosystems. Because of lengthy periods of time available for mutual adaptation, bouts of pestilence or outbreaks of disease usually have been limited in scope and impact. But globalization processes are mixing people and microorganisms on an unprecedented scale, thus causing major discontinuities in biological evolutionary processes. And as the industrial revolution spreads worldwide, patterns of human interaction are also changing. These shifts in the way that people live and behave are also dramatically transforming relationships between people and pathogens.

In an era when the United States is spending nearly $270 billion annually to protect people against *potential* threats from human adversaries, it is important to reflect on the comparatively feeble commitment to fighting these *actual* microbial threats to human well-being. In this chapter we suggest an 'ecological security' framework for thinking about the future of such defence allocations. We identify some historical and contemporary discontinuities in biological and sociocultural evolution that have increased and are increasing microinsecurity. We conclude by focusing directly on the biological and socioeconomic causes and consequences of one of the most serious contemporary challenges to microsecurity: the unfolding AIDS epidemic in sub-Saharan Africa.

Ecological security

Concern about the security of human societies has historically focused on minimizing the impact of armed conflict among them. Dabelko and Dabelko report that, 'At its most fundamental level, the term security has meant the effort to protect a population and territory against organised force while advancing state interest through competitive behaviour'.[6] Given the destruction that has been associated with violent conflicts among peoples since ancient times, it is understandable why security has been thus defined. Military threats have been vivid, understandable; and defences could, at least in theory, be mounted against them. While a plethora of other challenges to human survival – famines, plagues, pestilence and so forth – certainly have caused much greater human misfortune, there has been little under-standing of their causes and thus of possible defences against them. But advances in medical and environmental sciences are now yielding a much better understanding of the causes of these tragedies, thus opening up new opportunities to deal resolutely with these primary threats to human security.

While the cross-border machinations of neighbouring states have certainly been a cause of death and destruction throughout history, these other sources of insecurity have been much more destructive. But since these have been considered to be the work of God or of gods, and thus beyond human remedy, there has been little reason for security policies to deal with them. Thus, the 'Black Death' (Bubonic Plague) in the fourteenth century was certainly perceived by those afflicted to be a major source of insecurity, especially since nearly 40 per cent of those exposed to the disease perished. But the only 'defensive' actions that were perceived to be efficacious at that time were prayer, human sacrifices and self-flagellation.[7]

An ecological security approach to thinking about the welfare of human societies builds on the rather sensible notion that defence poli-cies ought to be designed to prevent the premature loss of human lives. At present, nearly 50 per cent of these premature deaths are caused by infectious diseases.[8] Throughout the twentieth century casualties from military engagements paled in comparison with human suffering and premature deaths due to famine and disease. While the eyes of the world were focused on the military horrors of World War I, for example, an influenza virus which originated in the United States spread around the world, exacting more than 20 million human casu-alties, many times the total of battlefield deaths.[9] It is estimated that all the wars of the twentieth century – 100 years – took the lives of some 111 million combatants and civilians, but infectious diseases are now killing more than 17 million people annually.[10]

This way of thinking about human security begins with the hum-bling consideration that *Homo sapiens* is but one species among mil-lions, albeit a very significant one. *Homo sapiens* has evolved within the changing constraints of physical environments shared among human populations, with various kinds of microorganisms, and with popula-tions of other species. These co-evolutionary processes have been at various times influenced by environmental changes, shifts in human behaviour, the growth and decline of populations of other species, the changing capabilities of pathogenic microorganisms and by techno-logical innovation.

This ecological perspective on human security thus moves well beyond worries about military force and weaponry and focuses on bal-ances in four continually co-evolving relationships critical to the well-being of the human race. Ecological security is enhanced when a balance or equilibrium is maintained in the following four relationships:

- Between human populations and the sustaining capabilities of the relevant physical environments (environmental security).
- Between human populations and those of other species (species security).
- Among human populations sharing the same ecosystems (military security).
- Between human populations and pathogenic microorganisms (microsecurity).

The environmental security of human populations is strengthened when their needs for resources and environmental services are met without weakening sustaining natural systems. Human populations, like those of other species, tend to expand until checked by resource limitations. From local firewood crises to global warming, there are now abundant signs of growing imbalances between the demands of people and the sustaining capabilities of ecosystems. In spite of the sometimes benevolent impact of new technologies, in many parts of the world the bulk of humanity still lives very close to the margin. For these people, living space is at a premium, environmental services are heavily burdened, and food and fuel supplies are problematic. The population explosion in the Global South and the growing resource demands of industrialization have already seriously stressed the rele-vant ecosystems, leading to land degradation, increased vulnerability to disease and, not infrequently, to violent conflict.[11]

Similarly, the well-being of human populations has been and still is very much influenced by interactions with other species. *Homo sapiens* doesn't possess many of the physical attributes, such as sharp claws and long legs, essential to competition in the wild, and for much of history large predators have represented a substantial threat. People still share their habitat with potentially dangerous animals in many parts of the world and are frequently in direct conflicts with them. Periodic and sometimes fatal rampages of elephants and tigers in 'humanised' parts of India or the nuisance activities of racoons, bears and deer in suburban areas of the United States, are evidence of continuing skirmishes between man and beast. But technological innovations, ranging from rifles to insecticides, have tipped this balance in favour of people in many parts of the world and threats from large predators are now much diminished. Smaller species, however, can still create problems. From biblical times to the present, plagues of locusts as well as many other pests have been a serious threat to food supplies.[12] On the other hand, growing human populations often threaten the extinction of large numbers of other species, possibly undermining ecological interdependence and rebounding to the detriment of all creatures.

Maintaining equilibriums among human populations is the third component of ecological security. This aspect of it is in some ways similar to traditional military security, but there are two significant differences. The state is no longer assumed to be the most important actor in many conflicts, and the breadth of security concerns expands to encompass socioeconomic and environmental well-being. In the contemporary world, military insecurity is less often the result of conflicts among states and much more frequently the result of quarrels among ethnic groups at the sub-national level. And troops are more frequently involved in refereeing disputes among ethnic groups or rebuilding societies after humanitarian or environmental disasters.

By far the most serious ongoing threat to ecological security, and the subject of the rest of this chapter, is the destabilization of the historically tenuous equilibrium between *Homo sapiens* and pathogenic microorganisms. *Homo sapiens* and a wide variety of microorganisms have coevolved over centuries and most of the time this relationship has been marked by peaceful coexistence. This equilibrium has been facilitated by the development of the human immune system, honed by centuries of encounters with pathogens. Periodically, however, this delicate truce has been disturbed in one way or another when human populations have come into contact with novel pathogens. For example, rats and their flea passengers travelling trade routes from China to Europe were a vector for the bubonic plague that struck previously unexposed Europeans during the Middle Ages. Similarly, the 'discovery' of the Americas opened up a two-way flow of microorganisms that wreaked havoc in both Europe and the Americas.[13] There is now considerable evidence that changes in biological and sociocultural evolution associated with globalization and changes in human circumstances are combining to make societies much more vulnerable to new and resurgent diseases. The next century could well see increasing microinsecurity caused by the outbreak of rapidly moving plagues brought about by changes in man–microbe relationships.[14]

Globalization and microsecurity

The original outward movement of *Homo sapiens* from North Africa and the Middle East eventually resulted in a world inhabited by thousands of geographically isolated human populations living within clans, tribes and small kingdoms.[15] These populations coevolved biologically with other species and microorganisms within the constraints of shared local ecosystems. But, over time, technological innovations in transportation and weaponry led to the merger of these groups into larger and often more powerful units. This long and steady historical trend has culminated in contemporary globalization and the large-scale mingling of human populations and the microorganisms that they carry.[16]

Throughout history, the integration of previously small and isolated populations into larger kingdoms and empires created significant discontinuities in biological and sociocultural evolution and exacted a tragic toll of deaths from both warfare and disease. William McNeill has observed that the expanding Roman Empire was repeatedly wracked by strange diseases. There were at least 11 microbial disasters in Republican times. A major epidemic struck the city of Rome in 65 AD, but that paled in comparison with a more widespread epidemic that began to sweep the Roman Empire in 165 AD. Mortality as a result of this latter plague was heavy: one-quarter to one-third of those catching the disease died.[17]

More recently, contact between expanding European populations and those in other parts of the world also had similar disease ramifications. By the year 1350, the various kingdoms of Western Europe had become large and dense enough to press against the carrying capacity of relevant ecosystems. Growing population density led to local European famines which were reported in most years between 1290 and 1350 AD.[18] At the same time, contacts and commerce among populations was increasing, even spreading out to lengthy trade routes between Western Europe and China. During this period of European population increase, urban growth and expanded commerce, significant numbers of people, including messengers, merchants and mercenaries, were moving among previously isolated human populations. And this increased contact resulted in the spread of new diseases from the Orient to Europe, the most infamous being *Pasteurella pestis*, also known as the Black Death. The arrival of the Black Death in Europe in 1346 began a lengthy pruning process through which successive waves of disease trimmed the region's population by nearly 40 per cent, with the highest mortality rates being in the urban areas.[19]

These contacts between peoples and unfamiliar microbes took another leap forward during the ensuing age of European exploration and colonization. The ships of Christopher Columbus, arriving in the Caribbean in 1492, were the first of a wave of European vessels which brought Europeans and the microorganisms that they carried into contact with indigenous peoples. And these microorganisms wiped out a significant portion of them. The military history of the period is replete with tales of miraculous conquests of huge numbers of Indians by mere handfuls of European troops. In reality there were few *bona fide* miracles. Epidemics, particularly of smallpox, unwittingly launched by the invaders, killed approximately two-thirds of the indigenous populations, leaving them in disarray and unable to muster the strength for a decent defence of their territories. As William McNeill has put it, 'From the Amerindian point of view, stunned acquiescence to Spanish superiority was the only possible response. ... Native authority structures crumbled; the old gods seemed to have abdicated. The situation was ripe for the mass conversions recorded so proudly by Christian missionaries.' The spread of smallpox was followed by measles and eventually by typhus, with diseases imported from Africa – such as malaria and yellow fever – being transplanted in the American tropics. By the time that these diseases had run their course, it is estimated that only one in twenty of the indigenous inhabitants in the affected areas survived.[20]

Deadly epidemics thus very frequently come from biologically naive human populations coming into contact with pathogens with which they have little experience. Obviously people who move into new ecosystems or disease environments are at substantial risk of contracting illnesses. This is why business people or scholars who have attended international conferences often come down with influenza or similar illnesses upon return, or why people who move from one coast of the United States to the other are frequently ill during their first year of residence. Well-travelled people (or animals) moving into new social environments can similarly bring microbial travellers with them, thus threatening these populations with potentially deadly diseases.

Pathogens lurking in previously uninhabited areas also can be a threat to people. Rapid population growth in tropical areas of the world is driving people to clear and occupy land at the edges of rain forests, thus liberating various kinds of microorganisms from their previous isolation within animal hosts. AIDS, Ebola, Marburg, and yellow fever viruses were probably first found in monkeys, Rift Valley fever in cattle, sheep, and mosquitoes, and Hantaan virus in rodents. Homer-Dixon found that, 'These pathogens lurked relatively undisturbed in their animal hosts in the tropics, jumping to humans only on rare occasions. They had little opportunity to adapt to humans, who usually were "dead end" host species, because the viruses would fizzle out once they swept through a small population at the edge of the forest.'[21] But now these and other viruses can make successful leaps from animals to larger human populations, thus putting deadly new diseases in motion. Between 1997 and 1999, for example, viruses were making leaps from monkeys to humans in Congo (Monkeypox), from chickens to humans in Hong Kong (influenza H5N1), and from pigs to humans in Malaysia (agent unknown).

Thus, epidemics that have transformed the biological and sociocultural nature of human societies have most frequently occurred when human immune systems have encountered pathogenic microorganisms with which they have had little evolutionary experience. The contemporary frenetic pace of industrialization and globalization is increasingly bringing previously separated people and pathogens into closer contact in many different ways, thus increasing microinsecurity and the potential for the rapid worldwide spread of new diseases.

Social transformation and microsecurity

While technological innovation, rapid growth of international travel, expansion of markets, and the associated globalization have combined to greatly increase the risk of the worldwide spread of disease, changes in the way that people live and behave have also increased such vulnerability. People now are living in more densely packed megacities, major changes are taking place in the way that food is grown, handled and marketed, economic conditions are stagnant in many parts of the world, and many people are engaging in biologically risky behaviour. All of these changes have negative consequences for microsecurity.

It is ironic that twentieth-century advances in medical and biological knowledge have been heralded as having the potential to wipe out most infectious diseases at the same time that traditional diseases are making a comeback and novel microbes are on the attack. Mark Lappe comments that 'At the root of the resurgence of old infectious diseases is an evolutionary paradox: the more vigorously we have assailed the world of microorganisms, the more varied the repertoire of bacterial and viral strains thrown up against us.'[22] Just as scientific discoveries have seemingly given *Homo sapiens* new weapons in the struggle against disease, changes in the human condition have opened up new opportunities for pathogenic microorganisms.

The large-scale demographic changes taking place in the contemporary world are well documented, but the epidemiological significance of these shifts is often neglected. A demographically and epidemiologically divided world has passed through the period of most rapid population growth, but there is still tremendous growth momentum on the southern side of the demographic divide. The current world population of six billion is projected to grow to 8.1 billion by the year 2025. At that time nearly seven billion people will reside in what is now the less industrialized world.[23] The largest portion of these people will be living under marginal conditions in densely populated megacities where disease organisms can spread rapidly. Large-scale urbanization in the less industrialized parts of the world is creating unmanageable slums in which diseases can rapidly spread among the victims of urban poverty. The larger the number of people living under conditions of squalor in densely populated cities, the greater the opportunities for viruses, bacteria and other microorganisms to prey on human beings.

This rapid population growth on the south side of the global demographic divide is accompanied, in many countries, by deteriorating economic circumstances. Between 1990 and 1997 there was a decline in gross domestic product per capita in 41 of the 136 countries for which adequate data are available.[24] In countries ranging from Middle Eastern oil exporters to impoverished states in sub-Saharan Africa, where rapid population growth has outstripped feeble economic gains, this traditional measure of economic progress has shown a decline. Even aggregate groups of countries showed signs of worsening conditions. Both the 'least developed countries' and 'Eastern Europe and former IS countries' showed substantial per capita economic declines during this period. And the 'sub-Saharan Africa' region experienced a steep 4.5 per cent decline over the period.

The causes of this increasing impoverishment are varied, but it is clear that the spread of the industrial revolution and its assumed benefits to many parts of the world is no longer guaranteed. More to the point, however, is the impact of poverty on human health. While annual per capita health care expenditures amount to nearly $3000 in the United States, in Zaire, Tanzania, Sierra Leone and Mozambique, five dollars or less is spent per person.[25] The recent impoverishment of the former Soviet Union has been associated with a significant increase in disease in that part of the world.[26] The latest innovations in biomedical technology and pharmaceuticals may mean little to afflicted people in countries that cannot afford to import costly medicines and vaccines produced in the industrialized countries.

Many aspects of technological innovation have proved to be beneficial forces for human progress, but technology also has a darker side. While progress in biomedical technology has led to considerable gains in the battle against pathogenic microorganisms, some other aspects of technological innovation seem to favour the microbes. Technology-induced changes in the production and distribution of food products, for example, can increase microinsecurity. Agricultural production, especially in the industrialized countries, now takes place on megafarms; processing is done in food factories; distribution is via megamarkets; and consumption often takes place in fast-food emporiums. Not surprisingly, in the United States, there are frequent large-scale outbreaks of disease from the resulting bacterial contamination of food. Widely distributed products, ranging from hamburgers to ice cream, have been responsible for debilitating outbreaks of illness. And the continuing globalization of food markets raises the spectre of more severe outbreaks of disease coursing through human populations.

Ironically, even the use of antibiotics against pathogens can be counterproductive. Large-scale use of antibiotics and other drugs is rapidly re-shaping the microbial world in both positive and negative ways. Since there are few limits on the use of these chemicals, their consumption by people and farm animals is becoming a major factor in changing the human–microbe equilibrium. Many microorganisms now are mutating into drug-resistant forms. The first apparent case of drug resistance was a strain of gonorrhea that emerged in the Philippines. More recently, new strains of tuberculosis resist most drugs previously used in treatment. And a growing list of other resistant microorganisms has emerged from encounters with antibiotics and other drugs, including tuberculosis, pneumonia and dysentery.[27]

Environmental transformation, whether or not caused by human activities, can also upset the delicate equilibrium between *Homo sapiens* and pathogens. There is ample evidence that global greenhouse warming is now a significant factor in the spread of diseases beyond their normal domains. Fatal outbreaks of hantavirus in the southwestern United States have been triggered by changes in rainfall which increased food availability and facilitated the growth of the rodent populations that carry the virus.[28] Mosquitoes bearing tropical diseases, such as West Nile fever, are passing on these exotic diseases to people in the northeastern portion of the United States, areas that were previously thought to be too cold for them to survive.[29]

There are three types of environmental change that could have a significant impact on the future evolution and spread of serious diseases: the multifaceted impact of global warming, the breakdown of the ozone layer and its associated greater penetration of ultraviolet radiation, and the creation of new kinds of polluted primordial soups within which various microbes can mingle, leading to the increasingly rapid exchange of genetic information between microbes which in turn allows for rapid mutation and adaptation into new 'resistant' and 'lethal' strains.

Projecting the future course and consequences of global warming is still an uncertain science and numerous estimates of future temperature increases have been made. But even small increases in temperature are likely to have a significant impact on regional weather conditions. Increased temperature or rainfall could lead microbe-carrying animals to range into new territories, and diseases that thrive in warm, wet climates, such as malaria or yellow fever, to make inroads into formerly cooler and drier regions.[30] An increase in ultraviolet radiation may well be related to a growing number of melanomas and cataracts, and also may have less obvious effects on the human immune system.[31] Last but not least, the waste products of human activities, ranging from sewage to chemicals, increasingly mingle in rivers, bays, streams and coastal ecosystems where mutations and recombinations among viruses and bacteria are constantly taking place.[32]

Changes in human sexual behaviour, at least partially a response to the availability of new contraceptives and medicines, have significantly increased the incidence of sexually transmitted diseases. Whereas only a few decades ago most of these diseases could be treated successfully with antibiotics, some of them are now fatal. Over the last three decades a worldwide sexual revolution has led to the proliferation of sexually transmitted diseases such as herpes, syphilis, gonorrhea, hepatitis and AIDS. More widespread use of recreational drugs, particularly those injected with shared needles, is another peculiar change in human behaviour that is tipping the security balance toward the microbes.

The ongoing worldwide AIDS epidemic offers a powerful example of these varied and growing challenges to microsecurity. Even though this particular disease is not unusually contagious, the inexorable spread of HIV to tens of millions of people has been facilitated by increased global travel, changes in sexual behaviour and an increase in intravenous drug usage. The disease has now spread to almost all parts of the world. While the origins of the AIDS epidemic are still somewhat obscure, its impact on microsecurity is not. This is particularly true in sub-Saharan Africa where endemic poverty, permissive sexual behaviour, and some traditional social customs have combined to create a major challenge to microsecurity.

Microinsecurity in sub-Saharan Africa

The conditions previously discussed – globalization, rapid population growth, urbanization, grinding poverty, behavioural changes and the resulting increase in disease – have a direct impact on political, economic and social life. There is no region of the world that has been more plagued by these conditions than sub-Saharan Africa. The sub-Saharan region has historically been ecologically insecure and challenged in a number of ways – the colonial experience, high birth rates, extreme poverty and a wide range of endemic infectious diseases. But some improvement in several indicators of progress over the last few decades encouraged hopes that the situation was finally changing. Even though the region retains one of the highest fertility rates in the world, between 1978 and 1998, annual sub-Saharan population growth declined from 3.9 per cent to 2.7 per cent. Infant mortality during that same time span declined from 121 to 91 per 1000 births.[33] Despite these improvements, however, average life expectancy in the region rose only slightly from 47 to 49 years, well below the global average of 66 years.[34] While several factors undoubtedly contribute to the persistence of low life expectancy, none is as dominant as that of infectious disease.

Of the myriad infectious diseases compromising microsecurity in sub-Saharan Africa, AIDS now stands apart as the most critical. While the prevalence of AIDS clearly varies among different sub-Saharan countries, the regional statistics indicate an alarming trend. As of 1997, 14 million people in the region were HIV positive – more than two-thirds of the world total.[35] In Zimbabwe, one-quarter of the adult population is currently infected, and more than 200 die every day. In Kenya, 12 per cent of the population is infected.[36] The scope of the AIDS problem is so severe that it has actually reversed life expectancy. In the nine countries where more than 10 per cent of the population is infected, the average current life expectancy is 48 years. In the absence of AIDS it would be 58.[37]

The rapid transmission of AIDS and the high prevalence rates in these countries is due to a number of factors, but economic privation and established social customs play a significant role. Poor women often turn to prostitution to earn a living. Lacking education and skills required for other employment, it is often the only option. Clients who become infected with HIV can pass it along to their partners. In some African societies cultural norms dictate that new widows become the responsibility and sex partner of a brother-in-law, and AIDS spreads accordingly. Thus, HIV is now firmly entrenched in many sub-Saharan populations, wreaking havoc as it spreads.

The growth of AIDS in countries already challenged by endemic disease has serious social, economic and political ramifications. Socially, the disease can sharpen divisiveness and increase group cleavages. Because HIV is primarily a behaviourally transmitted disease, moral condemnations are much more explicit than in the case of vector-borne diseases such as malaria or plague. Infected persons not only suffer from the diseases, but also may find themselves pariahs in the community. The AIDS epidemic can also exacerbate pre-existing social cleavages since one ethnic group may be targeted for blame by others.

While the HIV epidemic has generally exacerbated social tensions in the region as a whole, in Uganda it has actually begun to foster social activism. More than 1.8 million Ugandans have already died of AIDS. Out of a population of only 21 million, another 900 000 are currently infected with the virus.[38] Beginning in the late 1980s with an aggressive plan to contain the disease, the national government employed both its own agencies and enlisted NGO cooperation to achieve its goals. It has been noted that: 'The Uganda campaign succeeded by mobilising a wide spectrum of groups. A student heading home after class may well get an update of the latest information on avoiding HIV courtesy of her "boda boda" bicycle taxi driver, who has been trained by the Community Action for AIDS Prevention project. Or the local Muslim spiritual leader, or Imam, may stop by for a discussion of AIDS and Islam.'[39] The results of this expansive program indicate a drop in HIV prevalence and incidence of new cases. Between 1991 and 1996, the percentage of pregnant women testing positive for HIV in urban areas actually dropped from 30 per cent to 15 per cent.[40]

In addition to social consequences, AIDS has at least two major economic implications. First, the infection of a significant percentage of the labour force has negative consequences for the economy in terms of lost productivity and a contracting labour supply. This problem is worsened by the fact that half of all new AIDS cases in the sub-Saharan region occur in 15–24 year olds – a group supposedly entering the most productive phase of life.[41] Second, AIDS also has international ramifications – especially in attracting foreign direct investment. In situations where AIDS is known to be widespread, concerns over productivity and an uncertain labour supply may dissuade investors. And in cases where AIDS is not yet known by outsiders to be highly prevalent, governments may deliberately obfuscate data in order to ensure that investment does not decline. In the case of Kenya, for example, where tourism is a significant source of GDP, the government refused to admit the scope of the AIDS problem until late 1997, by which time more than a million Kenyans were already infected.[42] Disease surveillance in many less industrialized countries remains limited, and this could easily be repeated elsewhere.

Because AIDS is both socially and economically debilitating, it also has political repercussions. As the disease spreads, moving from limited and identifiable groups (prostitutes, drug users) to wider segments of the population, it requires a more active policy response. But in Africa that response is not always continuous, coherent or effective. Formal and informal institutional constraints, resource constraints and cultural norms may preclude leaders from making control of an AIDS epidemic a state priority. In Kenya, for example, interest group pressure and the large number of Christian voters have constrained the ability of President Daniel Arap Moi and other elected officials to pursue an aggressive programme to control the spread of HIV.[43] Because Moi's party enjoys only a slim majority in parliament, the sensitivity to interest group and voter pressure is acute.

AIDS threatens to weaken political institutions in other ways. While democracy has never had a vibrant history in most of sub-Saharan Africa, the AIDS epidemic clouds the outlook for its future development. The progress of the disease could provide justification for the political tightening of the autocratic noose. In Kenya, a society in which political corruption has been rampant, a recent demonstration concerning the epidemic indicated the scope of the problem. One protestor displayed a sign that addressed the 2003 elections: 'Don't worry about the elections, we'll all be dead.'[44] While such expressions of discontent may not necessarily yield a widespread political firestorm, they do demonstrate the extent to which the disease has implications for future political stability.

The political economy of AIDS in South Africa

Of all the sub-Saharan countries, the AIDS epidemic may have the greatest sociopolitical and economic impact on South Africa. According to current estimates, by 2005, more than six million South Africans will be HIV-positive. At present, more than three million are infected, and 1600 new cases occur each day – the highest infection rate in the world.[45] These high rates, however, are a relatively new phenomenon. Prior to 1994, when the apartheid system came to an end, only about eight per cent of the population was infected. As new investment began flowing in, and employment opportunities beckoned migrants from neighbouring countries, it rose to 18.6 per cent by 1998. It reached an amazing 30 per cent in the highly infected KwaZulu-Natal province.[46]

South African society is being devastated by the AIDS epidemic. Certain social practices, while making sense in a historical context, are now highly problematic. As in other countries in the region, new widows move in with their husbands' male relatives. If their husbands died of AIDS, the widows are likely to pass the disease on to others. The existing social order, which evolved under different circumstances, thus encourages the contemporary spread of disease. In the South African mining industry, workers spend long periods away from their wives. And when miners go home, they take the virus with them. Sometimes they infect their wives, sometimes women become infected through sexual contact with other men while their husbands are away. The role men traditionally played as head of the family has broken down. Boys grow up without fathers. Children are born HIV positive, and women are left impoverished and unprotected.[47] Additionally, because the social stigma attached to the disease is so great, there is a marked tendency not talk about it lest one be beaten or killed. This indeed happened to a woman who revealed her positive HIV status on a local radio show. She was subsequently stoned to death by a mob.[48]

The two major economic concerns associated with the AIDS epidemic in the rest of sub-Saharan Africa are also compromising the economy in South Africa. The mining sector, long the most important component of South Africa's GDP, has been hit especially hard by lost productivity and a shrinking labour supply. Dormitory living and prostitution near the mines have increased transmission rates among miners, and the consequences for the industry are severe. An official at Anglo Coal, one of the largest coal mining operations in the country, has stated that the number of shifts lost due to HIV-related illness has doubled in the last six years. He furthermore estimates that HIV/AIDS will cost the company an estimated R156 million ($25 million) over the next ten years.[49]

More pernicious, however, is the fact that the age distribution of those infected is expected to have a measurable effect on productivity over the next few decades. Sixty per cent of HIV infections in South Africa occur in the 15–25 age group.[50] The United Nations Development Programme has cautiously summarized the South African situation as follows: 'declining productivity, rising rates of absenteeism, and the loss of skilled and experienced labour over time may result in higher labour costs and weakened economic performance'.[51]

While these barriers to economic growth are sobering, they are complicated by the impact that HIV/AIDS has had on foreign investment. Since 1994, foreign investment has totalled less than ten billion dollars, well below previous expectations.[52] One of the reasons most frequently cited by corporate executives for the investment slowdown is the potential losses due to the AIDS epidemic.[53]

The AIDS situation in South Africa has also had other international ramifications. In one of South Africa's boldest moves, the government has taken on established principles governing intellectual property and encouraged the development of cheap, domestically produced, anti-AIDS drugs. Current costs of the recommended imported 'drug cocktails' in South Africa far exceed the ability of most South Africans to pay for them. Thus, the strategy is to produce domestic generic versions of drugs to counter the epidemic. While morally defensible, South Africa's action has triggered a decidedly negative response abroad. The US Trade Representative and Vice President, Al Gore, chairman of a bilateral commission on US-South African relations, have continued to press for protection of drug patents held by US and British companies and the eventual outcome now remains unclear.[54]

Reversing the economic slowdown and repairing the social fabric in South Africa depends to a great extent on political action. The disease has indeed elicited a government response, but that response has lacked the cohesion and coherence required to stem the tide of infection. As in many other sub-Saharan African countries, where the frank discussion of sexual practices and behaviour is largely absent from the political arena, cultural barriers have constrained leaders from openly advocating the practices required for prevention. Sporadic attempts to address the problem have been ineffective: musical theatre about HIV, for instance, and a failed attempt to promote an ineffective vaccine.[55] But in July 1999, new regulations made the notification of the government and immediate family members of any person who has AIDS compulsory.[56] Because the stigma attached to the disease is so great, many health professionals and activists worry that the policy will result in increased acts of violence against patients.[57] Whether this happens, and whether protest or other action will be directed at and weaken the government, remains to be seen.

In summary, the continuing AIDS epidemic in sub-Saharan Africa, and especially South Africa, illustrates the connections between globalization, changing social behaviour, disease and sociopolitical instability. Economic and social problems associated with the epidemic demand strong action by political authorities. But already weakened or failing state institutions in many cases cannot effectively respond. Thus, the AIDS tragedy, like many before it, continues to grind forward, weakening economies and political systems that hold the key to effective remedial action.

Notes

1. Ollson, Karen. 'We Must Eat, Drink, and Still be Wary'. *The Washington Post* September 6, 1998: C-1.
2. Chase, Marilyn. 'Hepatitis A Outbreaks in the US are Target of Vaccine Campaign'. *The Wall Street Journal* November 12, 1999: B-1.
3. Reported in 'As Food Imports Grow, Federal Inspections Lag'. *The Washington Post* May 12, 1998: A-2; See also Gerth, Jeff and Weiner, Tim. 'US Food-Safety System Swamped by Booming Global Imports'. *The New York Times* (World) September 29, 1997.
4. See Cohen, Jon. 'The Flu Pandemic That Might Have Been'. *Science* September 12, 1997; Vogel, Gretchen. 'Sequence Offers Clues to Deadly Flu'. *Science* January 16, 1998.
5. Richburg, Keith. 'Malaysia Slow to Act On Virus'. *The Washington Post* April 29, 1999: A-21.
6. Dabelko, Geoffrey D. and Dabelko, David D. 'Environmental Security: Issues of Conflict and Redefinition'. *Environmental Change and Security Project Report*. Spring 1995: 3.
7. For a more detailed description of early European responses to the plague see Watts, Sheldon. *Epidemics and History: Disease, Power and Imperialism*. New Haven: Yale University Press, 1997, 1–15.
8. World Health Organization figures published in Brown, David. 'WHO: Diseases that Kill Millions Can Be Stopped'. *The Washington Post* June 18, 1999: A-24.
9. See Crosby, Alfred. *America's Forgotten Pandemic: the Influenza of 1918*. Cambridge: Cambridge University Press, 1989.
10. Data from 'Millennium of Wars'. *The Washington Post* March 13, 1999: A-13.
11. See Homer-Dixon, Thomas F. 'Environmental Scarcity and Violent Conflict: Evidence from the Cases'. *International Security* Summer 1994; Homer-Dixon, Thomas F. and Blitt, Jessica. *Ecoviolence: Links Among Environment, Population, and Security*. Lanham, Maryland: Rowman & Littlefield, 1998.

12. In addition to its continuing economic and disease problems, Russia was also afflicted with a serious plague of locusts in 1999.
13. See Crosby, Alfred W. *Ecological Imperialism: the Biological Expansion of Europe, 900–1900.* Cambridge: Cambridge University Press, 1986.
14. See Garrett, Laurie. *The Coming Plague: Newly Emerging Diseases in a World Out of Balance.* New York: Farrar, Straus and Giroux, 1994; Morse, Stephen S., ed. *Emerging Viruses.* New York: Oxford University Press, 1993.
15. For more information on this early scattering see Cavalli-Sforza, Luigi and Cavalli-Sforza, Francesco. *The Great Human Diasporas.* Reading, MA.: Addison-Wesley, 1995:157–9.
16. See Pirages, Dennis and Runci, Paul. 'Ecological Interdependence and the Spread of Infectious Disease'. in Cusimano, MaryAnn, ed., *Beyond Sovereignty: Issues for a Global Agenda.* New York: St. Martin's/Worth, 1999.
17. McNeill, William. *Plagues and Peoples.* Garden City, NY: Anchor Press, 1976, 115–7.
18. Hobhouse, Henry. *Forces of Change: an Unorthodox View of History.* New York: Arcade Publishing, 1990, 11.
19. Hobhouse, op. cit., 11–23.
20. See McNeill, op. cit., 215 and references cited therein.
21. Gibbons, Ann. 'Where are New Diseases Born?' *Science* August 6, 1993: 680.
22. Lappe, Mark. *Evolutionary Medicine: Rethinking the Origins of Disease.* San Francisco: Sierra Club Books, 1994, 8.
23. Data from 'World Population Data Sheet 1999'. Washington: Population Reference Bureau, 1999.
24. United Nations Development Program. *Human Development Report 1999.* New York: Oxford University Press, 1999, Table 6.
25. Data from World Health Organization. *The World Health Report 1995.* Geneva: World Health Organization, 1995, Table A-3.
26. John Maurice. 'Russian Chaos Breeds Diphtheria Outbreak'. *Science* March 10, 1995.
27. See Levy, Stuart. 'The Challenge of Antibiotic Resistance'. *Scientific American* March 1998; Brown, David. 'Drug Resistance in Food Chain'. *The Washington Post* May 20, 1999: A-2.
28. James M. Hughes, *et al.* 'Hantavirus Pulmonary Syndrome: an Emerging Infectious Disease'. *Science* November 5, 1993.
29. Duke, Lynne. 'New York Outbreak Gets New Diagnosis'. *The Washington Post* September 28, 1999: A-3.
30. See Martin, Philippe H. and Lefebvre, Myriam G. 'Malaria and Climate: Sensitivity of Malaria Potential Transmission to Climate'. *Ambio* June 1995; Hopkins, Janic Tanne. 'Change in the Ecosystem Leads to disease in Humans'. *British Medical Journal* (Intl.) April 25, 1998; Chandra, Candace and Bright, Chris. 'Sick Planet, Sick People'. *World Watch* November 1997; Colwell, Rita R., 'Global Climate and Infectious Disease: the Cholera Paradigm'. *Science* December 20, 1996.
31. See 'Environmental Effects of Ozone Depletion'. Special issue of *Ambio* May 1995.
32. See Laurie Garrett. *The Coming Plague* New York: Penguin Books, 1995, 557–68.

33. World Health Organization. *World Health Report, 1999.* Geneva: World Health Organization, 1999, Statistical Annex.
34. Ibid.
35. World Health Organization. *World Health Report, 1997.* Geneva: World Health Organization, 1997, 124.
36. Caron, Mary. 'The Politics of Life and Death: Global Responses to HIV and AIDS'. *World Watch* May 1999: 30–8.
37. Statistics available from the World Health Organization. See *Demographic Impact of AIDS.* World Health Organization. <http://www.who.org>
38. Caron, p. 33.
39. Ibid., p. 33.
40. Ibid.
41. Ibid., p. 38.
42. Ibid.
43. 'AIDS in Kenya: Serial Killer at Large', *The Economist* Feb 7, 1998: 49.
44. Ibid., p. 49.
45. Shillinger, Kurt. 'Southern Africa Faces AIDS Catastrophe'. *The Gazette (Montreal)* October 16, 1999: The Review, B1.
46. Muwakkil, Salim. 'Africa Is Dying'. *In These Times* August 22, 1999: 17.
47. Shillinger, B1.
48. Key, Sandra, Daniel J. DeNoon and Salynn Boyles. 'Minister Predicts Six Million South Africans with HIV'. *AIDS Weekly Plus* September 6, 1999: 9–11.
49. Simon, Bernard. 'Employers Slow to Grasp Reality: Business and AIDS'. *Financial Times* September 20, 1999: Survey – South Africa, 5.
50. Baleta, Adele. 'South Africa Holds Crisis Summit on HIV'. *Lancet* May 19, 1998: 968.
51. Quoted in Simon, p. 5.
52. Jeter, Jon. 'South Africa's Image Problem Deters Investors'. *The Washington Post* October 17, 1999: A21.
53. Ibid.
54. Chenault, Kathy. 'Will the AIDS Plague Change US Trade Policy?' *Business Week* September 13, 1999: 58.
55. Cleary, Sean. 'South Africa: Mobilising All Possible Resources'. *World and I* April 1999: 72–3.
56. Key, *et al.*, p. 10.
57. Ibid.

11
Beyond the Traditional Intelligence Agenda: Examining the Merits of a Global Public Health Portfolio

Loch K. Johnson and Diane C. Snyder

> The traditional idea of intelligence is the spy who provides the enemy's war plans. Actually, intelligence is concerned not only with war plans, but with all the external concerns of our government.
>
> Senior intelligence analyst[1]

Since the creation of the Central Intelligence Agency (CIA) in 1947, the modern American intelligence community – comprised of 13 major federal agencies – has focused on a set of traditional requirements for collection and analysis. The pre-eminent targets have included foreign military capabilities and intentions, the politics and economics of other countries and worldwide mapping (mainly for military contingencies). Throughout the Cold War (1945–91), these topics as they related to the Soviet Union – the only unfriendly nation capable at the time of destroying the United States in a hail of nuclear missiles – understandably attracted a majority of America's intelligence resources.

With the break-up of the USSR, the focus of America's intelligence agencies shifted dramatically away from the former Soviet republics (which now draw only an estimated 15 per cent of this nation's intelligence resources[2]) and toward a host of other nations and factions that threaten the United States. These targets range from 'rogue' countries like Iraq and North Korea to terrorist groups and weapons proliferators.

In this new era, some government officials and outside experts have questioned whether the attention of the CIA and its companion agencies should remain fixed on traditional intelligence requirements. As the danger from Russian tanks and ICBMs has receded, they point to fresh perils, as well as to lingering threats never given adequate attention by policymakers during the Cold War. Thus, the debate has begun over how the pie should be divided with respect to finite intelligence resources in the post Cold-War era.[3]

This essay examines a slice of that debate, namely, whether the new intelligence agenda should include greater attention to global health issues. More specifically, we attempt here to appraise the desirability of channelling increased resources of the US intelligence agencies towards global disease surveillance and analysis – 'public health intelligence' for short – encompassing issues from the threat posed to American security by pandemics (at the macro-level) to the health of foreign elites whose governments are important to US interests (at the micro-level).

In search of a post-Cold-War intelligence agenda

In 1994, the US Congress joined with President Bill Clinton to create a Commission on the Roles and Capabilities of US Intelligence (the Aspin–Brown Commission, led initially by Les Aspin and, after he passed away, by Harold Brown, both former secretaries of defence). The enacting legislation required the commissioners to investigate:

> Whether the roles and missions of the intelligence community should extend beyond the traditional areas of providing support to the defence and foreign policy establishments, and, if so, what areas should be considered legitimate for intelligence collection and analysis, and whether such areas should include, for example, economic issues, environmental issues, and health issues.[4]

The Aspin–Brown Commission was only one of several panels of inquiry, public and private, to consider the question of intelligence options for the United States in the aftermath of the Cold War.[5] Although often referred to as the 'New Intelligence Agenda', the topics examined by these study groups were in fact not new at all to the intelligence agencies. Economic intelligence has been a subject of interest to policymakers and, therefore, to intelligence officers throughout the Cold War; and US intelligence had closely monitored Soviet dumping of radioactive wastes in the Arctic circle, the drying up of the Aral Sea between Kazakhstan and Kyrgyzstan, and a variety of other environmental concerns.

Nevertheless, non-traditional intelligence topics were largely relegated to the CIA's back burner during the Cold War. Intelligence managers dipped into this small budget to cope with their more immediate responsibilities for helping to contain the global communist threat. As the Cold War began to wind down, however, resources once targeted against the communist threat became increasingly available for the New Agenda. Yet the back burner is precisely where many critics (inside and outside the intelligence community) would like to banish the New Agenda priorities. From their point of view, military threats – the whereabouts of Russia missiles and warheads, Indian and Pakistani nuclear testing, Iraqi and North Korean nuclear weapons production, the sale of Chinese missiles to Pakistan – must remain the primary concern of officials responsible for the protection of the American people.[6]

Moreover, in reaction to the runaway defence spending of both superpowers during the Cold War, US government officials have turned to the challenge of bringing the budget back into balance and drawing down the national debt. This popular political movement toward a reduction in government expenditures mitigates against an expansion of intelligence requirements that lack a strong consensus in their favour and whose direct relationship to national security and foreign policy may not be as readily apparent as warheads and missiles in the hands of rogue nations. 'Just say no!' is the private declaration of many intelligence officers who feel overwhelmed by the list of fresh collection-and-analysis requirements that continues to grow without concomitant resources to fill them.

In sharp contrast, other observers maintain that Americans can no longer afford to define this nation's security in narrow, traditional terms. If the ozone layer erodes, if the rain forests vanish, if the Ebola virus spreads across continents, or, for that matter, if a large asteroid strikes the planet, the American people may be just as endangered – or dead – as they would have been under a massive Soviet nuclear attack during the Cold War. To define the nation's security strictly in terms of foreign military dangers is, so this argument runs, delusionary. An obsession with the USSR obscured our attention to these other dangers, but now they can be addressed; old-fashioned views of threat assessment must undergo new definition in the climate of uncertainty that charac-terizes the post Cold-War world.[7] As one specialist puts it with respect to public health intelligence, 'Infectious diseases are potentially the largest threat to human security lurking in the post-cold war world.'[8]

As for balancing the budget (continues the argument in favour of monitoring New Agenda threats), the fresh set of targets can be covered in part by reorienting technical systems – satellites, for instance – once directed toward the USSR. Many maintain as well that the United States has invested too much money in gold-plated collection systems ('platforms') equipped with every conceivable bell and whistle. An official at the National Security Agency (NSA), for instance, has accused the National Reconnaissance Office (NRO) of 'building Cadillacs' instead of smaller satellites that could just as well meet America's security needs.[9]

Better intelligence about the New Agenda items can actually save money, according to some reports. The President's Office of Science and Technology Policy has calculated that the lack of early warning about a resurgence of drug-resistant tuberculosis (TB) 'undoubtedly contributed to the more than $700 million in direct costs for TB treatment incurred [by the United States] in 1991 alone'. The Office adds that surveillance of this form of tuberculosis 'was not reinstated until 1993, by which time multi-drug-resistant TB had become a public health crisis and millions of Federal dollars had been allocated'.[10]

In the US, support for attention to non-traditional intelligence topics comes from the highest levels of government. In a report on 'The National Security Science and Technology Strategy', issued in 1996 under the guidance of the National Science and Technology Council (NSTC, a Cabinet-level panel), President Bill Clinton stated that 'no country is isolated from the consequences of newly emerging diseases, environmental degradation, or other global threats – even if the roots of these problems lie in distant parts of the world'. As an example, he offered 'the tragedy of AIDS [acquired immunodeficiency syndrome]'.[11]

This was not the first expression of presidential concern about the AIDS pandemic. In the mid-1980s, President Ronald Reagan issued a directive ordering federal agencies to develop a model that could predict the global spread of AIDS and its demographic effects. Working under the auspices of the State Department, the CIA led this research in cooperation with a number of other government entities (including the Departments of Energy and Defence).[12] The initial focus was on Africa (where the AIDS epidemic originated), as researchers sorted out the infected groups according to such standard demographic variables as age, gender and rural–urban residence. The model was subsequently expanded to include Latin America and Asia, taking into account as well infection by the AIDS virus (HIV) through intravenous drug use, homosexual transmission and blood transfusion.[13]

Clearly, the global resurgence of disease has failed to ebb, despite one's hopes in this age of advanced medical knowledge.[14] Yellow fever haunts Benin; viral meningitis has surfaced in Romania, polio in Albania, cholera in the Philippines; bubonic and pneumonic plague in India; and tuberculosis has undergone a worldwide resurgence. As reported by the World Health Organization (WHO, an arm of the United Nations), malaria, plague, diphtheria, cholera, yellow fever and dengue have re-emerged around the globe.[15] Moreover, at least 33 new disease-causing organisms have been identified since 1976, including HIV, hepatitis C, the Ebola virus, sabia virus and rotavirus, along with the development and spread of previously unseen strains of bacteria resistant to antibiotics.[16]

These diseases obey no border guards. As the White House has warned:

> Diseases affecting humans, plants, and animals are spreading rapidly as a result of trade and travel and, especially when combined with malnutrition, threaten public health and productivity on a broad scale. The rapidly growing human population, widespread pollution, and the deterioration of other environmental factors that contribute to the maintenance of good health, as well as the lack of dependable supplies of clean drinking water for fully a fifth of the world's people, contribute to the acceleration and spread of such diseases.[17]

It goes without saying that concern over world health risks must not diminish America's vigilance against potential military threats from abroad – priority No. 1 on the traditional intelligence agenda. We continue to live in a time when weapons of mass destruction remain plentiful; the spectre of swift and devastating carnage to entire civilizations still stalks the planet, as does the prospect of a terrorist attack using chemical or biological agents. Nor can the United States afford to ignore budget imbalances that have threatened bankruptcy of the American people.

Yet, concerns about new dangers to the United States cannot be ignored either. The topics mandated for investigation by the Aspin–Brown Commission are hardly inconsequential; they warrant close scrutiny by policymakers and the public they serve, if US officials are to make thoughtful judgements about competing intelligence resource priorities. Among these post-cold-war claimants for additional intelligence resources is one that is perhaps the least well understood of all: global public health intelligence.

The significance of global public health intelligence

At first sight, it is easy to dismiss public health intelligence as a topic of limited relevance. After all, the United States already has more medical journals and more Nobel laureates for medicine than any other country; the open literature, scientific and popular, on health threats is vast. Moreover, the Centers for Disease Control (CDC) and the Carter Center (both based in Atlanta) monitor and report on health conditions and threats throughout the world. So does the United Nations, as well as a scattering of private organizations like the Federation of American Scientists (FAS).

With all the open sources of information on possible threats to the physical well-being of Americans, why devote limited intelligence resources to this subject? Even the Aspin–Brown Commission, which endorsed the proposition that a 'legitimate role for intelligence' existed within the health domain, devoted only a quarter-of-a-page to the topic in a 151-page report and offered virtually no evidence to support its endorsement.[18]

Health intelligence scenarios

Nonetheless, as one begins to probe beneath the surface of the limited information available on this subject, one realizes that public health intelligence bears more serious attention than it has thus far received. Imagine the following scenarios:

1. A Third World nation with mineral resources important to the US industrial base has an alarming recent history of AIDS spreading throughout its population. Indeed, about one-third of the children born in the nation's capital city in the previous year began life with HIV in their bloodstreams. The National Security Council (NSC) is concerned about the stability of the regime (presently pro-US), since some of the ruling council appear to have symptoms of the AIDS disease. The President's national security adviser wants to know to what extent the higher echelons of the foreign government have been infected by AIDS and the likely effect this will have on the regime's stability.

The CDC does not collect information about foreign leaders; and, even if it did, many countries hide the truth about the prevalence of AIDS within their own borders – and certainly within their own ruling councils. Further, the CDC and its staff would lack the qualifications to write an accompanying analysis on the political, economic, and military implications.

2. The Secretary of State is concerned about widespread unrest in another Third World country that seems to be a result of extensive poverty and disease. Particularly disquieting is the near endemic nature of debilitating intestinal afflictions in its northern territories. The Secretary wants an analysis of what might be causing the illnesses. This information may be available somewhere in UN files, but she wants it right away and with an analysis that will explain the implications for American foreign policy. The Secretary is especially concerned about the potential of infected populations moving across national borders into neighbouring states, further spreading the disease.

3. American troops are ordered by the President to join a UN peacemaking mission in the heart of Central Africa. Among the responsibilities of the field commander is to ensure the safety of the troops against local contagious diseases. He requires up-to-date information on what to expect. Some of this data are available in the open domain, but part of the military action is apt to take place in a remote jungle where few Western medical experts have travelled. The commander needs to know what inoculations and other precautions are necessary to keep his troops healthy – and he needs to know immediately. His counterparts who will be dealing with humanitarian aid have the same concerns; their workers must also be protected from indigenous health risks.

4. The President has just read a techno-thriller about a member of a Middle East terrorist faction who leases a Twin Otter airplane from a small airport in the Virginia countryside, heads for Washington, DC, and drops a fine rain of anthrax spores out the window from a suitcase while flying at low altitude along the Smithsonian Mall in the nation's Capital. In the novel, the attack proves fatal within 48 hours to almost everyone inside the Beltway. The President wants to know how far-fetched this scenario is, along with a full report on anthrax and other biological materials that could cause death to Americans targeted by a terrorist attack. He also wants to know what can be done to guard against such contingencies, as well as the history of international agreements on the control of biological substances. He further charges the Department of Defence and the Federal Emergency Management Agency (FEMA) to determine

whether the US government is working to develop easily accessible antidotes available to the citizens in case of a terrorist strike using disease-inducing substances. These agencies in turn request from the intelligence community a full report on the threat of biological terrorism.[19]

5. The Secretary of State is expected to attend a worldwide conference on the health dangers to citizens and military combatants when environments are destroyed as a byproduct of warfare. Of particular interest to conferees is likely to be the effect of toxic gases released in the aftermath of environmental damage incurred during war, as took place during the Persian Gulf conflict in 1991. He requests an immediate intelligence report on the subject.[20]

6. The Secretary of Defence wants to know if his counterpart in a certain Asian nation is mentally unstable (as is rumoured), or in fact someone with whom he can deal. He wants, in short, a psychological profile of the foreign minister of defence, prepared before his meeting with him scheduled in a fortnight. For this mental-health information, the Secretary of Defence has no place to go except to the US intelligence agencies.[21]

One does not have to be neurotic to fret about these and related scenarios (although some are obviously more likely and immediate than others). After all, we have the recent history of an Ebola outbreak in Zaire (killing 240 people in 1995 alone), whose potential for spread alarmed US officials – and even the risk in 1989 of an Ebola outbreak in the United States from diseased monkeys housed in a medical facility in Reston, Virginia, near Washington, DC.[22] Moreover, we have experienced worldwide concern recently over an outbreak of 'Bird Flu' in Hong Kong (1997).[23] In addition, researchers have pointed to a relationship between a nation's health conditions and its degree of political stability. With respect to the AIDS pandemic, for instance, Garrett notes that as early as 1988 economists envisioned the creation of 'a global underclass' and 'an economic disaster' in Africa as a result of

the direct costs of AIDS care, HIV-testing costs, a year's supply of condoms, AZT (azidothymine) and other drugs for opportunistic infections (where such pharmaceuticals were at all available), and loss of net industrial and agricultural productivity due to deceased work force.[24]

Responding to the requirements – sometimes the urgent demands – of policymakers for accurate information on selected world health problems, the intelligence community has established a history of activity in this domain that predates the post-Cold-War New Agenda concerns about global disease surveillance and analysis. Policymakers understand that relying on media reporting alone with respect to world health problems is insufficient. Foreign governments will sometimes try to conceal health dangers from foreign correspondents, as witnessed recently in the cover up by Chinese military leaders and Communist Party officials of an allegedly AIDS-contaminated blood product (serum albumin) manufactured by a military-run factory in China.[25] The purpose of clandestine intelligence collection is to help ferret out such hidden information.

Macro-level health concerns

The intelligence agencies are expected to tackle the question of health conditions in entire countries and regions. Some observers believe, for example, that Russia's greatest challenge presently is not so much economic or military reform but the health of its citizens. Thanks in large part to a high rate of vodka consumption, Russia's male population is suffering high mortality rates, leading some analysts to predict that rampant alcoholism may prevent Russia from ever achieving the economic and political reforms to which it aspires.[26]

Long before discussion of a New Intelligence Agenda emerged in the wake of the Cold War, the intelligence community generated studies on country, regional, and indeed global health trends, supplementing UN, CDC and other public reporting with information from so-called all-source collection (that is, open as well as clandestine). One of the strong contributions made by government intelligence analysts is the skillful blending of open information (roughly 80 per cent of the total in most cases) with secret 'nuggets' from espionage channels – something no one else is in a position to do.

Separating the wheat from the chaff in the open information can be an enormously valuable – but often difficult – task in itself, validating what is truly reliable in the public record. Is a particular city in Bosnia actually under siege, as reported (let us say) by a European correspondent? What is an accurate population estimate for the city, counting fresh waves of refugees, so that the amount of humanitarian aid flown in will fit the city's needs without creating surpluses that will foster a black market? What is the quality of the drinking water in the city? Is the report of the European correspondent accurate about an outbreak of cholera in the city's main hospital? How much and what kinds of medicines are available in the hospital?

On the list of health topics analysed by the US intelligence agencies in the past have been studies on the access of foreign peoples in developing countries to safe drinking water and adequate sanitation. The underlying assumption is that a populace whose physical and mental well-being is under stress is vulnerable to radical political movements and other manifestations of social and political unrest that can shake the stability of a foreign regime and, therefore, possibly affect America's interests.[27] Another topic of increasing concern is the spread of HIV in foreign countries, which is so extensive that it may well begin to undermine the stability of some regimes. In Janeiro, Zaire, for instance, 23 per cent of the babies born in 1990 reportedly had the AIDS virus.[28]

American intelligence units have also gathered information from around the world on medical concerns related to peacekeeping and humanitarian operations, data that are shared with UN and NATO officials. Of recent special concern have been the preparation of assessments on the incidence and the effects of HIV and AIDS on foreign military forces with whom the United States must work shoulder-to-shoulder in the field, as well as possible hazards to American soldiers from having to handle HIV-infected prisoners of war or American civilians involved in the humanitarian aspects of peacekeeping missions.[29]

The intelligence agencies also keep tabs on environmental health dangers. The accident that occurred in 1986 at the Chernobyl nuclear plant, located in the Soviet Ukraine, provides an example. In the region near the stricken plant, cancer cases have doubled and calves are born routinely without heads and limbs. Radioactive particles from the Chernobyl melt-down have been tracked as far away as Scandinavia. One ranking UN official estimates that 'up to 40 potential Chernobyls are waiting to happen in the former Soviet Union and Central Europe'.[30] What if another Chernobyl were to occur? What are the health implications for US personnel and citizens travelling or living in Europe and for America's allies?

A related concern is biological warfare. While beyond the scope of this analysis, in the USA, the federal government is well aware of the serious risks faced by US troops abroad. 'Reversing earlier opposition, the nation's military chiefs have endorsed a plan to vaccinate all US forces against anthrax in what would be the Pentagon's first regular inoculation program against a germ warfare agent', reported the *Washington Post*. 'The about-face ... reflects heightened Pentagon concern about the prospect of biological attack. Iraq, Russia and as many as ten other countries are said by US officials to have at least the capability to load spores of anthrax into weapons, although no country is known is have released the bacteria on a battlefield.'[31]

While much information on global health threats is in the public domain, someone has to ferret it out of obscure UN documents and data bases or other archives (sometimes in difficult foreign languages) and collate it into a readable – ideally, an eye-catching – format that will attract and hold the attention of busy policymakers. As important, someone must ensure that the information addresses the current in-box demands on the most prominent desks scattered around Washington. The UN does not do this for Washington officialdom; the CDC and the Carter Center do not; the government's various hospitals do not; the Library of Congress does not; the Brookings Institution, RAND, the Heritage Foundation, the Aspen Institute, and the American Enterprise Institute do not. So when the information is needed, the intelligence community is expected to have it – and it must be accurate, timely, and focused on the latest problem or crisis.

Resources for public health intelligence

Despite all the hoopla over the New Intelligence Agenda, global health concerns have received only limited support. America's budget woes, for example, have resulted in significant reductions of US intelligence personnel overseas, along with the closing of many installations – especially in Africa, where many of the worst infectious diseases germinate. The United States in the post-Cold-War era has shifted from a condition of 'global presence' (eyes and ears in every country) to 'global reach', that is, a policy of mobilizing resources when necessary to 'surge' collection capabilities against targets of imminent concern.

In this time of budget reductions (at least for human intelligence collection, if not for the ongoing infatuation with expensive surveillance satellites – none of which can discern the spread of an infectious disease), health is a 'tasking' priority far down the list of intelligence collection concerns for Washington decision-makers. Nonetheless, by 1996, the CIA had established a Conflict Issues Division within the Intelligence Directorate's newly established office of Transnational Security and Technological Issues. Here, a dozen analysts track health and humanitarian issues, from the spread of global diseases to the (sometimes related) flow of refugees.[32]

From time to time the open media will report accurately on global health issues, as when Reuters documented that hundreds of Rwandan Hutu refugees had died daily of cholera in eastern Zaire during the summer of 1994.[33] Often, though, foreign correspondents are not in the right place at the right time, or they may fail to focus on the health side of a story and its implications for US security interests. Then collection and analysis by intelligence agencies become all the more important.

The US Army Medical Research Institute for Infectious Diseases (AMRIID) and the Armed Forces Medical Intelligence Center (AFMIC) play significant roles in monitoring global health conditions that may impinge upon peacekeeping operations, humanitarian and rescue missions, and other US military operations abroad (either alone or in coalition with UN or NATO forces).[34] Their primary missions are to identify health threats to the war fighter. Their funding is modest, too, and frequently their integration into the intelligence process is inadequate – particularly in terms of tasking (collection targeting) and subsequent sharing of information for the production of community-wide ('all source') reports.

While efforts have been made to upgrade the intelligence community's attention to health intelligence, sometimes the left hand has been unaware of what the right hand is doing – a persistent problem facing the vast and loosely connected intelligence bureaucracy spread out around Washington (the largest interagency cooperative venture in the government). In recognition of the more complicated nature of world affairs in the post-Cold-War era, the community has expanded its concentration on global and multilateral issues, including health concerns. The government's premier entity for intelligence analysis is the National Intelligence Council or NIC, which is located at CIA Headquarters but staffed by 'superanalysts – called National Intelligence Officers (NIOs) – recruited from throughout the community, as well as from some selected universities and think tanks.

In 1993, the NIC created a new NIO position for global issues, with health-related topics folded into the portfolio of the woman selected to handle this oversized basket of responsibilities.[35] The NIC has also produced from time to time National Intelligence Estimates or NIEs (the community's major research reports and forecasts on selected world issues) which have a health focus.[36]

The future of public health intelligence

In the grand scheme of things, health issues are in our view a less important focus for the intelligence community than traditional military, political and economic collection requirements. Foreign diseases, it is true, can infect soldiers in the field; but Russian missiles continue to have the capacity to annihilate an entire society (even if, for the moment, they may not be targeted in any one direction). Moreover, a resumption of fighting in Bosnia could spread throughout Central Europe and once again engulf the Western powers in a global war. Terrorists continue their attacks on civilian and military targets. Political unrest in Mexico can produce additional waves of immigrants across the Rio Grande. International economic conditions can directly affect the living standards of single nations.

Still, health risks to soldiers serving overseas can hardly be casually dismissed. Nor can one blithely push aside the other health concerns discussed in this study, even if limitations on available resources prohibit a full coverage of every possible risk to the health and well-being of any particular nation.

The need to keep public health intelligence in proper perspective, without ignoring its obvious importance, leads us to this central policy conclusion: in a time of government downsizing and budget reductions, it is vital to preserve the current levels of funding for health intelligence (as the Aspin–Brown Commission also concluded, however elliptically in the American case).

Again relating to the American situation, we also believe (and on this point the Aspin–Brown Commission was silent) that, without appreciable cost, some improvements can be made to provide better information to policymakers on global health risks to America's security interests. This will require cooperation among groups unaccustomed to working together – or even to being in the same room.

First, the CIA and the other intelligence agencies must take the health portfolio more seriously. The Directorate of Operations (home of the CIA's case officers who recruit and handle agents overseas) should report more regularly and systematically from the field on country and regional health trends – something that is presently neglected in the cable traffic sent back to CIA headquarters.[37] Case officers should pay closer attention to the spread of infectious diseases among foreign political and military elites.

The Operations Directorate cannot cover the international health beat alone, however. The Federal Bureau of Investigation (FBI), with an increased presence overseas to fight international crime,[38] should also be called upon to tap Bureau assets for information regarding global public health concerns, as well as the physical and mental status of foreign elites. This would represent an expansion of the FBI's traditional investigative mandate, yet only in the narrow sense of passing along to the CIA information on foreign health matters that have been picked up by Bureau assets abroad.

Second, the proper threshold for triggering collection on health matters – whether global, regional, national, group or individual in focus – requires further refinement. The system is presently too *ad hoc*; the intelligence community has yet to work out explicit and systematic triggering criteria that would indicate when a health issue has reached the level of national security significance, say, by virtue of disease lethality, proximity to US interests or communicability. As with every intelligence topic, analysts and managers throughout the intelligence community must redouble their efforts to learn what types of global health issues most concern policymakers right now.

Further, the integration of clandestine reporting and open-source material on world health conditions is presently inadequate. Since a considerable amount of health data surfaces in the public domain, the policymaker's request for information may be satisfied quickly by way of the community's capacity for open-source data searches, without engaging in clandestine collection methods. In the case of certain public health threats, WHO and the CDC already serve as important centres for what the intelligence community would refer to as 'indications and warning' (I&W) – quick alert on global health dangers. The intelligence community should monitor more closely the open publications of these and other health entities that have a global focus, turning to its own secret collection capabilities just for those topics that remain unreported (such as the health of specific foreign leaders, the presence of disease in potential battlefields or the risk of biological weapons use).[39]

A basic I&W question is: how much warning is enough? Just as for a missile attack, the rapid dissemination of accurate information about global health threats – a kind of 'viral telemetry' – is essential. Officials in the intelligence community responsible for tracking open-source information need to mine more effectively the data banks and eyewitness accounts of individuals who work on health-related missions abroad for non-governmental organizations and private volunteer organizations.

The community's relationship to private groups must be handled gingerly, though. As one FAS scientist has observed: 'We are in communication with DoD [Department of Defence] officials and are, of course, aware of the value of disease surveillance data to the intelligence community; [however], we – and they – recognize that any overt involvement by DoD or intelligence [in the data-collection activities of these civilian groups] would kill the effort to monitor effectively.'[40]

The intelligence community's health data bank is presently inadequate. The CIA's sophisticated in-house computer system charged with scanning the public-source literature (known as ROSE, for Rich Open Source Environment) fails to have among its machine-readable subscription lists many of the key specialized publications from private and international governmental organizations dealing with health and medical subjects. For very little investment, the ROSE system could be further enriched with open-source disease data useful for both an early warning and full understanding of global health dangers.

Third, the intelligence community should shift some resources from collection against conventional military targets towards the more probable danger (again, talking here of the United States) of a terrorist attack employing biological weapons. An inadequate number of human intelligence agents is currently targeted against foreign chemical-biological warfare capabilities and intentions. Further, more research on antidotes and the preparation of nationwide defences is necessary, with private industry, the Department of Defence and the intelligence agencies working in tandem (as they have so well in satellite and reconnaissance airplane development over the years). 'Our ultimate goal', states a recent White House report, 'is to foster the creation of a worldwide disease surveillance and response network'.[41] This laudable objective warrants more resources to match the rhetoric.

Fourth, the tasking and analytic integration of clandestine health intelligence cries out for better coordination. Several federal agencies have given some attention to public health intelligence, but the links between them are few and far between. The FBI, the Federal Emergency Management Agency (FEMA), and the US Public Health Service, for example, have put together a crisis-management plan to cope with a chemical/biological terrorist attack, but 'there has been relatively little emphasis on devising practical measures for protecting public health in the event of such an attack'.[42]

The current fragmentation of efforts could be alleviated by the creation of a Task Force on Global Disease Surveillance and Analysis, under the auspices of the Director of Central Intelligence (DCI). The Task Force might be expected to convene at least twice a year to review current world health issues and to determine how well the intelligence community has been sharing its responsibilities for collection, data analysis and final product dissemination related to these issues. Members of the task force might well include:

- the NIO for Global Issues (who would chair the panel and report directly to the DCI);

- a representative from the CIA's Directorate of Operations (DO) with knowledge of clandestine collection methods related to public health intelligence;
- a global-health analyst from the CIA's Directorate of Intelligence (DI);
- representatives from the National Security Agency (NSA) and the Defence Intelligence Agency (DIA);
- a representative from the Department of State;
- a representative from the FBI;
- a representative from the US Customs Service;
- a representative from both the Armed Forces Medical Intelligence Center and the US Army Medical Institute for Infectious Diseases;
- a representative from FEMA;
- a representative from the US Public Health Service;
- a physician/researcher from the Centers for Disease Control;
- an academic medical expert with extensive international experience; and,
- the NSC staff aide with responsibilities for global health issues.

One of the key issues for the Task Force to consider would be who needs to know what and when about potential disease threats, especially when the territory of the United States itself is threatened. That is, exactly who are the key potential consumers of this form of intelligence? The intelligence agencies must do a better job of informing policymakers about health dangers that have been uncovered by agents in the field, as well as what analytic reports are presently available on this subject.

As matters presently stand, often the wrong information is gathered because of inadequate communications between the consumers of intelligence (the policymakers) and its producers (the intelligence agencies). All too often in our research, we have come across evidence of one part of the government not knowing what another related part is doing, even at the level of the higher echelons. A senior NSC staffer, for instance, had never met the key NIO dealing with global health and environmental issues – even though both had been in their respective positions for almost a year.

At the heart of successful intelligence support to decision-makers on matters of global health – as for every other policy subject – lies the problem of dialogue. When dialogue exists, ideally with intelligence liaisons or analysts in attendance at the policymakers' morning staff meetings and afternoon coffee breaks, intelligence has a much better chance of meeting two of its most important obligations: relevance and timeliness.[43]

Further, while the United States already has procedures in place to deal with health threats when the warning comes from public sources, less adequately worked out is the manner in which clandestinely derived disease warnings should be disseminated to the civilian population in times of an emergency involving a health danger (such as a terrorist attack employing biological substances).

Conclusion

Foreign policy traditionalists will continue to focus on issues of balance-of-power with respect to the world's major military forces. This is a sensible concern, as it always has been since the advent of nation-states. International affairs, though, have become more complicated in recent years. The Clinton administration's first Secretary of State, Warren Christopher, had it right when he warned in 1996 that the greatest future threat to America's national security is likely to come from a host of 'transnational issues', among them environmental stress, population growth, narcotics flows and infectious diseases.[44]

While continuing to monitor weapons systems that can cause us great harm, America's intelligence agencies must also expand their responsibilities to include the New Agenda topics. President George Bush once referred to intelligence as America's 'first line of defence'.[45] Clearly, the first line of defence against the outbreak of infectious disease is global surveillance of health conditions. To be successful in this endeavour, the intelligence community must receive the necessary support – not from new monies in this time of economic belt-tightening, but through improved efficiencies along with the shifting of funds away from outdated Cold War activities and profligate spending on gold-plated collection platforms.

Notes

1. Analyst, Central Intelligence Agency (CIA), declassified mimeograph statement presented to the US Senate Select Committee on Intelligence Activities (the Church Committee), dated 21 February 1974, and provided to the Committee in September 1975, cited in Loch K. Johnson, *America's Secret Power: the CIA in a Democratic Society* (New York: Oxford University Press, 1989), p. 80.

2. Interview by Loch K. Johnson with Robert M. Gates, Washington, DC, 28 March 1994.

3. See Loch K. Johnson and Kevin J. Scheid, 'Spending for Spies: Intelligence Budgeting in the Aftermath of the Cold War', *Public Budgeting & Finance* 17, no. 4 (Winter 1997), pp. 7–27; and Loch K. Johnson, 'Reinventing the CIA: Strategic Intelligence and the End of the Cold War', in Randall B. Ripley and James M. Lindsay, eds, *US Foreign Policy After the Cold War* (Pittsburgh: University of Pittsburgh Press, 1997), pp. 132–59.

4. Intelligence Authorization Act for Fiscal year 1995, PL 103–359, Sec. 903(b)(2), signed by the President on 14 October 1994. The Commission began its work on 1 March 1995, and reported exactly one year later in a volume entitled *Preparing for the 21st Century: an Appraisal of US Intelligence*, Commission on the Roles and Capabilities of the United States Intelligence Community, Washington, DC, US Government Printing Office, 1 March 1996.

5. Among the most prominent were: John Hollister Hedley, *Checklist for the Future of Intelligence* (Georgetown University: Institute for the Study of Diplomacy, 1995); Report of an Independent Task Force, *Making Intelligence Smarter: the Future of US Intelligence* (New York: Council on Foreign Relations, 1996); Staff Study, *IC21: Intelligence Community in the 21st Century*, Permanent Select Committee on Intelligence, US House of Representatives, 104th Cong. (Washington, DC: US Government Printing Office, 1996); *In From the Cold: the Report of the Twentieth Century Fund Task Force on the Future of US Intelligence* (Washington, DC: Brookings Institution, 1996); and *Modernizing Intelligence* (Fairfax, VA: National Institute for Public Policy, 1997).

6. See, for example, the scepticism expressed by some intelligence officials about using America's secret agencies to monitor pollutants and other ecological dangers from outside the United States, cited in Loch K. Johnson, 'Smart Intelligence', *Foreign Policy* 89 (Winter 1992–93), p. 59.

7. See, for example, Laurie Garrett, *The Coming Plague: Newly Emerging Diseases in a World Out of Balance* (New York: Farrar, Straus, and Giroux, 1994); Thomas Homer-Dixon, 'On the Threshold: Environmental Changes as Acute Causes of Conflict', *International Security* 16 (Fall 1991), pp. 76–116; Thomas Homer-Dixon, 'Environmental Scarcity, Mass Violence, and the Limits to Ingenuity', *Current History* 95 (November 1996), pp. 359–65; Thomas Homer-Dixon and Valerie Percival, *Environmental Security and Violent Conflict* (Toronto: University of Toronto, 1996); Dennis Pirages, 'Microsecurity: Disease Organisms and Human Well-Being', *Washington Quarterly* 18 (Fall 1995), pp. 5–12; C.F. Ronnfeldt, 'Three Generations of Environment and Security Research', *Journal of Peace Research* 34 (November 1997), pp. 473–82; Jessica T. Mathews, 'Power Shift', *Foreign Affairs* 76 (January–February 1997), pp. 50–66; Myron Weiner, ed., *International Migration and Security* (Boulder, CO: Westview Press, 1993).

8. Pirages, 'Microsecurity: Disease Organisms and Human Well-Being', p. 11. Similarly, Col. Gerard Schumeyer, Director of the Armed Forces Medical Intelligence Center, writes that 'the medical threat may be the most serious threat to future [US military] operational deployments' ['Medical Intelligence: Making a Difference', *American Intelligence Journal* 17 (1996), p. 11].

9. Quoted by Walter Pincus, 'Military Espionage Cuts Eyed', *Washington Post*, 17 March 1995, p. A6.
10. 'The National Security Science and Technology Strategy', National Science and Technology Council, Office of Science and Technology Policy, Executive Office of the President (Washington, DC: US Government Printing Office, 1996), p. 55.
11. Foreword, President Bill Clinton, ibid., unpaginated.
12. Diane C. Snyder, interview with senior officer in the CIA's Directorate of Science and Technology, Washington, DC, November 1994.
13. Ibid.
14. On the threat of global disease, see two works by Laurie Garrett, *The Coming Plague* (cited earlier) and *Microbes Versus Mankind: the Coming Plague* (New York: Foreign Policy Association, 1996); Robin Marantz Henig, *A Dancing Matrix: Voyages along the Viral Frontier* (New York: Knopf, 1993); and Schumeyer, 'Medical Intelligence', pp. 11–15. A useful web site on this subject is: Program for Monitoring Emerging Diseases (ProMED), Federation of American Scientists, at http://www.fas.org/pub/genfas/promed.
15. See, for example, Susan E. Robertson, Barbara P. Hull, Oyewale Tornori, Okwo Bele, James W. LeDuc, and Karin Esteves, 'Yellow Fever: a Decade of Reemergence', *Journal of the American Medical Association* 276 (9 October 1996), pp. 1157–62.
16. World Health Organization, 'Emerging and Other Communicable Diseases (EMC)', http://www.who.ch/programmes/emc/news.htm, 2 October 1996; see, also, Sharon Begley, 'Commandos of Viral Combat', *Newsweek* 125 (22 May 1995), pp. 48–54.
17. 'The National Security Science and Technology Strategy', p. 43.
18. *Preparing for the 21st Century*, p. 26.
19. For a non-fictional account of this possibility, see 'Proliferation of Weapons of Mass Destruction: Assessing the Risks', Office of Technological Assessment, OTA-ISC-559, US Congress (Washington, DC: US Government Printing Office, August 1993), p. 53. Two authorities have recently concluded that the likelihood of terrorists using biological agents as weapons is 'probably increasing, as biological weapons proliferate and the stability of the cold war balance of power passes' [Robert H. Kupperman and David M. Smith, 'Coping with Biological Terrorism', in Brad Roberts, ed., *Biological Weapons: Weapons of the Future?* XV (Washington, DC: Center for Strategic and International Studies, 1993), p. 45]. An analyst in the Canadian Security Intelligence Service concludes similarly that 'the likelihood of future terrorist use of CB [chemical-biological] agents is both real and growing' (Ron Purver, 'Understanding Past Non-Use of C.B.W. by Terrorists', presentation to the Conference on 'ChemBio Terrorism: Wave of the Future?', sponsored by the Chemical and Biological Arms Control Institute, Washington, DC, 29 April 1996. See, also, Richard Betts, 'Weapons of Mass Destruction', *Foreign Affairs* 77 (January/February 1998), pp. 26–41, who calls for 'standby programs for mass vaccinations and emergency treatment with antibiotics' to increase protection or recovery from biological terrorist attacks (37); also, Jonathan B. Tucker, 'Chemical/Biological Terrorism: Coping with a New Threat', *Politics and the Life Sciences* 15 (September 1996), pp. 167–85 and accompanying commen-

taries by a host of experts. On 22 May 1998, President Clinton announced a series of measures to improve US defences against bioterrorism, including the stockpiling of antibiotics and vaccines (William J. Broad, 'How Japan Germ Terror Alerted World', *New York Times*, 26 May 1998, p. A1).

20. For an example of an intelligence report that examines the tie between warfare and public health issues, see 'CIA Report on Intelligence Related to Gulf War Illnesses', Central Intelligence Agency, Langley, Virginia (24 September 1996), 9 pp.

21. On the US intelligence community's psychological profiling of foreign leaders (a micro-health intelligence problem, in contrast to the macro-health issues that are the primary focus of this article), see Tom Omestad, 'Psychology and the CIA: Leaders on the Couch', *Foreign Policy* 95 (Summer 1994), pp. 105–22. The health of an individual foreign leader is a far narrower topic than the broader public health issues at the focus of this study; nevertheless, these individual health profiles are important to US officials as a form of political-risk analysis and the same intelligence agencies are expected to produce both micro- and macro-health reports.

22. See the account by Richard Preston, *The Hot Zone* (New York: Random House, 1994).

23. 'Another Sort of Asian Contagion', *The Economist* 345 (20 December 1997/ 2 January 1998), p. 125.

24. Garrett, *Microbes Versus Mankind*, p. 40.

25. Patrick E. Tyler, 'China Concedes that AIDS Virus Infected Common Blood Product', *New York Times*, 25 October 1996, p. A1. Garrett notes that many nations have deliberately tried to cover up their epidemics 'for political and economic reasons' (*Microbes Versus Mankind*, p. 19).

26. See, for example, Michael Specter, 'Deep in the Russian Soul, Lethal Darkness', *New York Times*, 6 June 1997, p. E1.

27. Andrew T. Price-Smith has written generally on the topic in 'Infectious Disease and State Failure: Developing a New Security Paradigm', paper, International Security Studies Section of the International Studies Association, Annual Meeting, 2 November 1996, Atlanta, Georgia.

28. This statistic is from an interview with hospital officials in Janeiro conducted by former President Jimmy Carter, 'State of Human Rights Address', the Carter Center, Atlanta, Georgia, 1991, p. 5.

29. Loch K. Johnson, interview with CIA analysts, Washington, DC, 26–27 September 1996.

30. Statement, Maurice Strong, secretary general of the United Nations Conference on Environment and Development, Brazil, 1992, reprinted in '40 Chernobyls Waiting to Happen', *New York Times*, 22 March 1992, p. E15.

31. Bradley Graham, 'Military Chiefs Back Anthrax Inoculations', *Washington Post*, 2 October 1996, p. A1.

32. Loch K. Johnson, interview with CIA analysts, Washington, DC, 26–27 September 1996.

33. See Reuters, 'Zaire Fighting Endangers Refugees, U.N. Says', *New York Times*, 25 October 1996, p. A7; see also, George A. Gellert, 'International Migration and Control of Communicable Diseases', *Social Science and Medicine* 37 (15 December 1993), pp. 1489–99.

34. Schumeyer, 'Medical Intelligence'.
35. Loch K. Johnson, interview with the NIC director, Langley, Virginia, 31 January 1995.
36. Ibid.
37. Loch K. Johnson, interviews with CIA analysts, Washington, DC, 26–27 September 1996.
38. See R. Jeffrey Smith and Thomas W. Lippman, 'FBI Plans to Expand Overseas', *Washington Post*, 20 August 1996, p. A1.
39. As Schumeyer notes, medical indicators can provide early warning with respect to an adversary's military intentions, say, by way of 'unusual acquisition or movement of medical resources, scheduled blood drives, and implementation of vaccination programs' (*Medical Intelligence*, p. 14).
40. Barbara Hatch Rosenberg, e-mail communication to Diane C. Snyder, 16 October 1996.
41. 'The National Security Science and Technology Strategy', p. 54.
42. Tucker, 'Chemical/Biological Terrorism', p. 177. For a plea to improve coordination of the broader US public health infrastructure in the fight against global infectious diseases, see Stephen S. Morse, 'Controlling Infectious Diseases', *Technology Review* 98 (October 1995), pp. 54–61.
43. See Loch K. Johnson, 'Analysis for a New Age', *Intelligence and National Security* 11 (October 1996), pp. 657–71. The third obligation of intelligence, and the most important, is truthfulness.
44. See Thomas W. Lippman, 'Success Stories, Symbolism Draw Christopher to Africa', *Washington Post*, 8 October 1996, p. A12.
45. Remarks by President George Bush at CIA Headquarters, Langley, Virginia, 12 November 1991.

12
The International Health Regulations in Historical Perspective

Simon Carvalho and Mark Zacher

Epidemics have always evoked political responses. As early as the fourteenth century, for example, city states established crude lazarettos, quarantine facilities for isolating sick passengers and sanitizing ships and goods. However, three major developments required that these initial efforts be modified: the growing number of pandemics, the consolidation of the nation-state as an actor capable of addressing the problem, and progress in medical science. As plague, cholera and yellow fever threatened Europe in subsequent periods, states scrambled to develop measures aimed at preventing their spread. They fashioned an International Sanitary Convention in 1903 which was frequently revised in the following decades. The World Health Organization's *International Health Regulations* (IHR), the modern version of this early agreement, are now again being altered in the face of changing epidemiological realities.

Efforts to regulate state behaviour are always controversial. Where disease is concerned, emotional responses by governments and the public often hinder international consensuses. In times of health crises, countries today often implement rules explicitly *in excess* of those permitted by the International Health Regulations. Such national measures are often based on inaccurate medical assumptions and do little to prevent transmission. In addition, they sometimes spark a pattern of retaliation as other states act in comparably inappropriate ways. This chain of responses can undermine the whole regulatory undertaking, itself long-criticized for being poorly designed from an epidemiological perspective.

This chapter traces the development of international health regulations from the late 1800s through the 1990s, focusing on the development of regulations requiring states to notify others in the event of outbreaks and to employ particular measures at ports and frontiers. Next it examines country submissions to WHO that comment on the functioning of the current regulations and, particularly, problems with their implementation. Finally, it assesses the current revisions of the Regulations as newly emerging diseases challenge old notions of how to respond to global health concerns.

This historical assessment illustrates the prominence of both state efforts to minimize the impact of the Regulations and disputes over the implementation of the rules. Both characteristics of the regime confirm that commercial considerations strongly influence regulatory efforts in the health regime and hinder substantial progress in this field. While these commercial motivations are very evident early in the history of the regime, they also exist in more recent years, albeit in more subtle forms. Ultimately, the revision process highlights the failure of the regime to prevent disease transmission around the globe as short-term economic self-interest and political inertia prevail over more far-reaching humanitarian and epidemiological concerns.

Regime formation and regulatory roots: 1851–1951

Historical background

Disease pathways have historically corresponded to those of human communication.[1] The most significant routes in this regard were between Europe and the Americas and among Asia, Europe and the eastern Mediterranean. Certain regions, like the Ganges Valley and parts of Africa, have historically been considered reservoirs of some diseases while other areas such as the Asian steppes, Mecca, Egypt and Malta have been important locales of secondary infection from which diseases spread to other, previously uninfected, parts of the world. In the nineteenth century, the routes between Asia and Europe were the conduits of many epidemics which prompted European powers to convene international conferences and draft regulations aimed at preventing the entry of plague, yellow fever and cholera into Europe.

A number of developments in the global and European economies promoted the international movement of people and consequently the spread of epidemic diseases. In particular, expanding trade routes between Europe and Asia created high-traffic corridors that facilitated the spread of many diseases.[2] Meanwhile, steel-hulled steamships, the telegraph and expanding rail networks all encouraged trade among far-flung areas, while the construction of the Suez Canal greatly increased interactions between Asia and Europe. Global migration also grew rapidly in this period: between 1815 and 1915 46 million people moved from Europe to other areas, mostly North America,[3] while 50 million left China and India in the nineteenth century and headed towards Latin America and Africa.[4]

Several diseases flourished in this environment. Plague had been a threat many times in the past but was not at the time a particularly serious problem. Cholera, on the other hand, thrived in countries with inadequate water and sewage systems, and replaced plague as the disease posing the greatest danger to European states.[5] The first of seven cholera pandemics in the late nineteenth century spread from India in the late 1820s and sped across Russia towards Europe. It also moved across the sea from India to the Middle East and Europe, carried in part by Muslim pilgrims travelling to Mecca. Yellow fever also spread quickly in this period, especially in Africa and Latin America.

The growth in international shipping meant that ship-owners and travellers were severely inconvenienced by the assorted quarantine rules imposed by port authorities in these and other regions. The regulations included forced confinement in lazarettos, comprehensive ship inspections and requirements of bills of health (documents regularly updated by ship's captains with information on health conditions on their ships as well as in the ports themselves).[6] While some early international organizations in Egypt, Constantinople, Tangiers and Tehran tried to coordinate actions on a regional basis, they were ineffective and short-lived. Generally, quarantine efforts around Europe were far from uniform, and states soon realized they needed to harmonize their policies.

Nineteenth century international sanitary conferences

States with particularly strong maritime interests called for international controls over the actions taken by port authorities in the nineteenth century and convened the first international sanitary conference in 1851. This meeting of 12 European states was notable for the conflict between two groups: Britain and some continental allies opposed the use of quarantine measures, while the Mediterranean states claimed the right to stop ships and travellers. The ensuing convention did not enter into force (only 3 states ratified it), but it did develop a number of important guidelines that influenced some states' actions in spite of this disagreement. These included sanitation standards for ships, inspections at ports and mandatory quarantine periods for infected carriers. Furthermore, the establishment of surveillance systems in Constantinople and Europe highlighted that European states primarily sought protection from other regions, as did a provision obligating states with territories in the Americas to report on yellow fever.[7] Despite these useful advances, states were on the whole very reluctant to support rules that might impede the flow of commerce. Furthermore, medical science was not particularly advanced in this period, and the lack of certainty concerning the transmission of diseases failed to inspire confidence in arguments for strict quarantine or inspection.[8]

A number of similar conferences were held throughout the nineteenth century. The second took place in 1859 and again saw Britain opposing quarantine and Turkey and Greece championing its use. The main point of contention was whether disease was caused by direct human contact (as the *contagionists* held) or by germs from filth and decaying matter (a view held by the *miasmatists*). Not surprisingly, states supporting strict controls over ships and travellers adopted the first approach, while those opposing them, like Britain, subscribed to the latter theory.[9] Interestingly, the miasmatists championed useful advances in sanitation in their own territories, but for the wrong reasons, believing that the major diseases like cholera were not in fact infectious.[10] The third conference was held in 1866, primarily in response to the 4th Cholera Pandemic which killed thousands of Mecca pilgrims.[11] At this meeting, Britain presented a list of sanitary improvements taken in Calcutta, Bombay and Madras in a tacit acceptance of their key role in preventing the spread of cholera from India.[12] Eight years later, Russia convened the fourth meeting in Vienna. Upset by restrictions on vessels exporting Russian goods from Black Sea ports, Russia joined several northern European states in once again opposing quarantines, only to be countered by the positions taken by the Mediterranean states.[13]

Additional congresses took place in the late nineteenth century, each motivated by a specific international health problem. An 1881 meeting, held in Washington DC, and attended for the first time by a number of western hemisphere states, dealt with yellow fever and plague. The main issue was the United States' controversial request that its own consuls stationed overseas be allowed to issue bills of health to vessels headed for the United States – a role to this point carried out by local authorities.[14] Next, the appearance of plague in several parts of Europe in 1883 led to an 1885 meeting in Rome at which many states (France in particular) grew annoyed with Britain's persistent unwillingness to establish quarantine procedures between the Mediterranean and Red Sea.[15] Participants at a conference held in 1892 discussed pilgrims returning from Mecca to their home countries and the need for mandatory disembarkation and inspections before proceeding through the Suez Canal.[16] Germany then called for a meeting the following year in response to a cholera outbreak, and parties agreed to ease the impact of regulations on commerce by forbidding land quarantines and ineffective train inspections. Interestingly, Britain for the first time admitted that its traditional position was wrong and that cholera was, in fact, spread from person-to-person. Finally, in what was a largely symbolic gesture, countries were requested to report the existence of cholera in their ports and territories.[17]

An outbreak among Mecca pilgrims led to an 1894 conference at which Britain agreed to carry out medical inspections and regulate conditions on pilgrim ships. Turkey, for its part, was unhappy with the agreement because of constraints on the Muslim pilgrimage. The country had an unusual ally in the United States regarding states' right to institute quarantine because the United States wanted to control the number of immigrants flooding its territory.[18] The final conference of the nineteenth century took place in 1897 and was a response to an outbreak of plague in Bombay which prompted a number of countries to impose very strict quarantine measures, including banning Muslims from travelling to Mecca. The 1897 convention required states to inspect ships and travellers leaving ports and implement both quarantine and medical examinations. Notwithstanding these efforts, however, the conference was like its predecessors, characterized by a widespread preference for freeing trade and shipping from immoderate restrictions.[19]

These conferences did not lead to widely accepted accords, and there is little evidence of compliance with the suggested rules. However, they introduced a number of key tools that are still used by states attempting to prevent the spread of disease. Not the least of these were sanitation requirements, medical inspections, and controls over pilgrims heading to and from Mecca. Furthermore, they fostered a sense of confidence in the utility of cooperation between states in achieving this goal. The disagreements among states and medical experts regarding the appropriate techniques to apply appear to have undermined the attempts to reach agreements. In fact, they really represent a process of learning which resulted in principles that remain influential over one hundred years later.

Many of the political disputes regarding the regulations were caused by medical uncertainty, and advances in medical science in the late nineteenth century altered the political dialogue to a certain extent and facilitated cooperation. For example, the discovery of the etiology of cholera in 1884 and the plague bacillus in 1894 promoted accords on these two diseases. In fact, it was progress in epidemiology that opened the door to several agreements in the 1890s and greater international coordination in the 20th century. That discoveries pertaining to plague, cholera and yellow fever coincided with the 'flurry of international conventions' preceding the 1903 convention speaks to this effect. However, the practical difficulty in preventing the spread of diseases and the commercial barriers to effective cooperation were ultimately more instrumental in shaping the regime.

The 1903 International Sanitary Convention and its revisions through World War II

The pace of international health cooperation continued to accelerate in the first decade of the twentieth century. While the nineteenth century treaties attracted a significant number of ratifications, the legal rules relating to international health issues remained unclear.

Furthermore, most states did not comply with the rules that did exist. As a result, both health and maritime interests were concerned about creating greater coherence and legitimacy for the regime in the form of a new integrated convention. An outbreak of plague in Nairobi and a cholera epidemic in the Philippines which killed 100 000 also heightened the sentiment that the international rules needed strengthening.[20] The resulting 1903 International Sanitary Convention of Paris combined the 1890s treaties and revised them on the basis of current scientific understandings. In addition, the French government called for the creation of an international health organization, *l'Office International d'Hygiene Publique* (OIHP), commonly called the Paris Office, which was subsequently approved in 1907. The 1903 agreement provided the basic elements of today's International Health Regulations. Still, the text is unclear as to whether states were *obliged* to apply certain measures in ports or only *had the right* to apply them.

The convention addressed only two diseases: plague and cholera.[21] Health authorities were required to inform each other of any outbreaks of these diseases and disclose the measures taken to combat them.[22] Other requirements involved ship inspection, isolation periods at suitably equipped ports and frontiers ranging from 5 to 10 days, disinfection, disinsection, deratting and bilge water expulsion.[23] Ships refusing to submit to inspections were permitted to leave ports, and those that had undergone measures earlier were exempt from submitting to the same at subsequent ports of call, provided they had not stopped in an infected area.[24] The convention had a host of regulations pertaining to pilgrim ships. In fact, 71 per cent of the 184 articles in the agreement dealt with places and events outside of Europe,[25] highlighting that the European states were primarily concerned with preventing the introduction of diseases from Asia, Africa and Latin America.

These 1903 regulations were not altered until a conference held in Paris in 1911–12 produced the International Sanitary Convention of 1911–1912.[26] The number of countries participating in this conference jumped from 20 to 40, largely because of the attendance of a large number of Latin American countries. Fourteen years later, the International Sanitary Conference of 1926[27] added some important new elements to this convention, as did the International Sanitary Convention for Aerial Navigation of 1933,[28] which provided rules on aircraft sanitation, inspection and certification, and the International Sanitary Convention of 1944,[29] which was overseen by the UNRRA. These agreements introduced changes in the following areas: diseases covered; epidemiological intelligence (reporting); measures implemented at ports; and general articles aimed at avoiding excessive measures.

Diseases covered

In 1912, the emerging yellow fever threat forced states to add that disease to the convention. (Articles 30–32) Then, in 1926, participants suffering from the post-World War I typhus epidemics that killed millions, inserted typhus and smallpox to the regulatory framework. (Articles 41 and 42–43) An interesting article in the 1944 convention showed noteworthy foresight regarding the importance of widespread surveillance efforts: it recommended that states notify others of the presence of *any* disease with the potential to threatening spread to other countries. (Article 1). However, states did not adopt this approach (which is the focus of the current revision process) and focused on the five specified diseases.

Epidemiological intelligence

Rules compelling states to report disease outbreaks are central, yet frequently understated, components of these conventions. Accordingly, the specific requirements relating to reporting changed more substantially than did other provisions. The 1912 Sanitary Convention legislated the first of a number of significant changes in this field, requiring states to submit weekly reports outlining the progress of notifiable diseases and to share information about steps taken to combat them. In 1926, a key step in the development of information sharing occurred with the requirements that states inform the Paris

Office of outbreaks and that the Paris Office disseminate disease information to all member states. Furthermore, the revised Convention stressed the importance of compulsory and increasingly detailed reporting of individual cases of cholera, plague and yellow fever, while actual epidemics were grounds for notification for smallpox and typhus (Article 8). The 1944 convention, meanwhile, instructed countries to notify UNRRA (which had assumed the role of the Paris Office) about current disease situations and outbreaks of designated diseases.[30] These developments demonstrate the regime's shift from quarantine harmonization to worldwide epidemiological surveillance[31] as developed countries used surveillance to respond to the threat of importation. Indeed, current revisions to the *International Health Regulations* illustrate that this transformation is now engrained.

Measures at ports and airports

States often disagreed on what measures health authorities could enforce against international travellers. Consequently, intense conflicts took place during the implementation of measures included in convention articles. Notwithstanding these conflicts, the revisions from one convention to the next were mostly insignificant and occasionally irrelevant. The requirement that ports of departure, not just arrival, take precautionary measures was probably the single most important contribution made by the 1912 convention and a key development in the regime (Article 10). A related provision held that measures enacted by authorities at points of arrival were to take into account procedures undergone at departure; another cut isolation and surveillance periods for plague in half, a measure which also lessened the burdens on ships and travellers (Articles 44, 22). Finally, the 1912 agreement also recommended that ships be deratted every six months (Article 26).

In 1926, several provisions again eased certain barriers to commerce. Specifically, port authorities were no longer allowed to disinfect healthy ships, and ships passing only through territorial waters (and not calling at a port) were exempt from sanitary measures (Articles 27, 33, 52). The convention also introduced deratization certificates which verified that ships were had undergone procedures to remove rats (Article 28). The 1944 International Sanitary Convention called for the elimination of bills of health. These certificates caused problems as they were often grounds for barring entry into ports and because port authorities were usually reluctant to fully disclose health problems in their ports.[32]

Excessive measures

Industrialized states were often concerned with the tendency of some regulations to impede the flow of commerce, although this anxiety was not quite as strong as it was in the nineteenth century. Consequently, some provisions in the convention did seek to discourage delays in travel and trade. The most significant provision in this vein was introduced in 1926, namely, that the measures established 'shall be regarded as constituting a maximum within the limits of which governments may regulate the procedure to be applied' (Article 15). This stricture against 'excessive measures' constitutes the normative hallmark of such a regime.

Despite the creation and frequent revision of the International Sanitary Convention, the burgeoning regime had relatively little impact for several reasons. First, the diseases subject to regulation were simply not serious threats over this period. The colonial powers managed whatever health problems arose in their territories and did not face major epidemics at home. Second, states did not report outbreaks for fear of excessive reactions from other countries, and there was neither regulated enforcement nor moral prohibitions to ensure compliance, especially regarding excessive measures. Finally, the increasing speed and volume of international traffic rendered border controls increasingly ineffectual in preventing the spread of disease.

Nonetheless, the regime experienced some success, most notably in the field of epidemiological intelligence. While the Paris Office had its critics, it as well as the Health Organization of the League of Nations did promote information-sharing during disease outbreaks. While the fundamental provisions regarding sanitation and inspection did not change appreciably after 1903, their regular assessment and occasional updating did ensure that government health authorities remained apprised of international health problems and controls.

Regulation experience and reform in the late twentieth century: 1951–95

The WHO was created as a specialized body of the United Nations in 1946, and assumed the responsibilities of the Paris Office. Before long, a 1947 outbreak of cholera in Egypt during which neighbouring states imposed severe measures such as refusing to accept travellers and turning back shipments of food and mail from Egypt, drew WHO's attention to the weakness of the stricture to avoid excessive measures.[33] During the 1949–50 discussions to revise the International Sanitary

Convention, some states wanted to establish rights to impose significant restrictions on ships and travellers, while others wanted tight restrictions on excessive measures by port authorities. Most developing countries like Egypt wanted significant latitude in managing ships and travellers.[34] France, on the other hand, criticized the tendency of countries to adopt excessive measures. This view represented the perspective of most developed states.[35] Interestingly, medical experts present at the proceedings generally opposed states' rights to restrict the movement of travellers. They argued that border controls were largely ineffective in controlling the spread of disease and that the improvement of national public health systems was a more effective strategy.[36] Clearly, the issues which characterized the nineteenth century conferences were still prominent in international health politics.

The first postwar revision of the International Sanitary Convention was the 1951 International Sanitary Regulations[37] (re-named the International Health Regulations in 1969).[38] This accord and subsequent revisions between 1952 and 1981 were not substantially different from the 1926 and 1944 versions, although the following revisions did take place.

Diseases covered

The conservatism characterizing the health conventions since 1903 did not preclude the addition and deletion of a few diseases subject to regulation. Most importantly, relapsing fever was added in 1951 with rules identical to those already in place for typhus. In 1969, however, both diseases were removed as diseases subject to regulation as they were no longer substantial threats. Smallpox too was deleted in 1981 after its global eradication. Following the example of the 1944 convention, the World Health Assembly requested in 1969 that states report on other serious communicable diseases and apply appropriate measures as permitted by the Regulations just as the 1944 convention suggested.[39] However, cholera, plague and yellow fever remained the only diseases on which states were required to report and they, in fact, seldom reported on other diseases.

Epidemiological intelligence

The 1951 alterations reflected a growing sophistication in the principles and techniques of surveillance and notification. For example, authorities were required to confirm disease outbreaks using laboratory tests and send information on such outbreaks to WHO. Furthermore, states were obliged to submit annual reports covering their vaccination requirements and responses to any outbreaks (Articles 6, 8–13). The

1981 Regulations added little, merely obliging states to notify WHO within 24 hours of cases of disease on ships and planes (Article 2). Despite a growing realization that accurate notification of outbreaks to other states was essential for controlling the spread of diseases, country reporting was generally superficial and sporadic, and controls at ports and airports remained the most prominent parts of the Regulations.

Measures at ports and airports

The port and frontier controls available to health authorities did not change significantly in the postwar conventions. The 1951 International Sanitary Regulations asked port authorities to reduce the number of rats in ports and, more importantly, to subject travellers leaving plague-infected areas to a 6-day isolation period (Article 16, 54). Cholera victims were no longer subject to some invasive examinations (Articles 61, 69); those suffering from typhus and relapsing fever were subjected to new measures (Articles 90–94); and yellow fever vaccinations gained greater legitimacy (Article 72). More generally, states were permitted to prevent the departure of those not only infected with disease, but also those suspected of being infected (Article 30). Those suspected of carrying an illness on arrival, meanwhile, were to be kept under surveillance but not detained unless the risk of transmission was 'exceptionally serious' (Article 39). The 1981 revisions included minor reductions in measures applied to travellers on arrival in certain situations (Articles 38, 45, 62, 63, 64, 66). In essence, the recommended measures differed remarkably little from those of the early twentieth century conventions.

Excessive measures

A little-used but important addition in 1951 was the provision allowing states to submit disputes regarding the implementation of the regulations to the Director General of WHO. If the Director General was unable to solve the dispute, he or she was given the power to forward it to a committee or *ad hoc* body for resolution (Article 106). This process took place only once. Finally, in keeping with long-standing attitudes, the 1951 and subsequent Regulations state that all prescribed measures are the maximum that can be applied to ships, planes and passengers (Article 23).

The functioning of the International Health Regulations

The 1951 Regulations required states to submit regular reports on their application to a body entitled the Committee on International Quarantine (re-named the Committee on International Surveillance of

Communicable Diseases in 1969). In the 1950s, this body met annually and roughly every other year in the 1960s and 1970s; in the 1980s and 1990s it met only sporadically. Country reports submitted to the Committee illustrate the continuing importance of many states' opposition to excessive measures and the facilitation of commerce in their valuation of the whole regulatory undertaking. Similarly, contributions from commercial shipping and air transport interests (ICAO, IATA) expressed either support or criticism of the Regulations in terms of their impacts on commerce.[40]

Country experiences with the Regulations as expressed through these reports varied greatly. Some states enjoyed relative success with them, whereas others – particularly those that experienced epidemic diseases quite frequently – had frequent conflicts with other states and complained about certain provisions. Overall, the reports and the WHO discussions illustrate implementation problems in three broad areas: excessive measures, inadequate notification and various practical problems in applying the provisions. These reports and deliberations speak to the Regulations' limitations – weaknesses that were to be particularly exposed with the recent emergence of new diseases.

A central feature of the international health regime from the 1940s through the 1980s was the tendency of countries to implement measures in excess of the regulations. Complaints to this effect started to become common by 1954. At the time, the WHO Committee overseeing the International Health Regulations stated that some countries, 'in a legitimate desire to protect their country against the importation of disease vectors, appear to have a tendency to take strict or more lengthy measures than formerly'. Few people involved in the administration of the Regulations denied their adverse impacts. For example, as early as 1951, the Director General admitted that even minor controls interfere with traffic.[41] Ironically, the very countries that took excessive measures against arrivals from infected areas themselves often failed to notify others about their own disease situations.

Countries violated terms of the Regulations in a number of ways. Some infractions were significant, like forbidding entry of travellers from infected states to a territory, while others were minor, such as charging excessive dues for issuing maritime sanitary stamps. Soon after the implementation of the Regulations, several countries in the Americas required presentation of a health certificate before allowing travellers to enter, but stopped this practice at the WHO's request.[42] The United States, meanwhile, reported that some authorities were requesting health certificates from travellers and refusing to accept valid smallpox vaccination certificates.[43] A more prominent case involved the Ecuadorean government reporting a case of excessive measures when two countries applied drastic measures following a 1955 plague outbreak on Puna Island (the disease was reportedly brought from fishermen from the north of Peru) even though the national plague control service controlled the disease quickly. Intervention by the Pan-American Health Organization led to a peaceful settlement of the dispute.[44]

Cholera outbreaks were especially notorious for leading to the imposition of excessive measures, some of which were implemented at the mere rumour of disease.[45] This tendency may be attributed to the long-standing stigma associated with the disease and, to a lesser extent, the relative ease with which it can be spread. With this in mind, states very commonly required cholera vaccination certificates, and did so as late as 1977.[46] During epidemics in India and Pakistan in 1958, travellers from both countries were not permitted to land in some foreign states, and were subjected to unnecessary extra doses of cholera vaccine. Similarly, Hong Kong and Taiwan were also guilty of imposing excessive measures against travellers from cholera-infected South Asia four years later.[47] One incident was referred directly to WHO for resolution under the official dispute resolution mechanism provision (Article 112). In this case, Turkey charged both Bulgaria and Romania with unnecessarily turning back goods at the border during a cholera epidemic. Turkey asked the Director General to resolve the dispute, and it was duly resolved with the assistance of the Quarantine Committee.[48]

Countries often overreacted because they failed to recognize that only small areas in a country, not the state as a whole, were infected. This happened principally when states failed to designate the local areas that were infected.[49] In responding to a complaint from five Asian countries infected with cholera, the Committee urged members to refer to Article 23 of the Regulations which holds that the sanitary measures in the Regulations were *maximum* measures applicable to international traffic. A component of this issue was the tendency of some countries to declare unilaterally local areas in other countries as infected. The Committee deemed that such announcements implied an intention to apply measures to arrivals from that area, and it urged states to cease this practice. WHO underlined its judgement on this matter by not publishing such declarations.[50]

Another persistent example of excessive measures involved countries persisting in demanding bills of health long after they were abolished. In particular, several South and Central American countries were identified as repeat offenders.[51] A number of states required bills of health and consular visas until domestic legislation officially suppressed their use. This lack of uniformity in state practice caused discord and sometimes led to situations that were 'illogical and embarrassing to the passenger'.[52] However, it probably did not seriously compromise the effectiveness of the regime itself since the number of problems noted by states and the number of revisions suggested by states declined markedly after the first set of country submissions to the committee.[53] A 1954 Committee Report noted that the Regulations were fitting well into existing national legislation and, more importantly, that when problems did arise they were dealt with internally or, when more than one country was concerned, by informal discussions.[54]

Poor notification, on the other hand, was a more serious and continuing problem. Authorities waited as long as six months before reporting cases of quarantinable diseases even when they had incontrovertible clinical evidence. In one instance, the WHO was informed of the presence of smallpox in a European port by two health administrations 1600 and 6600 miles away from the point of infection well before the country experiencing the outbreak itself reported the situation.[55] Additionally, health administrations were often slow to inform the WHO when yellow fever infected areas became free of the disease; and notification of yellow fever outbreaks that did not specify the local area involved resulted in authorities treating entire states as infected.[56]

As late as 1981 the Committee noted 'gross underreporting' of cholera cases.[57] Most states also did little to fulfil their regular reporting responsibilities to the WHO. In 1954, for instance, only 51 per cent of the 187 states and territories had established arrangements to receive the WHO's radio bulletins,[58] and as late as 1977, country annual reports were infrequently submitted. Over a three-year period reviewed by the Committee, only 33 countries submitted annual reports; 102 did so sporadically; and 52 submitted nothing at all.[59]

Sometimes states refused to report outbreaks because they feared exaggerated reactions (particularly in the form of embargoes on people and goods) from neighbours, but silence did nothing to guarantee against retaliation. Other states often took action based on incomplete media reports, action that target states could have avoided had they provided some information at the beginning of the outbreak.[60] Whatever the reason, states' reluctance to report outbreaks and their imposition of excessive measures had wide-ranging effects.

Finally, states had practical problems with implementing the surveillance provisions of the International Health Regulations. These included difficulties in carrying out surveillance,[61] the high costs of providing staff and high numbers of immigrants.[62] Non-compliance by airlines and poorly staffed ports were, however, the most serious problems in implementing the Regulations. Those involved with using the Regulations on a regular basis experienced difficulties quite regularly. Illiterate ship's captains and shipping-line agents often did not observe the Regulations, and they requested bills of health, expected instant approval of passage, or lacked proper vaccination or deratting certificates. In the words of an early Haitian submission, many of these cases of noncompliance were deliberate.[63] In other cases, pilots of small carriers or private aircraft and even international carriers sometimes lacked the necessary disinsecting equipment, and ports not officially recognized by the WHO issued invalid deratting exemption certificates or carried out negligent inspections.[64] Even personnel in embassies and consulates were on occasion unable to understand quarantine questions and interpret the Regulations, a situation the WHO Committee considered serious enough to urge health administrations to keep their diplomatic missions up to date on vaccination requirements.[65]

Several themes characterize of the evolution of the Regulations. First, only minor changes were made, and very few significant ones were even suggested. While a number of revisions (especially those dealing with vaccination requirements and medical exams) reflected advances in medical science, others really responded to states' unwillingness to burden travellers. Overall, states appeared to lack the sense of urgency required to effect significant change.

Second, states exhibited only a very modest concern regarding the spread of infectious diseases in the postwar era. Public health advances reduced developed countries' vulnerability to many epidemics originating in poorer regions, while increasing medical knowledge informed better responses to those diseases that were imported. By the early 1970s, public health professionals viewed infectious disease problems as of minor importance and turned their attention to the chronic diseases of the developed world and primary health care problems of developing countries.

In 1968, the Surgeon General of the US testified to Congress that it was time to 'close the book on infectious diseases'.[66] At the time there was a 'drug for every bug' and serious antibiotic resistance was not a concern. States were buoyed by Jonas Salk's effective polio vaccine in the 1950s, the global eradication of smallpox in 1977, and the development of antibiotics. States and international organization interest in communicable disease waned too, resulting in a loss of expertise in this field. For example, US surveillance of drug-resistant *Myobacterium tuberculosis* was discontinued in 1984 and only recently reinstated.[67] Scientific progress assisted states in eliminating some unnecessary quarantine measures, but unfortunately also reduced their states' interest in participating in efforts to reduce transmission.[68] By the early 1990s, however, the global disease situation worsened suddenly, prompting calls for regulatory reform.

Emerging diseases and new directions: reform in the 1990s

The global disease environment has changed dramatically in recent years, demonstrating that the supposed 'epidemiological transition' from communicable diseases to chronic health problems like heart disease has not occurred as previously thought. Moreover, global health programmes sponsored by states and international organizations such as the WHO have not significantly improved conditions in the developing world. Explosive outbreaks of new (or previously unseen) diseases like the haemorrhagic virus Ebola in Kikwit, Zaire in 1995 challenged the widespread political and medical complacency regarding epidemic disease. Rift Valley fever, Marburg fever, Hantavirus, and flesh-eating streptococcus had the same effect by terrifying the public in far flung areas and baffling medical experts, while BSE (mad cow disease) in the UK and Legionnaire's disease in the US alerted developed states to the new health threats. Similarly, the growing AIDS pandemic forced all states to reconsider what the real health threats were and rethink the usefulness of old techniques, many of which (like isolation) had their roots well before the first International Sanitary Conference in 1851. Seminal works such as the Institute of Medicine's *Emerging Infections: Microbial Threats to Health in the United States*, Laurie Garrett's *The Coming Plague* and Richard Preston's *The Hot Zone* helped alert the public to the new threats.

Accompanying the new diseases has been the re-emergence of old health threats like cholera and yellow fever, and the continuing predominance of age-old problems like plague, dysentery, tuberculosis, diphtheria (which ravaged the ex-Soviet Union in 1995) and malaria. The 1991 Peruvian cholera, 1994 Indian plague, and 1995 diphtheria outbreaks are the notable cases of re-emergence in recent years. Today, communicable diseases are the leading cause of death worldwide. They account for 43 per cent of all deaths in the developing world but only

1 per cent in developed countries, and although noncommunicable diseases are becoming increasingly important as causes of death, infectious diseases remain epidemiologically significant and the targets for international regulation through the International Health Regulations.[69] Equally dangerous to the public's health is growing antibiotic resistance: high public demand for antimicrobials and over-prescription by medical professionals has rendered even some of the most powerful antibiotics useless against minor colds and malaria and TB alike.

These recent epidemiological changes have been accompanied by a growing sentiment that new forms of international health cooperation are required. Specifically, states have realized the need for comprehensive reporting to track outbreaks of these new diseases and also rapid responses to disease outbreaks. The emergence of new diseases, and specifically the speed with which they can spread, highlight the weaknesses of the Regulations and challenge the long-standing complacency in both political and medical quarters. The rapid growth in international travel – seven million passengers made international flights in 1951 while 500 million did so in 1993[70] – dramatically increased the chances of transmission around the globe. Growing poverty in developing countries created conditions ripe for the proliferation of deadly viruses and bacteria which are transported by these travellers from these areas.

The implementation failings of the Regulations have been exposed in recent years more obviously than earlier in the WHO era. States rarely notify others when outbreaks occur; in addition, prescribed measures for dealing with such epidemics are ineffective. Even the supposed victory of improving conditions at ports and airports is a minor one since states have their own economic reasons for keeping these areas clean even in the hypothetical absence of any Regulations mandating such efforts.[71] The persistence of excessive measures, absence of enforcement mechanisms and epidemiolgical irrelevance of the diseases covered, are further fundamental defects of the existing regulations.

Despite their failings, some argue that the Regulations play an important 'moral and persuasive role'[72] and, further, supplement inadequate national surveillance networks. A convincing case may also be made that provisions pertaining to ship, plane, port and airport sanitation are major benefits of the Regulations, yet states would likely implement similar measures even without legislated duties.[73] Furthermore, the Regulations have succeeded in standardizing medical conditions in the shipping industry and indirectly creating certified yellow fever clinics. Their historical prominence also leads to continuing government funding for disease-related research that would not otherwise be available. Given the considerable attention paid to sudden outbreaks and the need for crisis response, though, more radical change is needed but difficult to achieve in the face of 'the heavy weight of tradition'.[74] The WHO's slowness in breaking from this tradition may be due to perceived lack of support from member countries or 'the failure of the IHR to uphold either maximum security or minimum interference'.[75] Emerging diseases and the availability of increasingly sophisticated tools for recognizing them, though, may help achieve slightly more security at a smaller cost than has been the case to date.

In responding to the recent disease and technological developments, the 1995 World Health Assembly, again stressing that 'the purpose of the Regulations is to ensure the maximum possible protection against infection with minimum interference in international traffic', recommended that member states participate in revising the current IHRs.[76] A 1995 WHO consultation about the Regulations produced a document which insisted that the fundamental principle – 'maximum security with minimum interference' – and basic structure of the existing Regulations remain valid. It did identify, though, two important shortcomings: the number of diseases covered by the Regulations and the limitations of existing notification practices. While participants in two Working Groups identified habit, routine and ease of response as the benefits of requiring states to report a limited number of diseases, they recognized that the existing system was too slow for reporting on the three diseases, restrictive, and difficult to implement in areas lacking suitable diagnostic capabilities.[77]

Consequently, they recommended that states report not a limited number of diseases but instead notify WHO of the appearance of 'syndromes' – general outward manifestations of disease. This technique allows health administrations to take action based on hints of serious disease, not just unassailable proof, facilitating a quicker response. On the notification front, they acknowledged that improved surveillance (and, also, interventions at the source) is more important than quarantine in preventing the spread of disease.[78] Despite this admission, they argued that interventions prior to, during and after travel are still useful.

The most recent 1998 draft regulations fulfil some of the promise of these early recommendations, but they also symbolize states' long-standing conservatism.[79] The most radical modification to the existing Regulations is the adoption of the syndrome approach. Instead of notifying the WHO of outbreaks of specific enumerated diseases, authorities are to report broad types of symptoms, as recommended in the 1995 consultation. These include hemorrhagic fevers and severe respiratory, diarrheal, jaundice and neurological problems in addition to other notifiable syndromes. Member states are obliged to report cases of acute hemorrhagic fevers immediately; they need only notify WHO of cases of the other syndromes if they have significant international public health implications (Appendix III).

This change in diseases subject to regulation is supplemented by changes to provisions regarding reporting. Authorities are to report cases of the above syndromes and the existence of agents that may cause or carry them. Supplementing this information-sharing is a new provision allowing WHO to request information from unofficial sources such as international organizations, other national authorities, and the public (Article 4). WHO then distributes information about syndrome occurrences to all health authorities, and it has a new role of commenting on incorrect information received from authorities. Furthermore, it should provide information on any inappropriate measures implemented by states (Articles 2.4; 9).

The draft Regulations, interestingly, both expand and restrict state capacity to act against diseases in ports and airports and at frontiers. While the draft explains, as did many preceding agreements, that the articles are the 'maximum measures applicable', authorities are given several exit clauses that may sanction excessive measures. One provision leaves open the types of measures applied against international arrivals with only a proviso that the measures be in accordance with 'expert consensus opinion' (Article 29.1). Most significantly, states may subject 'any' carrier and individual to health assessments and medical examinations (Article 32.1). This flexibility may be abused by states, especially during outbreaks. Moreover, states now have significant discretion in deciding which outbreaks to report and little incentive to report specific diseases in the absence of prohibitions of excessive measures.[80] Finally, states can also take additional health measures against migrants, nomads, seasonal workers or those participating in periodic mass congregations (a right they have possessed in the past) (Article 47.1) and require International Certificates of Vaccination for any syndrome diseases. Currently, they can request only yellow fever vaccination certificates.

A number of these state powers are, however, limited or balanced by new WHO authorities. Prior to implementing additional ('excessive') measures during emergencies, authorities must provide WHO with compelling scientific evidence of a threat to public health. Similarly, any new vaccination requirements and measures applied to ships and planes must be first cleared by WHO. More broadly, WHO assumes a more proactive role in these new Regulations, particularly by issuing specific instructions regarding the use of new measures in the control of serious outbreaks, by making statements on inappropriate or unnecessary measures (Article 44), and by offering to collaborate with states experiencing an outbreak or epidemic (Article 19). Finally, a new dispute settlement mechanism, although unlikely to be used, grants WHO new disciplinary authority. The Director-General can, if unable to solve a dispute, forward the disagreement to a new Committee of Arbitration. If any state fails to comply with the Committee's decision, the World Health Assembly can take punitive action which could include depriving states of voting rights (Articles 56.1, 56.3).

A number of modern surveillance techniques unrelated to the Regulations which strengthen state capacity to recognize and respond to disease outbreaks supplement these regulatory efforts. These include FLUNET, which disseminates information on emerging influenza strains; WHONET, a tool for tracking microbial resistance; GPHIN, a Canadian programme that scans the Internet for information on disease outbreaks and now provides WHO with between 20 and 40 per cent of all its disease outbreak information; ProMED-mail, which assembles disease information from health professionals around the world and publishes it on the Internet; and SatelLife, an NGO which uses radio and telephone networks in the pursuit of health information dissemination in developing countries. Furthermore, both major powers and a variety of NGOs have their own weighty intelligence networks. These surveillance tools which pick up on a many health threats in one sense weaken the existing Regulations by revealing the serious limitations of WHO rules. At the same time, they provide a great opportunity for bolstering a more flexible version of the regulations that are aimed at identifying disease outbreaks before they become too serious. More effective surveillance tools also make it very difficult for states to hide information on their disease situations, since information is easily accessible to NGOs, foreign governments, and international organizations. CNN's footage of people fleeing Surat in India during an outbreak of plague in 1994 is evidence of this greater transparency.

While the health regime may increasingly rely on epidemiological surveillance rather than border controls, measures at ports, airports and frontiers remain substantial elements of the draft Regulations. A number of these measures such as those requiring states to keep fresh food and water at crossings and conducting mosquito surveillance at airports are truly antiquated and not implemented by states. In addition, it remains to be seen how great an impact the WHO reporting system will have when so many other private, media, and state intelligence networks disclose outbreaks already. A WHO reporting system does lend legitimacy, formality and a sense of obligation to the practice, but it may not be of significant practical advantage considering the varied activities of NGOs, states and the media.

Furthermore, the attempts to provide stricter controls over inappropriate state conduct are confused by provisions granting states new powers to act independently during crises. The regime has been compromised in the past when states implemented excessive measures, and this situation is unlikely to change materially with only reference to the WHO for approval restraining states' discretionary actions. Ultimately, the real challenge is for the Regulations to balance flexibility and discipline. The proposed changes regarding diseases included in and notifiable under the regime do succeed in making it more relevant. However, the past and proposed provisions that increase the options available to health authorities encourage a kind of looseness. The potential success of the new rules, if they come into force, is currently difficult to predict. The history of the evolution and use of different agreements suggests, though, that the new Regulations will remain an imperfect, yet useful, tool for preventing the spread of disease.

Conclusion

From the *ad hoc* epidemic-driven conferences and conventions of the nineteenth century through the period of frequent yet minor changes in the International Health Regulations during the twentieth century, states have proven willing to tolerate an ineffective regime which dealt with only several diseases, used outdated control methods, failed to prevent excessive measures and did not ensure comprehensive reporting. While medical uncertainty exacerbated the inefficacy of the regime for some time, limitations in medical science are now only a minor factor in explaining the continuing conservatism characterizing the Regulations. Of greater import is the widespread unwillingness of states to impede the flow of commerce and to sacrifice their freedom of action to exclude travellers with diseases.

The continuing spread of diseases demonstrates, however, that border controls are patently ineffectual in preventing either epidemics or isolated outbreaks. This reality explains why most changes between 1903 and 1981 were minor, but it also suggests that the recent attempt to modernize the Regulations without questioning the usefulness of port and border controls may be misguided. It must be remembered, however, that the International Health Regulations rightly occupy only a minor role in overall international health cooperation. Just as many newly emerging diseases are diverting attention and resources away from public health infrastructures and traditional endemic diseases like malaria and tuberculosis, the International Health Regulations distract states from what ought to be the main emphasis of disease prevention: public health improvements in developing countries.

In 1960, the Assistant Director General of WHO said that the central goal of the Regulations is the 'freest possible movement of international traffic ... in the interests of world economic and social, including health, progress'.[81] Continuing references to the facilitation of commerce suggest that this object still motivates international health cooperation – especially that concerning port and border controls. Such controls are worthwhile if properly formulated, but they should not deflect attention from disease control programmes – especially in developing countries. Controlling the spread of communicable diseases is, in the final analysis, primarily a problem of reducing the incidence of such diseases in the developing world, and the industrialized countries are only likely to back new regulations and aid commitments if they address real threats of transmission that are susceptible to control through international action.

Notes

1. Siegfried, Andre, *Routes of Contagion* (New York: Harcourt, Brace, 1965), p. 16.
2. Foreman-Peck, James, *A History of the World Economy: International Economic Relations since 1850* (New Jersey: Barnes and Noble Books), p. 3.
3. Kenwood, A.G. and A.L. Lougheed, *The Growth of the International Economy 1820–1990* (London: Routledge, 1992), p. 44.
4. Schwarz, Herman, *States versus Markets: History, Geography, and the Development of the International Political Economy* (New York: St. Martin's Press, 1994), p. 125.
5. Fidler, David P., *International Law and Infectious Diseases* (Oxford: Clarendon Press, 1999), pp. 10, 29.
6. Goodman, Neville, *International Health Organizations and their Work* (Aylesbury: Churchill Livingstone, 1971), pp. 31–5; In: O. Schepin and

Y. Waldermar (eds) *International Quarantine* (Madison: International University Press, 1991), pp. 9–25.

7. Fidler, supra note 5, p. 29.

8. Conference Sanitaire Internationale, 1851, *Procès-verbaux* (Paris: Imprimerie Nationale, 1852); Goodman, ibid.; Schepin and Yermakov, ibid., p. 73.

9. Conference Sanitaire Internationale, 1859, *Protocoles* (Paris: Imprimerie Nationale, 1859); Goodman, ibid., p. 54; Howard-Jones, Norman, *International Public Health Between the Two World Wars – the Organizational Problems* (Geneva: WHO, 178), pp. 20–2.

10. Fidler, supra note 5, p. 33.

11. Conference Sanitaire Internationale, 1866, *Procès-verbaux* (Constantinople: Imprimerie Centrale, 1866); Goodman, supra note 5, pp. 54–8; Howard-Jones, ibid., pp. 23–34.

12. Fidler, supra note 5, p. 34.

13. Conference Sanitaire Internationale, 1874, *Procès-verbaux* (Vienna: Imprimerie Imperiale et Royale, 1874); Goodman, ibid., pp. 58–60; Howard-Jones, ibid., pp. 35–4; Schepin and Yermakov, supra note 5, pp. 95–101.

14. Goodman, supra note 5, pp. 61–3; Howard-Jones, ibid., pp. 42–5; International Sanitary Conference, 1881, *Proceedings* (Washington: Government Printing Office, 1881); Schepin and Yermakov, ibid., pp. 105–9.

15. Conference Sanitaire Internationale, 1885, *Procès-verbaux* (Rome: Imprimerie de Ministere des Affaires, 1885); Goodman, ibid., pp. 64–6; Howard-Jones, ibid., pp. 46–57; Schepin and Yermakov, ibid., pp. 111–21.

16. Conference Sanitaire Internationale de Venise, 1892, *Protocoles et procès-verbaux* (Rome: Imprimerie nationale de J. Bertero, 1892); Goodman, ibid., pp. 66–7; Howard-Jones, ibid., pp. 58–66; Schepin and Yermakov, ibid., pp. 131–3.

17. Goodman, ibid., pp. 67–8; Howard-Jones, ibid., pp. 66–70; Schepin and Yermakov, ibid., pp. 136–44.

18. Conference Sanitaire Internationale de Paris, 1894, *Procès-verbaux* (Paris: Imprimerie Nationale, 1894); Goodman, ibid., p. 68; Howard-Jones, ibid., pp. 71–5.

19. Conference Sanitaire Internationale de Venise, 1897, *Procès-verbaux* (Rome: Forzani et CIE. Imprimeurs de Senat, 1897); Cooper, Richard, 'International Cooperation in Public Health as a Prologue to Macroeconomic Cooperation', in *Can Nations Agree?* (Washington, DC: The Brookings Institution, 1989), pp. 212–13; Goodman, ibid., pp. 68–9; Howard-Jones, ibid., pp. 78–80.

20. Beck, Ann, *A History of the British Medical Administration of East Africa, 1900–1950* (Cambridge: Harvard University Press, 1970), p. 7; Ileto, Reynaldo C., in *Companion Encyclopedia of the History of Medicine* (London: Routledge, 1994), p. 127.

21. *International Sanitary Convention of Paris, 1903* (London: HMSO, 1904).

22. Ibid., Articles 1–10.

23. Ibid., Articles 37–45.

24. Ibid., Articles 29–36.

25. Fidler, supra note 5, p. 31.

26. *International Sanitary Convention of Paris, 1911–1912* (London: HMSO, 1919).

27. *International Sanitary Convention, 1926* (London: HMSO, 1928).

28. *International Sanitary Convention for Aerial Navigation, 1933* (The Hague, 1933).
29. *International Sanitary Convention, 1944* (Washington DC: UNRRA, 1945).
30. Goodman, supra note 5, pp. 71–4; Schepin and Yermakov, supra note 5, pp. 201–2; Howard-Jones, supra note 7, pp. 93–8.
31. Fidler, supra note 5, p. 43.
32. Goodman, ibid., pp. 141–6; Schepin and Yermakov, ibid., pp. 232–45.
33. WHO, *Draft International Sanitary Regulations* (WHO/Epid/48, 1950), p. 8.
34. WHO, *Draft International Sanitary Regulations* (WHO/Epid/44, 1950), pp. 51, 60.
35. WHO, *Draft International Sanitary Regulations* (WHO/Epid/44 Add.2, 1950), pp. 1, 3.
36. WHO, *Draft International Sanitary Regulations* (WHO/Epid/52, 1950).
37. WHO, *International Sanitary Regulations, 1951* (WHO: Geneva, 1951).
38. WHO, *International Health Regulations, 1981*, (WHO: Geneva, 1981).
39. World Health Assembly Resolution 22.47
40. WHO, *First Annual Report by the Director-General on the Working of the International Sanitary Regulations* (WHO/IQ/0 and Add. 1 and 2, 1953) at 20; WHO, *Third Annual Report by the Director-General on the Working of the International Sanitary Regulations* (WHO/IQ/26 and Add. 1, 1956), p. 31.
41. WHO OR, N.37, 1951, p. 330.
42. WHO, *Third Annual Report*, supra note 30, p. 12.
43. WHO, *Fourth Report of the Committee on International Quarantine* (WHO/IQ/48, 1956), p. 502.
44. WHO, *Third Annual Report*, supra note 30, p. 20.
45. WHO, 'Functioning of the International Health Regulations' (1980) 55 *Weekly Epidemiological Record*, p. 379.
46. WHO, 'Functioning of the International Health Regulations' (1978) 53 *Weekly Epidemiological Record*, p. 535.
47. WHO, *Sixth Report of the Committee on International Quarantine* (WHO/IQ/75, 1958), p. 463; WHO, *Eleventh Report of the Committee on International Quarantine* (A16/P&B/2, 1963), p. 37.
48. WHO, *Sixteenth Report of the Committee on International Quarantine* (A24/B/10, 1971), p. 123.
49. WHO, *Sixth Report*, supra note 37, p. 483.
50. WHO, *Ninth Report of the Committee on International Quarantine* (A16/P&B/2, 1963), p. 41.
51. WHO, *First Annual Report*, supra note 30, p. 20.
52. WHO, *Third Annual Report*, supra note 30, p. 19.
53. Leive, David M., *International Regulatory Regimes: Case Studies in Health, Meteorology, and Food, Volumes I & II* (Lexington: Lexington Books, 1976) at 102; WHO, ibid., p. 25; *Fifth Annual Report*, supra note 44, p. 405.
54. WHO, *Second Annual Report*, supra note 41, p. 6.
55. WHO, *Fifth Annual Report*, supra note 44, p. 400.
56. WHO, *Sixth Annual Report*, supra note 37, p. 476.
57. WHO, 'Functioning of the International Health Regulations' (1981) 56 *Weekly Epidemiological Record*, p. 387.
58. WHO, *Second Annual Report*, supra note 41, p. 8.
59. WHO, *Nineteenth Report*, supra note 45, p. 45.

60. WHO, 'Functioning of the International Health Regulations' (1986) 61 *Weekly Epidemiological Record*, p. 386.
61. WHO, *First Annual Report*, supra note 30, p. 21; WHO, *Second Annual Report by the Director-General on the Working of the International Sanitary Regulations* (WHO/IQ15/and Add. 1, 1954), p. 23.
62. WHO, *First Annual Report*, supra note 30, p. 21; WHO, *Seventh Report of the Committee on International Quarantine* (WHO/IQ/91, 1959), p. 42.
63. WHO, *Second Annual Report*, supra note 41, p. 20.
64. WHO, *Third Annual Report*, supra note 30, p. 25; WHO, *Fifth Report of the Committee on International Quarantine* (WHO/IQ/61, 1957), p. 405.
65. WHO, *Eleventh Annual Report*, supra note 37, p. 33; WHO, *Nineteenth Report of the Committee on International Surveillance of Communicable Diseases* (A30/26, 1977), p. 60.
66. Berkelman, Ruth L. and James M. Hughes, 'The Conquest of Infectious Diseases: Who are We Kidding?' (1993) *Ann Internal Medicine* 119, p. 426.
67. Ibid.
68. Fidler, supra note 5, p. 53.
69. WHO, *The World Health Report 1988* (Geneva: WHO, 1988), p. 44.
70. Fidler, supra note 5, p. 14.
71. Fidler, supra note 5, p. 67.
72. Black, Robert H. and David J. Sencer, 'The Long-Term Future of the International Health Regulations' (1978) 32 *WHO Chronicle*, p. 439.
73. Wahdan, M.H. 'Shortcomings in the current version of the International Health Regulations and difficulties in their implementation' (1995), *Informal Consultation to Review the International Response to Epidemics and Application of the International Health Regulations* (EMC/IHR/GEN/95.4), p. 4.
74. Dorelle, P., 'Old Plagues in the Jet Age' (1969) 23 *WHO Chronicle*, p. 110.
75. Fidler, David P., 'Return of the Fourth Horseman: Emerging Infectious Diseases and International Law' (1997) 81 *Minnesota Law Review* 4, p. 408.
76. World Health Assembly, Resolution 48.7
77. WHO, *Report of the Second WHO Meeting on Emerging Infectious Diseases* (WHO, CDS/BVI/95.2, 1995), p. 7.
78. Ibid., p. 14.
79. WHO, *Provisional Draft of the International Health Regulations* (Geneva: WHO, 1998).
80. Fidler, supra note 5, p. 73.
81. WHO, *Eleventh Annual Report*, supra note 37, p. 28.

Bibliography

Beck, A., *A History of the British Medical Administration of East Africa, 1900–1950* (Cambridge: Harvard University Press, 1970).
Berkelman, Ruth L. and James M. Hughes, The Conquest of Infectious Diseases: Who are We Kidding? (1993) *Ann Internal Medicine* 119, p. 426.
Black, Robert H. and David J. Sencer, The Long-Term Future of the International Health Regulations (1978) 32 *WHO Chronicle*: 437–40.

Conference Sanitaire Internationale de Venise, 1892, *Protocoles et procés-verbaux* (Rome: Imprimerie nationale de J. Bertero, 1892).

Conference Sanitaire Internationale de Venise, 1897, *Procés-Verbaux* (Rome: Forzani et C.ᴵᴱ Imprimeurs de Senat, 1897).

Conference Sanitaire Internationale, 1851, *Procés-Verbaux* (Paris: Imprimerie Nationale, 1852).

Conference Sanitaire Internationale, 1859, *Protocoles* (Paris: Imprimerie Nationale, 1859).

Conference Sanitaire Internationale, 1866, *Procés-Verbaux* (Constantinople: Imprimerie Centrale, 1866).

Conference Sanitaire Internationale, 1874, *Procés-Verbaux* (Vienna: Imprimerie Imperiale et Royale, 1874).

Conference Sanitaire Internationale, 1885, *Procés-Verbaux* (Rome: Imprimerie de Ministere des Affaires, 1885).

Cooper, Richard, International Cooperation in Public Health as a Prologue to Macroeconomic Cooperation, in *Can Nations Agree?* (Washington, DC: The Brookings Institution, 1989).

Dorelle, P., Old Plagues in the Jet Age (1969) 23 *WHO Chronicle*.

Fidler, David P., Return of the Fourth Horseman: Emerging Infectious Diseases and International Law (1997) 81 *Minnesota Law Review* 4.

Foreman-Peck, James, *A History of the World Economy: International Economic Relations since 1850* (New Jersey: Barnes and Noble Books).

Goodman, Neville, International Health Organizations and their Work (Aylesbury: Churchill Livingstone, 1971).

Howard-Jones, Norman, *International Public Health Between the Two World Wars – the Organizational Problems* (Geneva: WHO, 178).

Ileto, Reynaldo C., in *Companion Encyclopedia of the History of Medicine* (London: Routledge, 1994).

International Sanitary Conference, 1881, *Proceedings* (Washington: Government Printing Office, 1881).

International Sanitary Convention for Aerial Navigation, 1933 (The Hague, 1933).

International Sanitary Convention of Paris, 1903 (London: HMSO, 1904).

International Sanitary Convention of Paris, 1911–1912 (London: HMSO, 1919).

International Sanitary Convention, 1926 (London: HMSO, 1928).

International Sanitary Convention, 1944 (Washington DC: UNRRA, 1945).

Kenwood, A.G. and A.L. Lougheed, *The Growth of the International Economy 1820–1990* (London: Routledge, 1992).

Leive, David M., *International Regulatory Regimes: Case Studies in Health, Meteorology, and Food, Volumes I & II* (Lexington: Lexington Books, 1976).

Proces-verbaux (Paris: Imprimerie Nationale, 1894).

Schepin, Oleg, and Waldermar Yermakov, *International Quarantine* (Madison: International University Press, 1991).

Schwarz, Herman, *States versus Markets: History, Geography, and the Development of the International Political Economy* (New York: St Martin's Press, 1994).

Second Annual Report by the Director-General on the Working of the International Sanitary Regulations (WHO/IQ15/and Add. 1, 1954).

Siegfried, Andre, *Routes of Contagion* (New York: Harcourt, 1965).

Wahdan, M.H., Shortcomings in the Current Version of the International Health Regulations and Difficulties in their Implementation (1995), *Informal*

Consultation to Review the International Response to Epidemics and Application of the International Health Regulations (EMC/IHR/GEN/95.4).

WHO OR, N.37, 1951.

WHO, *Eleventh Report of the Committee on International Quarantine* (A16/P&B/2, 1963).

WHO, Functioning of the International Health Regulations (1978) 53 *Weekly Epidemiological Record.*

WHO, Functioning of the International Health Regulations (1980) 55 *Weekly Epidemiological Record.*

WHO, Functioning of the International Health Regulations (1981) 56 *Weekly Epidemiological Record.*

WHO, Functioning of the International Health Regulations (1986) 61 *Weekly Epidemiological Record.*

WHO, *Draft International Sanitary Regulations* (WHO/Epid/44 Add.2, 1950).

WHO, *Draft International Sanitary Regulations* (WHO/Epid/44, 1950).

WHO, *Draft International Sanitary Regulations* (WHO/Epid/48, 1950).

WHO, *Draft International Sanitary Regulations* (WHO/Epid/52, 1950).

WHO, *Eleventh Annual Report.*

WHO, *Fifth Report of the Committee on International Quarantine* (WHO/IQ/61, 1957).

WHO, *First Annual Report by the Director-General on the Working of the International Sanitary Regulations* (WHO/IQ/0 and Add. 1 and 2, 1953).

WHO, *Fourth Report of the Committee on International Quarantine* (WHO/IQ/48, 1956).

WHO, *International Health Regulations, 1981* (WHO: Geneva, 1981).

WHO, *International Sanitary Regulations, 1951* (WHO: Geneva, 1951).

WHO, *Nineteenth Report of the Committee on International Surveillance of Communicable Diseases* (A30/26, 1977).

WHO, *Ninth Report of the Committee on International Quarantine* (A16/P&B/2, 1963).

WHO, *Provisional Draft of the International Health Regulations* (Geneva: WHO, 1998).

WHO, *Report of the Second WHO Meeting on Emerging Infectious Diseases* (WHO, CDS/BVI/95.2, 1995).

WHO, *Seventh Report of the Committee on International Quarantine* (WHO/IQ/91, 1959).

WHO, *Sixteenth Report of the Committee on International Quarantine* (A24/B/10, 1971).

WHO, *Sixth Report of the Committee on International Quarantine* (WHO/IQ/75, 1958).

WHO, *The World Health Report 1988* (Geneva: WHO, 1988).

WHO, *Third Annual Report by the Director-General on the Working of the International Sanitary Regulations* (WHO/IQ/26 and Add. 1, 1956).

WHO, *Third Annual Report,* supra note 30.

WHO, *Third Annual Report,* supra note 30, p. 20.

World Health Assembly Resolution 22.47.

World Health Assembly, Resolution 48.7.

13
Public Health and International Law: the Impact of Infectious Diseases on the Formation of International Legal Regimes, 1800–2000[1]

David P. Fidler

Prior to the 1990s, the role of international law in efforts by states to control and prevent infectious diseases has not been frequently analysed by international lawyers or international relations scholars. International lawyers and international relations specialists historically generated a persistent lack of interest in public health issues. This historical scholarly neglect of the intersections between infectious diseases and international law is still curious given how much international law on infectious diseases has been developed from the mid-nineteenth century to the present day. Fortunately, the last decade has seen growing international relations and international legal interest in international public health issues generally and the global problems posed by infectious diseases specifically (Taylor 1992; Fidler 1996; Taylor 1997; Plotkin and Kimball 1997; Fidler 1997a; Fidler 1997b; Fidler 1997c; Fluss 1997; Zacher 1999; Fidler 1999a). This chapter provides a small glimpse of the many and complex aspects of the relationship between international law and infectious diseases. I briefly present a number of international legal regimes that directly and indirectly relate to the prevention and control of infectious diseases.

Although this chapter's specific focus is on international law and infectious diseases, I believe that this international legal analysis properly belongs within a more comprehensive study of how infectious diseases affect international relations. In writing on this topic, I have analysed the dynamics of what I call *microbialpolitik*, or the international politics of dealing with pathogenic microbes (Fidler 1998c; Fidler

1999a). The international legal regimes that I sketch in this chapter grew out of *microbialpolitik*, but they also have influenced in turn the dynamics of *microbialpolitik*. But I do not enter into the more comprehensive political examination required by the concept of *microbialpolitik* here. I believe that international law has played and will play a central role in *microbialpolitik*, making the various international legal regimes discussed in this chapter central concerns for those worried about the health of nations as the new millennium proceeds.

The globalization of public health and infectious diseases

Infectious diseases have burst back on to the world agenda under the rubric of 'emerging and re-emerging infectious diseases,' which the US Centers for Disease Control and Prevention and World Health Organization (WHO) define as 'diseases of infectious origin whose incidence in humans has increased within the past two decades or threatens to increase in the near future' (US CDC 1994: 1; WHO 1996b). New pathogenic scourges, such as HIV/AIDS, have appeared, while older, familiar killers, such as tuberculosis, have re-emerged to threaten human health on a global scale. The phenomenon of 'emerging and re-emerging infectious diseases' should be seen as part of larger problem for the health of nations, namely the globalization of public health (Fidler 1997; Yach and Bettcher 1998a, 1998b). Crudely defined, the globalization of public health refers to processes that are undermining the ability of the sovereign state to control public health in its territories. These processes include global travel, international trade, migrations, urbanization, war, civil unrest and environmental degradation. In the context of infectious diseases, the globalization of public health means that states today are constantly under threat from the international spread of infectious diseases while their sovereign capabilities for dealing with such threats have eroded. Recognizing the global nature of the infectious disease threat, national and international experts argue that only a global, coordinated response from states provides any hope of dealing with the threat of emerging and re-emerging infectious diseases (Fidler 1999a: 4–5).

What much of the contemporary literature about emerging and re-emerging infectious diseases does not adequately acknowledge is that the globalization of public health in connection with infectious diseases is not just a late twentieth century phenomenon. In fact, the globalization of public health existed in the mid-nineteenth century when European states realized that they could no longer control diseases, such as cholera, through national measures alone but had to engage in international cooperation to achieve that objective (Fidler 1997: 23–5). Hence, we witness the first International Sanitary Conference being held in Paris in 1851 (Goodman 1971: 42–50). The globalization of public health in the mid-nineteenth century produced the beginning of the era of international health diplomacy and international legal efforts on infectious diseases control.

The globalization of public health in the mid-nineteenth century had a certain 'pathology' that is important to understand. Two factors combined to produce the international concern about infectious diseases in the mid-nineteenth century: (1) the increasing power of travel and trade to spread pathogenic microbes internationally; and (2) the inadequate or non-existent public health systems in European and non-European countries (Fidler 1997: 25). By 1800, most European States attempted to deal with diseases, such as the plague, through national quarantine systems. But the cholera pandemics in Europe started around 1830, and the fear and frustrations of these recurrent waves of cholera weakened faith in quarantine as a national protective measure. In addition, increasing volume and speed of trade by land and sea also meant that national quarantine measures were growing economic burdens for merchants. Concerns about health and economics converged to produce the beginnings of the long line of international sanitary conferences that would stretch well into the twentieth century.

The globalization of public health at the end of the twentieth century has a more complicated pathology, but strong echoes of the earlier age remain. Five factors can be identified as characterizing the globalization of public health in the era of emerging and re-emerging infectious diseases:

- International trade and travel remain effective, very potent, means through which infectious diseases spread globally. In the twentieth century, improvements in transportation technologies and growing volumes of trade and travel have globalized germ pools and rendered them more volatile.
- Governmental complacency and/or lack of resources has produced deteriorating or non-existent national public-health capabilities, including the declining effectiveness of antimicrobial drugs, in both the developed and developing world.
- Despite notable successes, the internationalization of public health programmes through international health organizations has largely

failed to reduce materially the health gap between rich and poor nations, which has resulted in great opportunities for infectious diseases.

- The development of deeply rooted social, economic and environmental problems in developed but especially developing countries has provided pathogens with fertile conditions.
- Globalization has generally weakened the state's ability to control its domestic economy, and thus its ability to address public health needs and the social, economic and environmental problems (Fidler 1997: 33–4).

The implications of the contemporary pathology of the globalization of public health are grim because the pathology represents a depressing menagerie of human ills for which there is no easy solution. But, as in the nineteenth century, international law is at the centre of efforts to deal with the infectious disease threats emanating from the processes of the globalization of public health. Before analysing the contemporary importance of international law to national and international infectious disease control, I want to examine more precisely how states used international law in connection with infectious diseases in the nineteenth and early twentieth centuries.

Brief history of international law on infectious diseases

As mentioned earlier, infectious disease control between 1800 and 1851 was a matter of national law only. Infectious diseases did not become the subject of international diplomacy until 1851. But even during the first 50 years of the nineteenth century, states were starting to realize the limits of the traditional quarantine strategy, as evidenced by calls in 1834 and 1843 by France and Britain respectively to convene an international conference in connection with the cholera problem (Goodman 1971: 42; Howard-Jones 1975: 11).

Once infectious diseases became a subject of international diplomacy in 1851, frequent efforts began at international cooperation on infectious diseases over the course of the next century, culminating in WHO's establishment. A central feature of this international cooperation was the creation of international law on infectious disease control. Table 13.1 provides a glimpse of the intensity and scope of the international legal activity between 1851 and 1951. Not only is the number of treaties impressive but so also is their range of subject matter – human, plant and animal diseases are all subjects of treaty law. This list also

Table 13.1   Non-exhaustive list of international conferences and conventions on infectious disease control, 1851--1951

Year	Conference and/or convention
1907	Conference for the Creation of an International Bureau of Public Health in Rome adopted the Rome Agreement Establishing the Office International d'Hygiène Publique.
1912	International Sanitary Conference in Paris adopted the 1912 ISC; revised by 1926 ISC.
1914	Argentina, Brazil, Paraguay, and Uruguay adopt an International Sanitary Convention.
1923	League of Nations adopted the Scheme for the Permanent Health Organisation of the League of Nations.
1923	Poland, and the Russian, Ukrainian, and the White Russian Socialist Soviet Republics adopt a Sanitary Convention.
1924	Pan American Sanitary Conference in Washington, DC adopted the Pan American Sanitary Code.
1924	International Agreement for the Creation at Paris of the Office International des Epizooties.
1924	Agreement Respecting Facilities to be Given to Merchant Seamen for the Treatment of Venereal Disease adopted.
1926	International Sanitary Conference in Paris adopted the 1926 ISC; revised by 1938 ISC and 1944 ISC.
1927	Additional Protocol to the Pan American Sanitary Code adopted.
1928	Pan American Sanitary Convention for Aerial Navigation adopted.
1929	International Convention for the Protection of Plants adopted.
1930	Convention Concerning Anti-Diptheritic Serum adopted.
1930	Syria, Lebanon, and Egypt enter into an Exchange of Notes Constituting an Agreement Regarding the Measures to be Taken Against Dengue.
1933	ISC for Aerial Navigation adopted; revised by 1944 ISC for Aerial Navigation.
1934	International Convention for Mutual Protection Against Dengue Fever adopted.
1934	International Agreement for Dispensing with Bills of Health adopted, and International Agreement for Dispensing with Consular Visas on Bills of Health adopted.
1935	International Convention for the Campaign Against Contagious Diseases in Animals adopted.
1935	International Convention Concerning the Transit of Animals, Meat, and Other Products of Animal Origin adopted.
1935	International Convention Concerning the Export and Import of Animal Products (Other than Meat, Meat Preparations, Fresh Animal Products, Milk, and Milk Products) adopted.
1938	Convention amending 1926 ISC adopted.

Table 13.1 Non-exhaustive list of international conferences and conventions on infectious disease control, 1851--1951 *(continued)*

Year	Conference and/or convention
1944	ISC Modifying 1926 ISC adopted.
1944	ISC for Aerial Navigation Modifying the 1933 ISC for Aerial Navigation adopted.
1946	Protocol to Prolong the 1944 ISC adopted.
1946	Protocol to Prolong the 1944 ISC for Aerial Navigation adopted.
1946	Constitution of the World Health Organization adopted.
1951	World Health Assembly adopts the International Sanitary Regulations.
1951	International Plant Protection Convention adopted by Conference of the UN Food and Agriculture Organization.

Source: Fidler, 1999a: 22–23.

contains large multilateral treaties as well as bilateral treaties. Table 12.1 captures at a glance a body of international legal material that has largely been ignored by international lawyers and international relations specialists.

But merely listing lots of treaties tells us nothing about their substance or effectiveness. Evaluating all of these treaties is beyond the scope of this chapter, but four central objectives states tried to achieve through international law in the 1851–1951 period deserve highlighting.

Protecting Europe from 'Asiatic' diseases

One of the initial objectives of many of these treaties was to protect Europe from 'Asiatic' diseases, or diseases originating outside Europe, such as cholera, plague and yellow fever, that posed threats to populations in Europe. This objective reflects the reality that much of the international law in the 1851–1951 period was not humanitarian in nature and had much to do with European fears and prejudices concerning non-European peoples (Fidler 1999a: 28–35).

Harmonizing quarantine measures

A second initial goal of much of the international legal activity was to harmonize national quarantine measures. Behind this objective were, of course, concerns about the burdens quarantine systems placed on international trade and travel. The harmonization strategy aimed to rationalize quarantine regulations in order to facilitate trade.

States were not successful, however, at achieving this harmonization until the scientific work of Robert Koch and Louis Pasteur provided the foundations for the triumph of 'germ theory'. Prior to this scientific progress, states and their scientists waged a futile battle of contagionists against non-contagionists. Contagionists argued that diseases such as cholera were transmissible from human to human, which required the maintenance of national quarantine measures to break the chain of transmission. Non-contagionists, led for most of the nineteenth century by Great Britain, believed that diseases arose from local conditions, such as foul air or soil, and were not imported from abroad. Under this position, quarantine measures were useless as a health matter and burdensome as a trade matter; and the proper remedy was national reform of sanitation and hygiene.

Until science demonstrated that diseases were transmissible and that traditional quarantine was not effective, no progress was made in concluding any negotiated treaty on infectious disease control. Science was critical as a catalyst for the development of international law on quarantine harmonization because it provided the basis on which to build sound quarantine systems (Fidler 1999a: 35–42).

Creating an international surveillance system

The third objective that can be discerned in the international legal efforts of the 1851–1951 period is the creation of an international surveillance system for infectious diseases. The need for surveillance grew over the course of the latter half of the nineteenth century into a primary objective of international health diplomacy, eventually rivalling in importance the goal of quarantine harmonization. The triumph of 'germ theory' boosted the importance of surveillance as quarantine looked more and more suspect as an effective strategy for controlling infectious diseases. The 1903 International Sanitary Convention provided, for example, that each contracting party had to 'immediately notify the other governments of the first appearance in its territory of authentic cases of plague or cholera'. Obligations to notify other states parties, and later international health organizations, of specific disease outbreaks became one of the most important features of the treaties negotiated in the first half of the twentieth century (Fidler 1999a: 42–7; see also Zacher 1999: 272–3).

Creating a permanent international health organization

The fourth central objective for states became the creation of a permanent international health organization. The creation of such an entity became extremely important as states realized that *ad hoc* international conferences on infectious diseases, usually convened in response to an epidemic, were inefficient and ineffective. In addition, as surveillance grew in importance, the need for a central organization to coordinate information gathering, analysis and dissemination became clear. In the first 25 years of the twentieth century, four permanent international health organizations were established – the Pan American Sanitary Bureau (1902), the Office International d'Hygiène Publique (1907), the Health Organization of the League of Nations (1923), and the Office International des Epizooties (1924) (Fidler 1999a: 47–52).

As this overview of a century of international health diplomacy demonstrates, states used international law extensively to achieve infectious disease control. The process received its biggest boost from the development of better scientific knowledge about pathogenic microbes, which allowed states to harmonize quarantine more rationally, construct international surveillance systems and build permanent international health organizations. This history of international legal development was seen, at WHO's creation, as a precursor for a vibrant role for international law in connection with global health in the second half of the twentieth century.

The international health regulations[2]

At its creation, WHO was charged with unifying the patchwork of treaties on infectious disease control created prior to 1945 into a single, universal code. The WHO Constitution in Article 21 gave the World Health Assembly (WHA) the power to adopt binding regulations in connection with preventing and controlling the spread of infectious diseases (WHO 1946). As a matter of international law, this regulatory power was innovative, and was designed to allow WHO to keep international law on infectious diseases scientifically up-to-date. The WHA used this regulatory power to adopt the International Sanitary Regulations in 1951, which were renamed the International Health Regulations (IHR) in 1969 (WHO 1983).

According to WHO, the IHR are the only set of international legal rules on infectious disease control binding on WHO member States (WHO 1996a: 10). As such, they occupy a central place in the formation of international legal regimes relating to global public health. The purpose of the IHR, as stated in its text, 'is to ensure the maximum security against the international spread of diseases with minimum interference with world traffic' (WHO 1983: Foreword). The IHR seek the 'maximum security' objective by imposing duties to (1) report outbreaks of diseases subject to the IHR (i.e. cholera, plague and yellow fever); (2) maintain certain types of health-related capabilities at ports and airports to prevent the spread of infectious diseases; and (3) follow specific science-based rules for handling each of the diseases subject to the IHR (Fidler 1999a: 61–3).

The IHR seek the 'minimum interference' objective by establishing the maximum measures that a WHO Member State can take against travellers and merchandise moving in international commerce (Fidler 1999a: 63–5). The maximum measures are based on scientific principles, meaning that Member States may only restrict world traffic for infectious disease control purposes when it is scientifically justified to do so.

Unfortunately, WHO officials and public health experts agree that the IHR have been a failure as an international legal regime for infectious disease control. The maximum security objective has not been achieved largely because (1) WHO Member States have failed to support the global surveillance system by not notifying WHO of outbreaks as required by the IHR; and (2) the IHR only apply to three diseases (cholera, plague and yellow fever), a list that has long been considered inadequate given the international threats posed by many other infectious diseases (Fidler 1999a: 65–6). WHO failed to utilize its innovative international legal powers to keep the IHR relevant to the infectious diseases threat facing the world.

The minimum interference objective has likewise not been achieved largely because many WHO Member States repeatedly applied excessive measures to trade and travellers coming from countries suffering disease outbreaks. The real threat of excessive measures encouraged WHO Member States not to report outbreaks, creating a vicious circle of excessive measures and failures to report; and thus the entire regime collapsed from both ends (Fidler 1999a: 67–8).

Interestingly, all the weaknesses in the IHR were recognized and acknowledged long before the crisis of emerging and re-emerging in the 1990s (Dorolle 1969; Roelsgaard 1974). In essence, the IHR were largely moribund as an international legal regime when the world re-awakened to the threat from infectious diseases. This re-awakening has prompted WHO to undertake a revision of the IHR to make it more useful and effective in the face of globalization of public health and the threat from emerging and re-emerging infectious diseases.

The IHR revision process began in 1995 when the WHA instructed the WHO Director General to prepare a revised set of IHR in light of the new infectious disease threats (WHO 1995). In February 1998, WHO released to its Member States, other international organizations, and non-governmental organizations (NGOs) the IHR Provisional Draft – its first draft of a new international legal regime on infectious diseases (WHO 1998). In November 1998, WHO reviewed comments received on the IHR Provisional Draft from Member States (WHO 1999). The IHR Provisional Draft is itself currently undergoing revision based on input from WHO Member States, international organizations, and NGOs. Thus, it is premature to discuss in any detail the contents of this new international legal regime because the revision process remains fluid.

One change does, however, seem fairly certain. Rather than requiring surveillance of only three diseases, WHO has proposed requiring syndrome reporting, namely reporting of acute hemorrhagic syndrome, acute respiratory syndrome, acute diarrhoeal syndrome, acute jaundice syndrome, acute neurological syndrome and other notifiable syndromes (WHO 1998: Annex III). How syndrome reporting would work is too complicated to try to explain here, but the significance of the move to syndrome reporting is to require much more comprehensive surveillance of infectious diseases, which is more in keeping with addressing the threat pathogenic microbes pose to the world today.

Part of the story behind the rise and fall of the IHR as an international legal regime has been WHO's disinterest in international law as an instrument for pursuing global public health. I explore this problem at length elsewhere (Fidler 1998a), but one of the questions hanging over the IHR revision process is whether WHO has the international legal capabilities to revise and implement a radically different set of IHR. The timetable for completing the new IHR has slipped from the original deadline of May 1999 to May 2002 (WHO 1999).

Infectious diseases and international trade law

Even though the IHR represent the only international legal rules on infectious disease control binding on WHO Member States, the IHR do not represent the only international legal regime relevant to infectious diseases. In fact, infectious diseases affect a host of international legal regimes that stretch across virtually every aspect of international relations. This chapter briefly analyses how international trade law, international human rights law, international humanitarian law, international law on arms control and international environmental law play important roles in dealing with infectious disease threats today.

As seen in the nineteenth century objective of quarantine harmonization and the IHR's objective of minimum interference with world traffic, international law on infectious disease has always been attached to concerns about trade. International trade law, as developed primarily under the General Agreement on Tariffs and Trade (GATT), has come to include an increasingly sophisticated (and controversial) set of rules that apply, *inter alia*, to the threat of infectious diseases moving through the international trading system. Historically, the biggest infectious disease threats posed by trade came from the international movement of plants, animals and food-borne pathogens. International trade law has developed disciplines on a sovereign state's power to apply sanitary and phytosanitary (SPS) measures to imported goods.

Under GATT, a GATT Member State could violate GATT principles in order to protect human, animal or plant life or health if the protective measures (1) were necessary; (2) did not constitute arbitrary or unjustifiable discrimination; and (3) were not disguised restrictions on trade (GATT 1994: Art. XX(b)). Over GATT's history, GATT contracting parties often relied on Article XX(b) to justify trade-restrictive measures designed to prevent the importation of infectious diseases, such as foot-and-mouth disease and cholera. During the same period of time, however, many GATT parties also applied what appeared to be excessive or unnecessary (from a scientific viewpoint) SPS measures to the trade of other GATT contracting parties. Some of these problems arose in connection with infectious diseases (for example, the 1991 cholera outbreak in Peru), or from other types of purported health threats (for example, nuclear radioactive fallout from Chernobyl). By the time GATT contracting parties started the Uruguay Round negotiations in the mid-1908s, general consensus existed on creating tighter disciplines on states applying SPS measures. This consensus resulted in the negotiation and adoption of the Agreement on Application of Sanitary and Phytosanitary Measures (SPS Agreement), one of the mandatory side agreements under the World Trade Organization (WTO) (Fidler 1999a: 121–33).

The SPS Agreement requires all SPS measures to be based on a risk assessment, be supported by scientific principles and evidence, and be the least trade-restrictive measure possible (SPS Agreement 1994: Arts. 2(2), 5(1), and 5(6)). The SPS Agreement also requires WTO Member States to base their SPS measures on international standards developed by relevant international organizations (SPS Agreement 1994: Art. 3(1)). WTO Member States can apply SPS measures that set higher levels of protection than the relevant international standards, but they must demonstrate the scientific justification for such higher standards

(SPS Agreement 1994: Art. 3(3)). To the familiar trade-related discipline of the least trade-restrictive measure possible, the SPS Agreement imposes new scientific disciplines on the application of SPS measures.

Like the WHO under the IHR, the WTO under the SPS Agreement has made science central to an international legal regime on health matters. This elevation of science in international law relating to health I have called the 'science paradigm' (Fidler 1997d: 314). Under the science paradigm:

- Science becomes the standard against which national measures are evaluated under international law.
- Science sets the standards for the international harmonisation of public health measures under international law.
- The medical and legal role of science becomes institutionalized in international organisations responsible for health and for international trade; and these international organizations bear the responsibility of maintaining the integrity of the use of science in the attempts to balance public health and trade (Fidler 1999a: 135).

While the SPS Agreement applies to all SPS measures, it has been applied specifically in infectious disease contexts, as evidenced by the 1998 Australian Salmon Import Case between Canada and Australia (Salmon Import Case 1998). A complete analysis of the dynamics and problems of the SPS Agreement is beyond the scope of this chapter (see Fidler 1999a: 133–53), but the above analysis suggests that international trade law is very important to infectious disease control in the era of the globalization of public health. Perhaps one of the most important aspects of the SPS Agreement is that it is plugged into the powerful WTO dispute settlement system. Unlike under the IHR, WTO Member States can seek redress for 'excessive measures' in connection with trade-restricting health measures. As of this writing, the WTO Dispute Settlement Body has found the European Community, Australia and Japan to be in violation of the SPS Agreement through the application of scientifically unjustified SPS measures (Beef Hormones Case 1998; Salmon Import Case 1998; Japan Agricultural Products Case 1999). A number of other claims under the SPS Agreement are working their way through the WTO dispute settlement system (EC Asbestos Case 1998).

The SPS Agreement is not the only piece of international trade law relevant to infectious diseases. The protection of intellectual property rights under the WTO's Agreement on Trade-Related Aspects of Intellectual Property Rights (TRIPS) is also relevant because of the importance of the protection of intellectual property rights to the development of new antimicrobial drugs (TRIPS 1994; Fidler 1999a: 163). TRIPS attempts to harmonize the protection for intellectual property rights, including patents, among WTO Member States. WTO Member States that fail to comply with TRIPS are subject to the WTO dispute settlement process, and cases involving pharmaceutical patents have already been brought before the WTO Dispute Settlement Body (India Patent Case 1998; Canada Patent Case 1997). Many developing countries and NGO groups believe, however, that TRIPS adversely affects access to essential drugs in developing countries by raising the price and/or restricting availability through strengthened patent rights for pharmaceutical companies (Pécoul *et al.* 1999: 366).

Infectious diseases and international human rights law

International human rights law is another important international legal regime to consider in connection with infectious disease control. The importance of human rights law came to the forefront of infectious disease control efforts during the HIV/AIDS pandemic (Gostin and Lazzarini 1997), which forced public health experts and human rights lawyers to work together on a public health/human rights tragedy of global proportions. While the link between HIV/AIDS and human rights has dominated the relationship between human rights and infectious diseases, the relationship is both more complex and more comprehensive.

Within international human rights law, infectious disease control implicates both civil and political rights and economic, social and cultural rights. In the area of civil and political rights, international law recognizes that governments may restrict their enjoyment to protect public health but only if strict criteria are met: the restrictive measure: (1) must be prescribed by law; (2) must be applied in a non-discriminatory manner; (3) must relate to a compelling public interest (for example, the protection of public health); and (4) must be necessary to achieve the compelling public interest, meaning that the measure has to be proportional to the interest sought to be protected and the least trade restrictive measure possible to achieve the public interest in question (Fidler 1999a: 172–9).

Most of the controversy about the protection of civil and political rights in the infectious disease context has arisen in connection to the HIV/AIDS pandemic. Government policies on AIDS around the world violated many different civil and political rights, including the rights to liberty, integrity of person and privacy (Gostin and Lazzarini 1997: 12–27; Fidler 1999a: 200–9). Discriminatory policies and practices were also very common. While the scale of human rights violations has been enormous, HIV/AIDS-related human rights litigation before international bodies has pushed the boundaries of jurisprudence on civil and political rights, as witnessed by (1) the declarations of the UN Human Rights Commission that discrimination in the protection of rights on the basis of health status violates human rights law (UN Human Rights Commission 1995, 1996), and (2) the ruling of the European Court of Human Rights that the deportation of an AIDS patient back to a developing country lacking adequate public health would constitute inhuman or otherwise degrading treatment in violation of the European Convention on Human Rights (Case of *D. v. United Kingdom* 1997).

In the area of economic, social and cultural rights, infectious diseases raise many issues relating to the human right to health. The right to health is an enormously problematical concept; and experts still have difficulty defining exactly what it means, even though it can be found in a number of human rights treaties, including the European Social Charter (1961), International Covenant on Economic, Social, and Cultural Rights (1966), African Charter on Human and Peoples' Rights (1981), and the United Nations Convention on the Rights of the Child (1985). The rhetorical power of the concept means that it is frequently invoked; but, as a matter of international legal analysis, it is very difficult to discern much coherency in this human rights norm (Fidler 1999a: 181–3).

One of the largest obstacles to a constructive approach to the right to health is the principle of progressive realization. This principle provides that states may achieve the right to health progressively depending on their level of economic development (Fidler 1999a: 183–5). Thus, the right to health varies from country to country, as does a government's responsibilities to fulfil the right. The principle of progressive realization contributes significantly to the indeterminacy of the norm. Attempts to give the right to health some minimum core meaning often founder on any number of aspects of the right. In my 1999 book, *International Law and Infectious Diseases*, I try to find a minimum core meaning for the right to health centred on infectious disease control; but my attempt still leaves much to be desired because of the enormity of the challenge of even basic infectious disease control and the lingering problem of the principle of progressive realization (Fidler 1999a: 187–97).

The above analysis of civil and political rights and economic, social and cultural rights indicates that, though full of difficulties, international human rights law has a central role in global infectious disease control. The objective of more scientific, rational and humane public health responses to infectious diseases may be a little closer because of the application of human rights principles in the public health debate about HIV/AIDS, but it still remains a very distant goal. The fusion of public health and human rights fostered by HIV/AIDS promises to be a troubling feature of infectious disease control for decades to come.

Infectious diseases, war and weapons

War and pestilence make up two of the four horsemen of the apocalypse; and for good reason – they are old allies. War has long been a prolific creator of opportunities for the spread of infectious diseases. War disrupts the normal, peacetime relationship between humans and microbes decidedly in favour of the microbes. This powerful synergy between war and infectious diseases explains why infectious diseases factor prominently in international law on arms control and armed conflict.

In the area of arms control, international law prohibits the use, development, production and stockpiling of biological weapons. The use of infectious diseases as an instrument of war has been banned since the Geneva Protocol (1925). The Biological Weapons Convention (BWC) banned the development, production and stockpiling of biological weapons (BWC 1972). Currently, negotiations are ongoing to strengthen the BWC by creating a compliance regime. These negotiations have been stimulated by fears about the proliferation of biological weapons in the international system and the growing threat of biological terrorism. Whether these negotiations will ultimately be successful, or whether successful negotiations will produce an effective arms control regime, remains uncertain at the moment.

As for conventional weapons and infectious diseases, I have analysed whether certain types of conventional weapons can be considered to inflict superfluous injury or unnecessary suffering in violation of international humanitarian law because of the infectious diseases they cause (Fidler 1999a: 231–3). Although all wounds caused by any conventional weapon usually become contaminated and thus susceptible to infection, it could be argued that conventional weapons, such as land mines, that cause large wounds worsen the infectious disease burden to such an extent that superfluous injury or unnecessary suffering results. The link between large wounds and infectious diseases in connection with the concept of superfluous injury or unnecessary suffering is weak as no data have been gathered to support the hypothesis.

International humanitarian law contains a comprehensive set of rules that directly and indirectly seek to prevent and control infectious diseases during armed conflict. International humanitarian law does this by regulating targets for military attack (for example, objects indispensable to the survival of the civilian population, such as drinking water installations, cannot be attacked); the treatment of wounded and sick combatants; the treatment of prisoners of war; and the treatment of civilians in occupied territories (Fidler 1999a: 233–8).

Unfortunately, this comprehensive set of international humanitarian rules have been comprehensively violated in most wars of the past half-century. This lack of compliance raises questions about treating soldiers and officers who endanger health as war criminals. The concept of a 'war crime' has long been sufficiently comprehensive to cover violations of the laws of war that support infectious disease control. The Nuremburg, Far East and Yugoslavia war crimes tribunals have all considered violations of health-protective rules as punishable war crimes. In keeping with this history, the statute of the new International Criminal Court also defines war crimes to include violations of rules of international humanitarian law designed to protect health and control infectious diseases (Fidler 1999a: 238–42).

Sadly, the international law that supports infectious disease control and public health during armed conflict has so far proved no match for the violence and chaos of war. Another sobering thought is that most contemporary warfare occurs in developing countries, where infectious disease control in peacetime is often non-existent. This observation points to a tragedy that dwarfs the war-disease synergy: the everyday condition of public health in developing countries.

Infectious diseases and international environmental law

Public health experts often argue that environmental degradation and change play significant roles in the emergence and re-emergence of infectious diseases. Environmental conditions and alterations affect the human–microbe relationship in so many ways that it is necessary for environmental health to be on the infectious disease control agenda. The role played by the environment in infectious disease occurrence makes international environmental law a relevant international legal regime for infectious disease control.

Many kinds of environmental degradation cause infectious disease problems. Air pollution causes respiratory infections. Water pollution causes problems with many types of water-borne diseases, such as cholera. Marine pollution contributes to infectious disease problems created by algal blooms. Deforestation brings humans into contact with new pathogenic microbes, alters ecosystems so that disease vectors (for example, mosquitoes, rats) multiply, and destroys biodiversity that could be critical to the development of new antimicrobial products. The depletion of the ozone layer, some experts believe, will lead to ultraviolet radiation damaging the human immune system, thus creating more opportunities for infectious diseases. Global warming might lead to an increase in the habitat of disease vectors, such as mosquitoes, and contribute to increases in water-borne diseases (Fidler 1999a: 246–52).

International environmental law has developed in each of these areas of environmental degradation, making it a pertinent body of law for infectious disease control purposes. But it would be a mistake to pretend that infectious diseases played (or play) major roles in the development of international environmental law. The contribution of international environmental law to infectious disease control remains also suspect. International environmental law does, for example, address transboundary air and water pollution but does not address local air and water pollution, which are the biggest sources of infectious diseases that kill in the developing world. International environmental law on marine pollution is quite weak. States have not been able to agree on a treaty on deforestation, and the Convention on Biological Diversity (1992) remains mired in controversies between the North and South. While the international legal regime on ozone depletion has achieved some success, its progress remains fragile. Finally, the acrimonious negotiations of the Kyoto Protocol (1997) indicate how far the international community is from dealing effectively with the threat of climate change. Because environmental degradation factors powerfully into infectious disease occurrence, the state of international environmental law is not a source of public health confidence (Fidler 1999a: 252–74).

Future international legal challenges

Infectious diseases will continue to present new and disturbing threats in international relations that may require international legal action to address. Three developing threats are the infectious disease problems potentially created by the international trade in blood products and human organs (Tomasevski 1995: 886–9), the development of antimicrobial resistance (Fidler 1998; Fidler 1999b) and xenotransplantation (Fidler 1999a: 308).

International trade In blood and human organs

Despite the general problem of blood-borne diseases and the HIV/AIDS pandemic, Tomasevski noted in 1995 that '[i]nternational legal protection of blood safety is ... still lacking' (Tomasevski 1995: 888). International trade in human organs has also not been the subject of international legal activity within WHO despite calls by some countries to regulate trade in human organs internationally (Tomasevski 1995: 888–9). As pressure mounts on the supply of blood and human organs, the problems seen in the past in these areas will only continue.

Antimicrobial resistance

The development of antimicrobial resistance in many pathogenic microbes also raises many national and international legal issues (Fidler 1998b; Fidler 1999b). These issues arise in connection with the use of antimicrobials both in human medicine and in food animal health and production. One of the most controversial problems in this context is whether to regulate the use of antimicrobials that have human applications as growth promoters in food animal production. Many public health officials in the United States and Europe believe that the use of human-relevant antimicrobials as growth promoters in food animal production encourages the development of resistant organisms in humans, thus constituting a threat to public health. In late 1998, the European Union banned the use of four antibiotics in food animal production because of public health concerns; and Pfizer Animal Health, a producer of one of the banned antibiotics, challenged this ban in a claim for interim relief before the European Court of Justice in 1999. In late June 1999, the Court of First Instance denied Pfizer the interim relief it desired (Pfizer Case 1999). Although this decision only related to the claim for interim relief, with the main case, judged on its merits, still to come, the case illustrates the relevance of international law to addressing the problem of antimicrobial resistance.

Xenotransplantation

Xenotransplantation involves transplanting animal organs into humans. Interest in this technique of organ replacement has grown because of the shortage of human organs available for transplant candidates. Public health officials have raised concerns that xenotransplants may introduce into human populations zoonotic pathogens that could create public health concerns. Like antimicrobial resistance, xenotransplantation raises a host of national and international legal issues that governments and international organizations have only just begun to address (Institute of Medicine 1996; Nuffield Council on Bioethics 1996; Council of Europe 1997; WHO 1997).

Conclusion: the concept of global health jurisprudence

This chapter has highlighted, albeit briefly, the scope and nature of the international law that has developed to deal with infectious diseases. The impact of infectious diseases on human life can be glimpsed in all the various international legal regimes sketched above. It is, in fact, difficult to identify many other global issues that touch upon so many areas of international law. Infectious diseases have indeed left their mark on international law.

At the same time, we are left to wonder about the nature of the international legal mark left by infectious diseases. After all, this has been an area of international law that has been largely neglected until the past few years. In addition, the many and various problems noted with these international legal regimes above demonstrate that infectious diseases have not miraculously rescued international law from all the normal obstacles and limitations it confronts in an anarchical system of states.

In reflecting on the role of international law in infectious disease control specifically and public health more generally, I believe there is a greater role that international law can play in contributing to international stability and development. But this greater role fits into a larger legal framework that I call *global health jurisprudence*. Global health jurisprudence is a concept I developed to integrate legal efforts at the national and international levels to strengthen law's contribution to the public's health in the global era (Fidler 1998a: 1116–26). Central to the global health jurisdiction concept is the idea that national law and international law are interdependent when it comes to public health. Simply creating more rules of international law on infectious disease control will not advance the fight against infectious diseases much unless the international legal effort is accompanied by coordinated action at the national legal level. But often national legal reform will not take place unless international legal regimes take shape and catalyse the process of change. So intense legal activity is required at both the national and international levels to produce global health jurisprudence.

But let me be clear. Neither global health jurisprudence nor international law is a panacea for the global crisis in infectious diseases. It can be only one part of the overall strategy and solution, and it is not even the most important part. To pretend that humankind can achieve global health through global law would be a disservice to the value of health embedded within international scientific, public health, medical and legal communities.

Notes

1. This chapter is based on David P. Fidler's book, *International Law and Infectious Diseases* (Oxford: Clarendon Press, 1999) with grateful acknowledgement to the publisher.
2. See also Chapter 12 by Simon Carvalho and Mark W. Zacher in this volume for additional analysis on the International Health Regulations.

References

African Charter on Human and Peoples' Rights. 1981. International Legal Materials 21: 58.
Beef Hormones Case. 1998. EC Measures Concerning Meat and Meat Products (Hormones), Appellate Body Report, adopted Feb. 13, 1998, WTO Doc. WT/DS26/AB/R and WT/DS48/AB/R.
BWC. 1972. Convention on the Prohibition of the Development, Production, and Stockpiling of Bacteriological (Biological) and Toxin Weapons and on Their Destruction. *International Legal Materials* 11: 309.
Canada Patent Case. 1997. Canada – Patent Protection of Pharmaceutical Products, complaint by the European Communities, Dec. 19, 1997, WT/DS114/1.
Case of *D. v. United Kingdom*. 1997. European Court of Human Rights, <http://www.dhcour.coe.fr/eng/D.JUD.html>.
Convention on Biological Diversity. 1992. *International Legal Materials* 31: 818.
Council of Europe. 1997. Recommendation No. R (97) 15 of the Committee of Ministers to Member States on Xenotransplantation, Sept. 30, 1997.
Dorolle, P. 1969. Old Plagues in the Jet Age: International Aspects of Present and Future Control of Communicable Diseases. *WHO Chronicle* 23: 103–11.
EC Asbestos Case. 1998. EC – Measures Affecting the Prohibition of Asbestos and Asbestos Products, complaint by Canada, May 28, 1998, WT/DS135.
European Social Charter. 1961. United Nations Treaty Series 529: 89.
Fidler, D.P. 1996. Globalisation, International Law, and Emerging Infectious Diseases. *Emerging Infectious Diseases* 2: 77–84.

Fidler, D.P. 1997a. The Globalisation of Public Health: Emerging Infectious Diseases and International Relations. *Indiana Journal of Global Legal Studies* 5: 11–57.

Fidler, D.P. 1997b. Return of the Fourth Horseman: Emerging Infectious Diseases and International Law. *Minnesota Law Review* 81: 771–868.

Fidler, D.P. 1997c. The Role of International Law in the Control of Emerging Infectious Diseases. *Bulletin de l'Institut Pasteur* 95: 57–72.

Fidler, D.P. 1997d. Trade and Health: the Global Spread of Diseases and International Trade. *German Yearbook of International Law* 40: 300–55.

Fidler, D.P. 1998a. The Future of the World Health Organization: What Role for International Law? *Vanderbilt Journal of Transnational Law* 31: 1079–1126.

Fidler, D.P. 1998b. Legal Issues Associated with the Development of Antimicrobial Drug Resistance. *Emerging Infectious Diseases.* 4: 169–77.

Fidler, D.P. 1998c. *Microbialpolitik*: Infectious Diseases and International Relations. *American University International Law Review* 14: 1–53.

Fidler, D.P. 1999a. *International Law and Infectious Diseases*. Oxford: Clarendon Press.

Fidler, D.P. 1999b. Legal Challenges Posed by the Use of Antimicrobials in Food Animal Production. *Microbes and Infection* 1: 29–38.

Fluss, S.S. 1997. International Public Health Law: An Overview, in *Oxford Textbook of Public Health* (R. Detels *et al.*, eds). Oxford: Oxford University Press, pp. 371–90.

GATT. 1994. In 1995 Documents Supplement to Legal Problems of International Economic Relations (J.H. Jackson *et al.*, eds) Minneapolis: West Publishing, 15–78.

Geneva Protocol for the Prohibition of the Use in War of Asphyxiating, Poisonous or Other Gases and of Bacteriological Methods of Warfare, June 17, 1925, League of Nations Treaty Series 44: 65.

Goodman, N.M. 1971. International Health Organizations and Their Work, 2nd edn London: Churchill Livingstone.

Gostin, L. and Lazzarini, Z. 1997. *Human Rights and Public Health in the AIDS Pandemic*. Oxford: Oxford University Press.

Howard-Jones, N. 1975. *The Scientific Background of the International Sanitary Conferences 1851–1938*. Geneva: WHO.

India Patent Case. 1998. India – Patent Protection for Pharmaceutical and Agricultural Chemical Products, Appellate Body Report, adopted Jan. 16, 1998, WTO Doc. AB-1997-5.

Institute of Medicine. 1996. Committee on Xenograft Transplantation, Xenotransplantation; Science, Ethics, and Public Policy. Washington, DC: Institute of Medicine.

International Covenant on Economic, Social, and Cultural Rights. 1966. United Nations Treaty Series 993: 3.

Japan Agricultural Imports Case. 1999. Japan – Measures Affecting Agricultural Products, Appellate Body Report, issued Feb. 22, 1999, WTO Doc. WT/DS76/AB/R.

Kyoto Protocol to the U.N. Framework Convention on Climate Change. 1997. UN Doc. FCCC/CP/1997/L.7/Add. 1.

Nuffield Council on Bioethics. 1996. Animal-to-Human Transplants: Ethics of Xenotransplantation. London: Nuffield Council on Bioethics.

Pécoul, B. *et al.* 1999. Access to Essential Drugs in Poor Countries: a Lost Battle? *Journal of the American Medical Association* 281: 361–7.

Pfizer Case. 1999. Pfizer Animal Health SA/NV V. Council of the European Union, Case T-13/99 R, Court of First Instance, June 30, 1999.

Plotkin, B.J. and Kimball, A.M. 1997. Designing an International Policy and Legal Framework for the Control of Emerging Infectious Diseases: First Steps. *Emerging Infectious Diseases* 2: 1–9.

Roelsgaard, E. 1974. Health Regulations and International Travel. *WHO Chronicle* 28: 265–8.

Salmon Import Case. 1998. Australia – Measures Affecting Importation of Salmon, Appellate Body Report, issued Oct. 20, 1998, WTO Doc. WT/DS18/AB/R.

SPS Agreement. 1994. Agreement on the Application of Sanitary and Phytosanitary Measures. MTN/FA II-A1A-4, 1994.

Taylor, A.L. 1992. Making the World Health Organization Work: a Legal Framework for Universal Access to the Conditions for Health. American Journal of Law & Medicine 18: 301–46.

Taylor, A.L. 1997. Controlling the Global Spread of Infectious Diseases: Toward a Reinforced Role for the International Health Regulations. *Houston Law Review* 33: 1327–62.

Tomasevski, K. 1995. Health. In United Nations Legal Order, vol. 2 (O. Schachter and C.C. Joyner eds) Cambridge: Cambridge University Press, pp. 859–906.

TRIPS. 1994. Agreement on Trade-Related Aspects of Intellectual Property Rights. MTN/FA II-A1C, 1994.

UN Convention on the Rights of the Child. 1985. International Legal Materials 28: 1456.

UN Human Rights Commission. 1995. Resolution on HIV/AIDS, Res. 1995/44.

UN Human Rights Commission. 1996. The Protection of Human Rights in the Context of Human Immunodeficiency Virus (HIV) and Acquired Immune Deficiency Syndrome (AIDS), Res. 1996/43.

US Centers for Disease Control and Prevention. 1994. Addressing Emerging Infectious Disease Threats: a Prevention Strategy for the United States. Washington, DC: US Department of Health and Human Services.

WHO. 1946. Constitution of the World Health Organization. In WHO Basic Documents, 40th edn, 1994. Geneva: WHO.

WHO. 1983. International Health Regulations, 3rd ann. edn Geneva: WHO.

WHO. 1995. Revision and Updating of the International Health Regulations, WHA Res. 48.7, May 12, 1995.

WHO. 1996a. Division of Emerging and Other Communicable Diseases Surveillance and Control Strategic Plan 1996–2000. WHO/EMC/96.1.

WHO. 1996b. World Health Report 1996: Fighting Disease, Fostering Development. Geneva: WHO: 15.

WHO. 1997. Report of WHO Consultation on Xenotransplantation. WHO/EMC/ZOO/98.2.

WHO. 1998. Provisional Draft, International Health Regulations. Geneva: WHO.

WHO. 1999. Revision and Updating of the International Health Regulations: Progress Report, Report by the Secretariat, WHO Doc. A52/9, Apr. 1, 1999.

Yach, D. and Bettcher, D. 1998a. The Globalisation of Public Health, I: Threats and Opportunities. *American Journal of Public Health* 88: 735–7.

Yach, D. and Bettcher, D. 1998b. The Globalisation of Public Health, II: The Convergence of Self-Interest and Altruism. *American Journal of Public Health* 88: 738–41.

Zacher, M. 1999. Epidemiological Surveillance: International Cooperation to Monitor Infectious Diseases, in *Global Public Goods* (I. Kaul, M. Stern and I. Grunberg eds). Oxford: Oxford University Press, pp. 268–85.

Index